Professionalism in Health Care

A Primer for Career Success

Professionalism in Health Care

A Primer for Career Success

5TH Edition

Sherry Makely, PhD, RT(R)
President, Pine Ridge Publications, Bloomington, Indiana

Vanessa J. Austin, RMA, AHI, (AMT), M.Ed.
Medical Assistant Instructor,
Ross Medical Education, Cincinnati, Ohio
Contributing Author, The Practicum Experience, Chapter Seven

Quay Kester, PhD
President, Evoke Communications, Indianapolis, Indiana
Content Contributor, Cultural Competence, Chapter Five

PEARSON

Boston   Columbus   Indianapolis   New York City   San Francisco   Amsterdam
Cape Town   Dubai   London   Madrid   Milan   Munich   Paris   Montréal   Toronto
Delhi   Mexico City   São Paulo   Sydney   Hong Kong   Seoul   Singapore   Taipei   Tokyo

Publisher: Julie Levin Alexander
Publisher's Assistant: Sarah Henrich
Portfolio Manager: Marlene Pratt
Program Manager: Faye Gemmellaro
Program Management, Team Lead: Melissa Bashe
Project Management, Team Lead: Cindy Zonneveld
Editorial Assistant: Lauren Bonilla
Development Editor: Sandra Breuer
Marketing Manager: Brittany Hammond
Senior Marketing Coordinator: Alicia Wozniak
Full-Service Project Management: SPi Global

Product Strategy Manager: Amanda Killeen
Senior Operations Specialist: Mary Ann Gloriande
Digital Program Manager: Amy Peltier
Media Project Manager: Lisa Rinaldi
Art Director: Mary Siener
Cover Image: Comaniciu Dan/Shutterstock
Composition: SPi Global
Printing and Binding: RR Donnelley/Crawfordsville
Cover Printer: Phoenix Color/Hagerstown

Notice: The authors and the publisher of this volume have taken care that the information and technical recommendations contained herein are based on research and expert consultation and are accurate and compatible with the standards generally accepted at the time of publication. Nevertheless, as new information becomes available, changes in clinical and technical practices become necessary. The reader is advised to carefully consult manufacturers' instructions and information material for all supplies and equipment before use, and to consult with a health care professional as necessary. This advice is especially important when using new supplies or equipment for clinical purposes. The authors and publisher disclaim all responsibility for any liability, loss, injury, or damage incurred as a consequence, directly or indirectly, of the use and application of any of the contents of this volume.

Credits and acknowledgments borrowed from other sources and reproduced, with permission, in this textbook appear on page.

Library of Congress Cataloging-in-Publication Data
Names: Makely, Sherry, author. | Austin, Vanessa J., author. | Kester, Quay, author.
Title: Professionalism in health care : a primer for career success / Sherry Makely ; contributing authors, Vanessa J. Austin, Quay Kester.
Description: 5th edition. | New Jersey : Pearson Education, [2017] | Includes bibliographical references and index.
Identifiers: LCCN 2016011578| ISBN 9780134415673 | ISBN 0134415671
Subjects: | MESH: Professional Competence | Health Occupations | Interprofessional Relations | Ethics, Professional | Career Mobility
Classification: LCC R725.5 | NLM W 21 | DDC 610.69—dc23
LC record available at http://lccn.loc.gov/2016011578

1 16

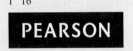

ISBN 10:   0-13-441567-1
ISBN 13: 978-0-13441567-3

Contents

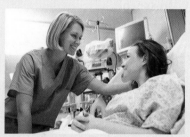

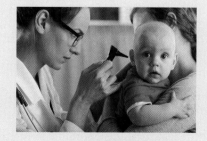

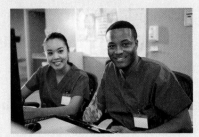

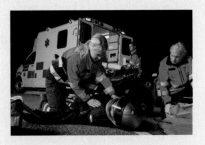

Chapter Five   Cultural Competence and Patient Care   124

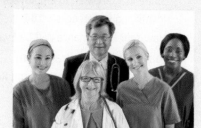

Chapter Six   Professionalism and Your Personal Life   157

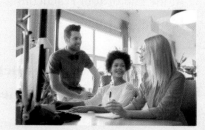

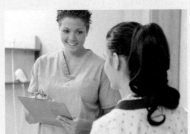

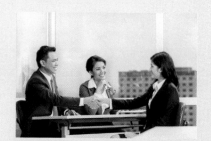

Preface

Who This Book Is For and Why It's Important

Professionalism in Health Care: A Primer for Career Success, 5th Edition, is designed for students enrolled in nursing and health sciences educational programs in colleges and universities, vocational-technical schools, hospitals, high schools, and on-the-job training programs. This book is also beneficial in orientation sessions for new employees and for in-service and refresher classes for experienced health care workers. Text information is applicable to all health careers and all types, sizes, and locations of health care settings.

This book provides information that is essential to the success of today's health care workers. Hands-on technical skills remain a high priority, but good character, a strong work ethic, and excellent personal and professional traits and behaviors have become more important than ever before. Statistics indicate a growing concern with theft, fraud, and behavioral problems in the workplace. Poor attendance, interpersonal conflicts, disregard for quality, and disrespect for authority all too often lead to employees being fired from their jobs. The inappropriate use of cell phones, digital devices and communication, and social media are causing major concerns.

With a growing emphasis on customer service, the patient experience, cultural competence, quality improvement, patient safety, and corporate compliance, health care employers are increasingly seeking workers with strong "soft skills" and "people skills"—people who communicate appropriately, work well on teams, respect and value differences, use limited resources efficiently, and interact effectively with coworkers, patients, and guests.

Regardless of job title or discipline, every health care student and worker must understand the importance of professionalism and the need to perform in a professional, ethical, legal, and competent manner. Developing and strengthening professional traits and behaviors has become a major challenge for both health care educators and employers. *Professionalism in Health Care: A Primer for Career Success* helps meet that challenge. It describes the professional standards that apply to all health care workers—the common ground that everyone shares in providing the highest quality of health care and service excellence for patients, visitors, and guests.

What This Book Covers

Professionalism in Health Care: A Primer for Career Success discusses in detail the following topics:

- The key elements of professionalism
- The health care industry and your role
- Your work ethic and performance

- Personal traits of health care professionals
- Relationships, teamwork, and communication skills
- Cultural competence and patient care
- Professionalism and your personal life
- The practicum experience
- Employment and professional development

New to This Edition

This 5th edition includes updated, expanded, and new content, photographs, and special features.

In response to growing concerns among instructors, employers, and patients, a new *Professionalism Online* feature has been added in each chapter of the text. Feature topics include: Digital Communication and Social Media, Digital Communication and Privacy, Your Reputation Online, Digital Communication and Etiquette Online, Diversity in Social Media and Online Resources for Patients, Health and Safety Concerns with Social Media, Complying with Your Practicum Site's Protocol, and Establishing a Professional Online Presence. These features provide extensive discussions regarding the advantages and disadvantages of social media and digital communication; the appropriate use of cell phones and other digital devices; and how the posting and sharing of content on social media sites can impact the privacy of patients, the confidentiality of health information, and the professional reputations of health care workers and their employers.

Each chapter has five new features: *Hot Topics*, *By the Numbers*, *Trends and Issues*, *The More You Know*, and *Professionalism Online*. These sections provide a wealth of interesting and supportive information on diverse topics that include: Obesity in America, Medicare Scams and Fraud, Personal Values and Ethical Conduct, Using Resilience to Deal with Change and Adversity, Multiple Chronic Diseases on the Rise, Contending with Conservative Dress Codes, From Prescription Painkillers to Heroin, and Making the Most of Your Time Off, to name just a few.

A new *Case Study* in each chapter picks up where the 4th edition left off. The case study follows the professional career of Carla, a fictional medical assistant, as she becomes a supervisor and deals with a variety of real-life behavioral issues in a large physician practice.

Additional enhancements in the 5th edition include the following:

- Chapter One, *The Health Care Industry and Your Role*, has been updated to include recent developments in health care reform and the Patient Protection and Affordable Care Act, along with other current trends and issues that impact health care workers, employers, and patients.
- Chapter Two, *Your Work Ethic and Performance*, has a new section discussing the importance of self-awareness, mindfulness, and acting with intent.
- Chapter Three, *Personal Traits of the Health Care Professional*, has a new section discussing negligence, malpractice, civil and criminal law, libel, slander, and other legal aspects.

- Chapter Four, *Relationships, Teamwork, and Communication Skills,* has been expanded with new content including: The Essential Elements of Communication, Factors that Influence Your Communication with Others, and Barriers to Communication. Additional new topics include Health Literacy and Hearing Loss.
- Chapter Five, *Cultural Competence and Patient Care,* has new content on patient consent, patient rights and responsibilities, and online patient portals. The Case Study involves a transgender patient who believes she has been disrespected by office staff.
- Chapter Six, *Professionalism and Your Personal Life*, has a new section on Self-Care for Health Care Workers with information on nutrition and a healthy diet, personal risk factors, and the importance of resilience. Text covering the standards for appropriate attire (dress codes) and the importance of exercising caution in after-hours behavior has been updated and reinforced.
- Chapter Seven, *The Practicum Experience*, has been expanded to include a new section on Safety at Work and a discussion about drug testing in states that have legalized the medicinal and recreational use of marijuana.
- Chapter Eight, *Employment and Professional Development*, has been reorganized and updated to emphasize the increasing use of Internet job boards and online job applications. New content provides resources for researching labor trends and projections, and reinforces the importance of leadership skills and participation in professional associations.

Additional changes in the 5th edition include the following:

- The *For More Information* sections in each chapter have been updated and expanded to provide additional resources.
- A new section, *Closing Thoughts*, has been added at the end of the text to summarize the key concepts that students need to think about and remember as they complete their education and join the health care workforce.
- The *Objectives, Reality Checks, Key Points, Chapter Review Questions, What If? Scenarios*, and *Appendices* have been updated and expanded.
- More than 55 new terms and definitions have been added to the *Glossary*, for a total of 318 terms.
- The *Instructor Resource Manual* has been revised to reflect updated, expanded, and new content in the text.

Information for Students

Students should read each chapter in the textbook and complete the end-of-chapter learning activities prior to moving on to the next chapter. The end-of-chapter learning activities include *Chapter Review Questions* and *What If? Scenarios*.

Information for Instructors

This textbook is designed for use in classroom and online courses. The book may also be used for personal reading, for orienting and training new health care workers, and for in-service and continuing education sessions for experienced health care workers.

The textbook may be incorporated into introductory, core curriculum, or capstone courses; used as preparation for practicum experiences; and used for workshops on topics such as Employment Strategies, Career Development, and Work Readiness. Instructors may choose to use this text in a general introductory course and then supplement learning later on through an advanced, discipline-specific course.

All ancillaries for this textbook including the Instructor Resource Manual, Power Point slides, and the Test Bank are accessible for download through the Pearson catalog as well as through the new MyHealthProfessionsLab for customers who purchase the digital solution. The new 5th edition MyHealthProfessionsLab features interactive activities that include self-assessments, preparatory materials for job interviews, role-playing exercises, video-based critical-thinking scenarios, and gradable homework questions.

In Closing

We hope you find *Professionalism in Health Care: A Primer for Career Success,* 5th Edition informative, thought-provoking, and beneficial.

Reviewers

About the Authors

Sherry Makely, PhD, RT(R) Textbook Author

Dr. Makely created and managed health sciences educational programs and workforce development initiatives in hospitals and universities for more than 42 years. She has a bachelor's degree in Radiologic Technology, a master's degree in Education, and a doctorate degree in Human Resources. Dr. Makely served as Director of Education for the School of Radiologic Science, and Manager of the Employee Education and Development Department for Methodist Hospital, Clarian Health, and Indiana University Health for 38 years. She has authored textbooks on professionalism for health care workers for more than 15 years for Pearson Education.

Vanessa J. Austin, RMA, AHI, (AMT), M.Ed. Contributing Author, Chapter Seven: The Practicum Experience

With more than 20 years experience as a Medical Assistant, Clinical Education Coordinator, and Program Director, Ms. Austin serves as Medical Assistant Instructor for Ross Medical Education in Cincinnati, Ohio. With a bachelor's degree in Health Care Management and a master's degree in Higher Education, she served as President of the Indiana State Society of American Medical Technologists and gives presentations on Professionalism in Health Care for state and national medical assisting conferences.

Quay Kester, PhD Content Contributor, Chapter Five: Cultural Competence

Dr. Quay Kester, President of Evoke Communications, specializes in diversity and inclusion initiatives to build cultural competence and confidence in health care, academic, and corporate organizations. Her avid commitment to learning about cultures and customs has taken her around the world and within various economies. Her national and international experience makes her a sought after speaker, leader, and facilitator. Dr. Kester has served as adjunct faculty at Indiana University, DePauw University, and as Visiting Professor at the University of Cape Coast, Ghana. With a doctorate degree from Indiana University, she is a Master Practitioner of Neurolinguistic Programming and a Certified Medical Illustrator. She serves on numerous boards including the Diversity Roundtable of Central Indiana.

Acknowledgments

A special Thank You! is extended to the following people for their expertise and time in developing this 5th edition:

Content Consultants

Frances Klene, RDMS, MS
Learning & Development Consultant
Franciscan Health Indianapolis
Indianapolis, Indiana

Jasmine Laseter, EMT-B
Emergency Medical Technician
TransCare Ambulance
Indianapolis, Indiana

Jennifer Olson, MS
Director of Education
Franciscan Health Indianapolis
Indianapolis, Indiana

Health Care Professionals

Recognition as a health care professional is something that has to be earned—a reputation that's developed and maintained each and every day you come to work. Professionalism is a state of mind, a way of "being," "knowing," and "doing" that sets you apart from others. It gives direction to how you look, think, and act. It brings together who you are as a person, what you value, how you treat other people, what you contribute in the workplace, and how seriously you take your job. Professionals don't just work to earn a paycheck. Income is important, but professionals view their work as a source of pride and a reflection of the role they play in society.

Health care professionals are good at what they do—and they like doing it. They enjoy helping others and knowing they've made a difference. Professionals have their "act together"—and it shows. They set high standards for their performance and achieve them. They see the "big picture" in health care and know where they fit in. Professionals care about quality and how to improve it. They treat everyone they meet with dignity and respect. And they continually strive to grow and to learn.

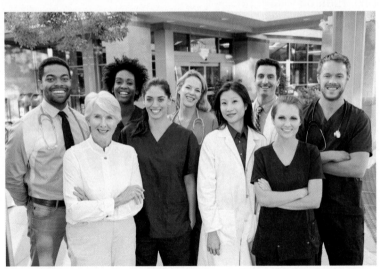

(*Monkey Business Images/Shutterstock*)

Introduction

Opportunity is missed by most because it is dressed in overalls and looks like work.

Thomas Alva Edison, Inventor, 1847–1931

Recognition as a Health Care Professional

There's no doubt about it. When you're sick or injured, or when a family member or friend needs health care, you want to be certain that you and your loved ones are cared for by **professionals** (people with experience and skills who are engaged in a specific occupation for pay or as a means of livelihood). Thinking back to the times when you've had a doctor's appointment, visited an **outpatient** clinic (a facility for care outside of a hospital) or emergency department, or been hospitalized for tests or treatments, you probably encountered many different types of health care workers. Although most of these workers performed their duties in a professional manner, you may have encountered a few who did not. We would like to think that everyone who works in health care functions as a professional, but experience has shown that this is not always the case.

What is a professional? How can you recognize a professional when you see one? What does "taking a professional approach" to one's work mean? Why is professionalism important? What must you learn as a student to prepare for future recognition as a health care professional yourself?

According to *Webster's New World Dictionary of the American Language, College Edition*, a *professional* is a person "with much experience and great skill in a specified role" who is "engaged in a specific occupation for pay or as a means of livelihood." As we look around us, we see many examples of professionals in different walks of life. In sports, for example, professional status is awarded to gifted athletes who have surpassed amateur events and moved into high-paying, major league competitions. In medicine, law, and science, people like doctors, lawyers, and engineers are considered professionals because of their expertise, college education, and special **credentials** (a letter or certificate given to a person to show that he/she has the right to exercise a certain authority) such as **licenses** (a credential from a state agency awarding legal permission to practice to a person who meets preestablished qualifications) and **certifications** (a credential from a state agency or a professional association awarding permission to use a special professional title to a person who meets preestablished competency standards). But truck drivers, hair stylists, and photographers consider themselves professionals too, as do bankers, insurance underwriters, and investment counselors. Exactly what is a professional and who is qualified to be one?

Occupations are sometimes divided into "professional" and "nonprofessional" categories based on criteria such as:

- unique and exclusive **scope of practice** (boundaries that determine what a worker may and may not do as part of his or her job)
- minimum educational standards and **accreditation** (certified as having met set standards) of educational programs
- minimum standards for entry into practice
- required credentials such as licenses or certifications
- **professional associations** (organizations composed of people from the same occupation) with codes of ethics and **competence** (possessing necessary knowledge and skills for a given occupation or task) standards.

When we apply these criteria to the health care workforce, then doctors, registered nurses, pharmacists, physical therapists, medical assistants, surgical technologists, dental assistants, radiographers, and the like are all classified as professionals. But that leaves other types of health care workers such as insurance processors, food service workers, housekeepers, and equipment repair technicians in the nonprofessional classification. Not making the list of professionals can be demeaning to people who work hard and make their jobs a top priority in their lives.

So in health care it's important to acknowledge another set of criteria that gives all health care workers the opportunity to be viewed as professionals whether they provide direct patient care or function in a support role behind the scenes: It's not *the job you do* that makes you a professional, it's *how you do your job* that counts.

Every health care worker has the opportunity—and the obligation—to strive for professional recognition. So regardless of how other people may classify your job as professional or nonprofessional, always remember that it's what you contribute in the workplace that really matters.

Professional recognition isn't something that's automatically bestowed upon a person when he or she completes an educational program, obtains a degree or certificate, or secures a license to practice. It's not dependent on a person's socioeconomic status, income, age, gender, race, job title, or position within the **hierarchy** (a group of people or units arranged by rank) of an organization. After all, we've all known people with college degrees, special credentials, and impressive job titles who don't behave in a professional manner.

Recognition as a health care professional is something that has to be earned—a **reputation** (a person's character, values, and behavior as viewed by others) that's developed and maintained each and every day you come to work. Professionalism is a state of mind, a way of "being," "knowing," and "doing" that sets you apart from others. It gives direction to how you look, think, and act. It brings together who you are as a person, what you value, how you treat other people, what you contribute in the workplace, and how seriously you take your job. Professionals don't just work to earn a paycheck. Income is important, but professionals view their work as a source of pride and a reflection of the role they play in society.

If you're serious about a career in health care, viewing yourself as a professional and being recognized as such by other people will be a major key to your success. Professionalism is something every organization looks for in its employees. How can you spot a health care professional when you see one? It's easy.

Health care professionals are good at what they do—and they like doing it. They enjoy helping others and knowing they've made a difference. Professionals "have their act together"—and it shows. They set high standards for their performance and achieve them. They see the "big picture" in health care and know where they fit in. Professionals care about quality and how to improve it. They treat everyone they meet with **dignity** (worth, merit, honor) and **respect** (a feeling or showing of honor or esteem toward another). They continually strive to grow and to learn.

Spotting a health care professional may be easy—but becoming one yourself is another matter. It's something you have to concentrate on every day—but it's worth it. To *be* a professional, you must *feel like* a professional. In our society, the amount of education a person has and what he or she does for a living have become important contributors to an individual's **self-esteem** (belief in oneself; self-respect) and sense of **self-worth** (a sense of one's own importance and value). *What we do* has become *who we are*. When you graduate from an educational program, earn a degree, or obtain a license or certification, you experience the exhilaration of knowing you've accomplished something worthwhile. Being recognized by others as a professional brings value and meaning to your efforts. It reminds you that what you do really counts. This is true whether you care for patients, process specimens, prepare meals, clean public areas, or work in any one of hundreds of different health care jobs. It's also true whether you work in a hospital, physician office, dental practice, clinic, rehab facility, or some other type of health care organization. No matter what your role involves, how you view your work and how you approach it can have a tremendous impact on your own life as well as on the lives of those you serve.

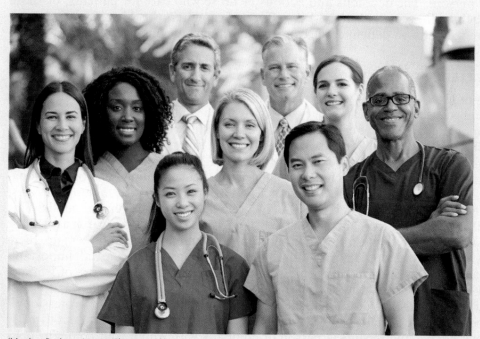

(*Monkey Business Images/Shutterstock*)

Why Health Care Needs Professionals

When you are sick or injured, health care can become a basic need for survival. Each year, millions of Americans receive health services in doctors' offices, hospitals, clinics, mental health facilities, and in their homes. Patients rely on health care professionals to provide affordable, state-of-the-art **diagnostic** (deciding the nature of a disease or condition) and **therapeutic** (an activity or method of treating or curing a disease or condition) procedures to help them overcome illness, injury, and other abnormalities that impact their health and quality of life.

But as you will learn in Chapter One, health care is a business, too. Finding ways to provide health care for more patients, using fewer resources, while achieving better outcomes has become a major challenge for health care **providers** (those who perform or enable a service such as a doctor, health care worker, or health care organization) and **payers** (a person or group that covers the expense of received goods or services). Meeting these challenges requires a cadre of health care workers who are committed to quality care, customer service, and cost effectiveness. People who fail to take a professional approach to their work are often late, absent, unreliable, and sloppy. Their actions may endanger patient care, customer service, safety, and the efficient use of limited resources.

Working in health care requires special skills and an **attitude** (a manner of acting, feeling, or thinking that shows one's disposition or opinion) that supports service to others. Patients seek health care services during some of the most vulnerable times in their lives, when they're sick, injured, and "at their worst." Each patient–worker interaction must build confidence and **trust** (confidence in the honesty, integrity, and reliability of another person). The decisions and actions of those who care for patients, or those who work behind the scenes to support the efforts of **caregivers** (health care workers who provide direct, hands-on patient care), can have an immediate and lasting impact.

The Importance of Every Job and Every Worker

Regardless of what type of job you are preparing for, you will play an important role in health care, because every job and every worker is important. Let's face reality—if a job weren't important it wouldn't exist. Everyone knows that the roles of doctors, nurses, pharmacists, and physical therapists, for example, are important. But patients and the general public may not be as familiar with the roles of other caregivers such as medical assistants, radiographers, EKG technicians, nuclear medicine technologists, occupational therapists, and sonographers, just to name a few. People who work in support roles, often behind the scenes, may be even less known to patients and the general public. This includes billing clerks, instrument technicians, biomedical engineers, research assistants, and social workers whose roles are also vital. Depending on how you add them up, there are several hundred different jobs in health care organizations and they are all important. Large urban hospitals and medical centers employ so many different types of workers they begin to resemble small towns.

If your job will involve direct patient care, it should be obvious that professionalism is important. The same holds true with other jobs where workers interact directly with visitors, guests, and **vendors** (a person or company with whom your company does business) such as customer service agents, telephone operators, purchasing agents, and billing clerks. But what about the large percentage of health care workers in support roles behind the scenes? Is professionalism really important in those jobs, too? What might happen if environmental services workers (housekeepers) miscalculated the dilution of an antiseptic cleaning fluid or used the wrong floor wax in a busy hallway? What if food service workers put the wrong items on a special-diet patient tray or spilled hot grease near an open flame in the kitchen? What if central service technicians failed to replace outdated stock or operated sterilizers at the wrong temperature?

It should be obvious that professionalism is vital in every job. Your challenge is to pull together the mixture of knowledge, skills, compassion, and commitment required to make you the very best employee you can possibly be. If you can meet this challenge every day on the job, then you've earned the privilege of being recognized as a health care professional. Nothing less is acceptable.

The information in this text will help guide your journey to professional recognition. It's important to start developing your reputation now while you are still a student. Apply yourself, take your studies seriously, learn to manage your time, and hone your communication skills. Make thoughtful decisions, encourage and support your fellow classmates, and find ways to balance the priorities in your life. Remember that everything that you hear, observe, learn, and experience will be important at some point in your health career. If your educational program includes a **practicum** (a "real-life" learning experience obtained through working on-site in a health care facility while enrolled as a student; also known as a clinical, an externship, an internship, a hands-on experience, or the like), you'll be interacting with health care workers, physicians, and patients to gain hands-on experience even before you graduate.

Expect some changes along the way, plan to continue your learning after you've graduated from school, and always strive to do your very best. You and the patients will someday serve deserve nothing less.

Professionalism in Health Care

A Primer for Career Success

The Health Care Industry and Your Role

1

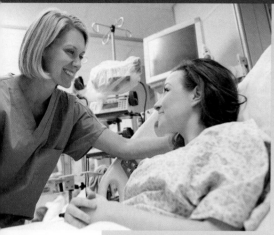

(Monkey Business Images/Shutterstock)

In a world that is constantly changing, there is no one subject or set of subjects that will serve you for the foreseeable future, let alone for the rest of your life. The most important skill to acquire now is learning how to learn.

John Naisbitt, international best-selling author

CHAPTER OBJECTIVES

Having completed this chapter, you will be able to:

- List four benefits of working in the health care industry.
- Explain the difference between *soft skills* and *hard skills*.
- List two reasons why health care workers must be aware of current trends and issues in the health care industry.
- List three reasons why health care is expensive and the costs continue to rise.
- Identify two ways that the Baby Boomer population will impact the health care industry.
- Describe two controversial issues associated with health care reform.

- Define *continuous quality improvement*.
- List two quality improvement goals.
- Define *sentinel event*.
- Explain the connection between sentinel events and patient safety.
- Identify two trends in the supply and demand of health care workers.
- List two advantages of electronic health records.
- Define *social media*.
- Give two examples of social media sites.

KEY TERMS

accountability

accountable care organizations

acute

advanced practice providers (APPs)

adverse effects

alternative medicine

apps

Baby Boomers

baseline data

blog

breach

chronic

cognition

complementary medicine

confidentiality

consumers

continuity

continuous quality improvement (CQI)

digital communication

disabled

discipline

diverse

electronic health record (EHR)

emoji

emotional intelligence quotient (EQ)

empowered

error

gatekeepers

geriatric

gross domestic product (GDP)

hard skills

health care exchanges

hospice services

individual mandate

infant mortality rate

intelligence quotient (IQ)

interpersonal skills

Lean Sigma

legibility

life expectancy

Medicaid

medical homes

Medicare

metrics

mistake

multiskilled

obese

outcome data

out-of-pocket expense

palliative care

people skills

personality

perspective

preexisting condition

prenatal

preventive

primary care

process

readmission

root cause

sentinel event

single-payer system

smartphones

social media

soft skills

specialists

staffing level

stakeholders

traits

transferable skills

work ethic

Working in Health Care

Whether you are preparing for your first job or gaining the knowledge and skills you need for career advancement, you've made a good decision choosing a health care occupation. Working in health care offers lots of benefits and opportunities.

Health care employs about 10% of all American workers. Job opportunities both now and in the future appear excellent. While the recent recession eliminated millions of jobs throughout the United States, jobs in the health care sector grew steadily. In fact, the past 14 years have seen unprecedented job growth in health care. Thirteen of the 20 fastest-growing occupations in the United States are in health care and this trend is likely to continue due to the rapid growth of the elderly population, expansion of health care information technology, and increases in the rates of **obese** (weighing more than 20% above a person's ideal weight) and **disabled** (having a condition that damages or limits a person's physical or mental abilities) Americans. Health care is one of the fastest-growing sectors in the U.S. economy. It's projected to generate more than 4 million new jobs between 2012 and 2022—more than any other industry.

The health care industry offers **diverse** (differing; varied) employment opportunities, ranging from small-town physician practices with one medical assistant to large, urban academic medical centers and health systems employing thousands of workers. Many employers offer flexible work schedules and most provide valuable benefits such as health and life insurance, paid vacation time and holidays, tuition assistance, and a retirement plan.

With so many different occupations from which to choose, health care workers have an abundance of opportunities for career advancement. You can:

- Earn advanced degrees and additional professional certifications
- Move up the ladder in your original **discipline** (a branch of knowledge or learning such as nursing, medical assisting, surgical technology, and so forth)
- Become **multiskilled** (cross-trained to perform more than one function, possibly in more than one discipline)
- Apply your **transferable skills** (skills acquired in one job that are applicable in another job) to train in a different discipline
- Advance into leadership, teaching, sales, or research jobs

One of the best benefits of working in health care is the opportunity to improve the quality of people's lives. As mentioned in the Introduction, when you are sick or injured, health care can become a basic need for survival. People seek health care services during some of the most vulnerable times in their lives. Premature babies struggle to survive, injured athletes strive to regain strength, people with **acute** (severe but of short or limited duration) and **chronic** (occurring frequently over a long period of time) ailments try to lead normal lives, and terminally ill patients face end-of-life decisions. Health care workers are at their patients' sides from cradle to grave, providing crucial diagnostic and therapeutic procedures, compassionate care, and helpful encouragement and support. It's a privilege to work in health care and touch the lives of everyone you serve.

As a service industry, health care requires superb **people skills**, also known as **soft skills** (personality characteristics that enhance one's ability to interact effectively with other people). Your **personality** (distinctive qualities of a person; patterns of behavior and attitudes) and your **interpersonal skills** (the ability to interact with other people) enhance your relationships, job performance, and career prospects. Sometimes referred to as your **emotional intelligence quotient (EQ)** (the ability to perceive, assess, and manage your own emotions and other people's emotions), soft skills relate more to *who you are* than *what you know*—your **intelligence quotient (IQ)** (the mental ability to learn and understand). Once you've graduated from your educational program and obtained credentials to practice, employers will assume you are competent to perform the hands-on, technical, **hard skills** duties of your job. Hard skills can be learned and improved over time, but soft skills are part of your personality and much more difficult to acquire and change. Employers are increasingly screening, hiring, paying, and promoting for soft skills to ensure that their employees work harmoniously with other people.

This book focuses on the soft skills you need to achieve success in health care. The following chapters discuss:

- **Work ethic** (attitudes and behaviors that support good work performance)
- Personal and character **traits** (characteristics or qualities related to one's personality)
- Relationships and communication skills
- Working with patients and customer service
- Professionalism and your personal life
- The practicum experience
- Employment and career advancement.

Before addressing these topics, we must first focus on another important step in preparing for a role in health care: learning as much as you can about the industry's current trends and issues. As a health care worker, you'll be part of the nation's fastest-growing industry.

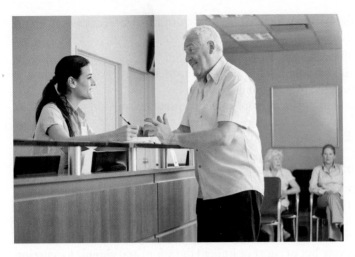

Figure 1-1 Patient checking in at registration (*Tyler Olson/Shutterstock*)

CONSIDER THIS

AMERICANS WITH DISABILITIES

More than 20 years after passing the Americans with Disabilities Act, research shows that more than 57 million people, nearly one out of every five American adults, has a disability. Disabilities include difficulty with vision, mobility, **cognition** (knowing, understanding), self-care, and independent living. The highest rates of disabilities are among adults with the lowest levels of education, income, and employment. People at least 80 years of age are eight times more likely to become disabled than people 15 years or younger. About 40% of disabled people ages 21–64 are employed, versus 79% of people who aren't disabled.

About 8 million people have vision problems, 2 million of whom are blind. More than 7 million people have difficulty hearing and 5.6 million use hearing aids. More than 30 million people report difficulty walking or climbing stairs, with many of them relying on canes, crutches, wheelchairs, and walkers. Seven million adults suffer with depression or anxiety issues that interfere with their normal daily activities.

As more Americans become older, the number of patients requiring medical care for disabilities will continue to rise, placing an even greater strain on the U.S. health care system.

- How much do you know about the health care industry?
- Are you up to speed with current topics and where health care is headed?
- Do you know enough about local and national health care issues to discuss them intelligently with other people?

Everyone is affected by the health care industry and many Americans have opinions about what's wrong with health care and how to fix it. This is especially true today because health care has become very expensive. All Americans, and especially health care workers, need to be actively involved in finding ways to make improvements.

If you want to be viewed as a health care professional, you need to be aware of what's going on in your industry. This doesn't mean you have to know everything about all of the issues under debate. But you do need to keep up with current trends and issues and consider how they might impact your job, your patients, your personal health, and your career. Be on the lookout for information from a variety of sources. Read articles about health care and watch the news for special programs about health care issues. Attend health care seminars and conferences when you get the opportunity and become active in your discipline's professional organizations. Speak with people who are current on the latest trends and join in conversations to discuss the issues.

By deciding to work in health care, you have chosen an industry like no other.

- Workers are dealing with life and death situations on a daily basis, 24/7/365.
- Things are changing rapidly; new devices, drugs, and medical procedures are under development every day.
- Hospitals and doctors are forming networks, restructuring organizations, and redesigning jobs and job duties.
- Population trends, especially the aging of **Baby Boomers** (people born in the United States between 1946 and 1964), are driving major changes in health care.
- An insufficient supply of doctors and health care workers in rural areas and economically depressed urban areas are leaving large segments of the population medically underserved.

When you consider all of these factors, it becomes clear that change is the name of the game in health care. It's a fast-moving train. You need to climb onboard or risk being left behind. You must know what's going on and where things appear to be headed, so you can be well informed and prepared for the future ahead.

Health care has become one of the most controversial industries in recent years, with new laws and regulations. What's the best way to retool our health care system so that everyone who needs health care can access medical services at an affordable cost? Health care is a business. As a health care professional, it's important to know about the business side of your industry and where you fit in.

TRENDS AND ISSUES

MULTIPLE CHRONIC DISEASES ON THE RISE

Approximately two-thirds of American older adults have more than one chronic disease and about 15% of them (4 million people) have at least six chronic conditions. Chronic diseases include diabetes, heart disease, depression, asthma, high cholesterol, high blood pressure, arthritis, and Alzheimer's disease. More than 41% of **Medicare** (a government program that provides health care primarily for people age 65 and older) funding is spent on seniors who are much sicker than those of past generations. **Life expectancy** (the statistical number of years of life remaining at any given age) is longer for today's seniors, so many of them will struggle with their diseases for decades to come, placing a major strain on Medicare funding.

Consider these statistics:

- Every day about 10,000 people reach age 65 and become eligible for Medicare.
- Seniors with five or more chronic ailments see about 13 doctors and take about 50 prescription drugs over a year's time.
- The average cost of caring for a patient with one chronic disease is three times greater than caring for a patient with no chronic disease.
- The cost of caring for a patient with five or more chronic diseases is 15 times more than caring for a patient with no chronic disease.
- One billion dollars in Medicare funding was spent on just 10,000 older patients in 2010.
- Seventy-five percent of the most expensive Medicare cases involve Alzheimer's disease.

(continued)

- Alzheimer's is the most difficult and expensive disease to treat because it complicates other conditions and requires long-term care.
- Nursing home care and related expenses can add up to $100,000 a year per person.

Helping patients with multiple chronic diseases manage their prescriptions and coordinate care among a dozen doctors presents an enormous challenge. Hospitals are responding by employing care coordinators and redesigning areas of the ER for seniors. As patients become sicker, the goal is to intervene quickly and provide them with helpful services without admitting them to the hospital. When patients require hospitalization, teams of people from area doctor's offices, rehab facilities, home care agencies, pharmacies, and nursing homes meet to discuss cases and coordinate discharge procedures so that details don't fall through the cracks. This type of teamwork, communication, and coordination will become more common in the future as an effective approach to helping seniors manage multiple chronic diseases.

Health Care as a Business

Most of what you learn here relates to working in a patient care environment—the service side of the health care industry. But understanding the business side of health care is very important, too. Health care is expensive, it's a necessity of life, and it affects everyone including **consumers** (purchasers or users of a product or service), taxpayers, employers, businesses, government, and other **stakeholders** (people with a keen interest in a project or organization; may be end-users of a product or service). Consider the following:

- As patients, everyone is a consumer of health care. When the need arises, consumers want the best health care available regardless of the cost.
- As taxpayers, everyone pays for health care through programs such as Medicare and **Medicaid** (a government program that provides health care for low-income people and families and for those with certain disabilities).
- The United States spends about $2.5 trillion per year (about $8,500 per person) on health care, significantly more than any other developed nation, and the cost is rising.
- Unpaid medical bills account for about 60% of all personal bankruptcies in the United States.
- Health care costs account for about 20% of the nation's **gross domestic product** (GDP; the total market value of all goods and services produced in one year) and is rising.

So when it comes to health care, everyone is a stakeholder with concerns and opinions to voice.

Providing health care for everyone who needs it at a reasonable expense is an enormous challenge. The cost of health care in the United States is growing faster than the cost of most other goods and services. Cost increases result from:

- The need to recruit, pay, and retain highly competent doctors and health professionals
- Medical research to develop new drugs, devices, and procedures
- The rising cost of medical equipment, supplies, and utilities
- Building construction, remodeling, and maintenance
- The expense of training future doctors, nurses, and other health professionals.

As the cost of health care increases, Americans continue to debate the best way to pay for it. People who have health insurance typically receive coverage through their employer, a government program such as Medicare or Medicaid, or an individual or group policy. Each patient has a **primary care** doctor who provides the initial or basic medical care needed. The primary care doctor then refers the patient to a variety of **specialists** (people who are devoted to a particular occupation or branch of study) depending on the additional services required. With primary care doctors acting as **gatekeepers** (people who monitor the actions of other people and/or control access to something), the goal is to:

- Encourage **preventive** services (actions taken to avoid contracting a medical condition) such as vaccinations, flu shots, and health screenings
- Provide medical care in the least expensive settings such as doctors' offices, outpatient clinics, and the patient's home
- Avoid unnecessary or duplicate tests and treatments
- Coordinate services from different providers to ensure **continuity** (the quality of being continuous, uninterrupted, and connected) in care and the best outcomes for the patient.

Controlling the cost of health care is just one of the problems. Ensuring adequate access to health care services is also an issue. Millions of Americans don't have health insurance or a primary care doctor. They go without medical care or rely on hospital emergency departments where the cost of caring for patients is very high. They go without prescription drugs, which makes their conditions more difficult and expensive to treat in the long run. Pregnant women forego **prenatal** (before birth) care, which can cause major problems later on.

When patients are unable (or unwilling) to pay their medical bills, the providers must write off the loss as charity care or unreimbursed services. Since hospitals and doctors have to cover their expenses to remain in business, this loss of income drives up the cost for other patients who do have health insurance and who do pay their bills.

The lack of doctors and medical facilities in rural areas and in medically underserved urban areas also limits access to health care services for many Americans. Many doctors and health care professionals prefer to live and work in attractive urban areas, making it difficult to recruit and retain a sufficient labor supply in other parts of the country.

Before examining some of the new laws and current efforts to improve America's health care system, let's examine what to expect as Baby Boomers age and place increased demands on the industry.

BY THE NUMBERS

OBESITY IN AMERICA

At a cost of $147–$210 billion per year, obesity has become a major concern in the health of Americans. Obesity leads to several types of preventable chronic diseases and life-threatening conditions including type 2 diabetes, hypertension, arthritis, heart disease and stroke, and obesity-related cancer. More than 75% of patients with hypertension and a third of cancer deaths can be linked to insufficient physical activity and/or obesity. In 1994, 7.8 million people were diagnosed with diabetes. By 2014 that number had grown to almost 26 million. Today, nearly 40% of people ages 40–59 are obese.

Obesity rates vary from state to state. Every state has an obesity rate above 20%, and 23 states have rates at 25% or more. Adult obesity is highest in Mississippi and West Virginia at 35% while Colorado has the lowest rate at 21%. States with the highest rates are in the South or the Midwest. States in the Northeast and West have the lowest rates. Between 2012 and 2013, six states had sharp increases in their obesity rates: Alaska, Delaware, Idaho, New Jersey, Tennessee, and Wyoming.

As of 2013, nearly 14% of high school students were obese and almost 17% were overweight. The rates were highest in Kentucky at 18% and lowest in Utah at just above 6%. Obesity rates among children ages 10–17 range from about 10% in Oregon to almost 22% in Mississippi.

(continued)

Obese adults spend 42% more on direct health care costs than nonobese patients. Obesity is associated with lower productivity at work, increased number of sick days, and higher medical claims. Reducing obesity and related chronic conditions will likely become a high priority in the future. Although obesity rates appear to be stabilizing somewhat, it's projected that by the year 2030 about 42% of Americans will be obese, seeking treatment in oncology, cardiology, and primary care offices throughout the country.

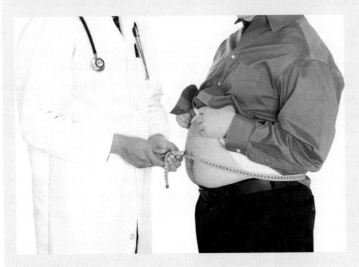

Figure 1-2 Obese patient being assessed by his doctor (*PathDoc/Shutterstock*)

Impact of the Baby Boomer Population

The older population in the United States is growing rapidly due to the aging of the Baby Boomer population—the 78 million people born between the years 1946 and 1964. Here are some things to consider about this large population:

- The over-65 population will almost double in the coming years.
- The first Baby Boomer reached 64 in 2010; it will take another 21 years for the last one to reach that milestone.
- When compared with previous generations, Baby Boomers have higher education levels, use more online Internet resources, and are more directly involved in their health care.
- Almost 20% of Baby Boomers are minorities, requiring more attention to cultural differences.
- Baby Boomers possess 75% of the nation's disposable income but worry about covering their health care and retirement expenses.
- Thanks to joint replacements and other medical advancements, Baby Boomers are more physically active than seniors in the past and suffer from fewer disabilities.
- Seventy percent of baby boomers subscribe to **complementary medicine** (combining alternative medical approaches with traditional medical practices) and/or **alternative medicine** (healing arts that are not part of traditional medical practice in the United States) such as massage therapy, chiropractic care, meditation, and acupuncture.

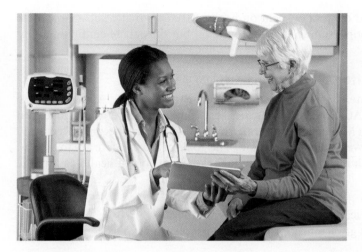

Figure 1-3 Baby Boomer patient consulting with her nurse practitioner *(Monkey Business Images/Shutterstock)*

Baby Boomers are predicted to have an unprecedented long-term impact on the health care industry, consuming far more medical services than any older population in the past. Baby Boomers will live longer than their predecessors. In fact, half of all of the people who have ever lived to age 65 are alive today. By the year 2030, 6 out of 10 seniors will have at least one chronic condition, 1 out of 3 will be considered obese, 1 out of 4 will have diabetes, and 1 out of 2 will be living with arthritis. More than 25% of the total health care spending for each patient occurs in the final years of his or her life. By the year 2030, 4 out of 10 adult visits to doctors' offices will be baby boomers, 55 million lab tests per year will be needed for diabetic seniors, eight times more knee replacements will be performed than today, and 4 million more emergency department visits will be logged than today.

Efforts are already underway to prepare for the impact of this large patient population. New medicines, monitoring equipment, and surgical techniques are in development. With new technology, seniors will be able to monitor more of their conditions from home and communicate remotely with physicians and specialists. Hospitals are remodeling to offer the more personalized care and convenience that baby boomers expect, including more private rooms with sound-reduction materials and in-room computers for patient use.

These are just a few examples of how health care providers are preparing for the arrival of this large population of older patients. But much more needs to be done to improve the nation's health care system for all patients.

Improving the Nation's Health Care System

As large numbers of Baby Boomers interact more frequently with the health care system, they will likely become even more engaged in improvement efforts. In doing so, they will join the increasing number of lawmakers, employers, business leaders, providers, consumers, insurance companies, drug manufacturers, and other groups involved in health care reform. There's no question that the United States has one of the best health care systems in the world, but Americans lag behind other countries in life expectancy, **infant mortality rate** (the number of infants that die during the first year of life), preventive care, and other common measures of health and well-being. Studies indicate that as much as one-third of what is spent on health care isn't really necessary. Most everyone agrees there are ample opportunities for improvement but the debate continues about the best way to proceed.

Health Care Reform and the Affordable Care Act

After many months of heated debate and negotiation, the Patient Protection and Affordable Care Act (PPACA), also known as the ACA (Affordable Care Act) and Obamacare, was signed into law by President Barack Obama in March 2010. Several provisions of the law became effective in 2010 while others have rolled out over a four-year period. The goals of Obamacare are to expand access to affordable, quality health insurance and to reduce the rising cost of health care in the United States.

The Affordable Care Act:

- Increases the number of Americans covered by health insurance.
- Offers tax credits and expands government programs for people who can't afford to pay for health insurance.
- Establishes **health care exchanges**, open marketplaces through which buyers and sellers of health insurance can come together to help consumers compare and shop for health insurance coverage.
- Prevents insurance companies from cancelling policies or denying coverage to people with a **preexisting condition** (a medical condition that a patient has prior to applying for health insurance).
- Mandates that all qualified insurance plans must offer the ACA's 10 essential medical benefits necessary to prevent and treat health conditions.
- Provides annual checkups, immunizations, and preventive testing with no **out-of-pocket expense** (costs not covered by insurance that patients have to pay themselves).
- Prohibits insurance companies from charging more based on gender or health status.
- Prohibits plans that put annual or lifetime dollar amount limits on health care benefits.
- Includes an **individual mandate**, a requirement that everyone must have health insurance or be subject to a penalty tax.
- Allows parents to keep children on their health insurance policies up to 26 years of age.

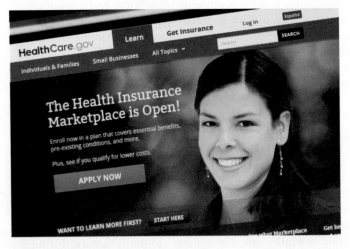

Figure 1-4 Healthcare.gov website (*Sjscreens/Alamy*)

As a result of the new law, the rate of uninsured Americans has dropped significantly. The cost of health care continues to grow but at a slower pace. Efforts are underway to restructure health care delivery systems to improve efficiency, cost-effectiveness, and quality of care. But many stakeholders don't support the ACA and are taking steps to change it or repeal it. Some feel the law went too far in involving the government in what should be a private health insurance marketplace. Others feel the law didn't go far enough and would prefer a **single-payer system** (a universal health care system where a single-payer fund, rather than private insurers, pays for health care costs), as found in other developed countries. So far the law has withstood multiple legal challenges including cases brought before the Supreme Court, but the debate continues.

Many health care organizations are undergoing major change as a result of the ACA. Hospitals in particular are experiencing a great deal of pressure in the new world of health care reform. Mergers and buyouts among U.S. hospitals doubled between 2009 and 2012, resulting in layoffs and closures. Since millions of people have gained health insurance through the ACA, hospitals must provide care for more patients at the same time they face cuts in payments for services. The ACA provides financial incentives when patients receive care in outpatient settings or in the patient's home instead of in hospitals. As a result, over the past few years, jobs in outpatient settings and home health companies have grown by 9% while jobs in hospitals have grown by less than 1%.

Several new approaches have emerged aimed at enhancing health care services through better coordination among health care providers. Patient-centered **medical homes** are organizations that provide comprehensive, coordinated health care to patients who are members. First proposed in 2007, this concept strengthens the partnership between a patient and his or her primary care doctor and strives to improve access to care as well as quality and safety. Health care providers receive financial incentives for service improvements.

Accountable care organizations are composed of several medical homes. Often referred to as medical neighborhoods, ACOs are networks of health care providers that work together and share responsibility and **accountability** (accepting responsibility and the consequences of one's actions) for a large group of patients. Primary care doctors, specialists, home health companies, rehabilitation centers, and hospitals all collaborate to eliminate duplicative tests and procedures, focus on prevention, manage diseases, share medical information, care for patients in the least expensive settings (outpatient clinics and doctor's offices as opposed to emergency departments), and reduce medical **errors** (something done incorrectly through ignorance or carelessness). Under this new plan, accountable care organizations receive financial incentives to reduce costs while achieving quality outcomes—thereby getting paid more to keep their patients healthy and out of the hospital. ACOs that fail to meet performance and financial expectations can face financial penalties. The ACO approach is quite different from the current fee-for-service model where providers receive payment based on hospitalized patients and the number and types of diagnostic tests and treatments they order and perform. The advent of ACOs is already having an impact on the American health care system as providers rush to form or enlarge their networks and adopt strategies to become integrated systems.

The goals of a concept called Triple Aim go even further. Through the Institute for Healthcare Improvement (IHI) and as the framework for the National Quality Strategy of the U.S. Department of Health and Human Services (HHS), Triple Aim is based on the belief that no single industry or sector of the country can change the health of the U.S. population on its own. Therefore health care organizations, social service agencies, school systems, employers, and public health departments are challenged to work together to tackle three overriding goals: improving the population's health, improving the patient's experience of care, and reducing the per capita cost (the cost per patient). First proposed in 2008, Triple Aim initiatives are now underway not only in the United States but around the world as diverse organizations work and learn together to share innovative approaches and valuable data.

As stakeholders debate the Affordable Care Act and as people throughout the country and the world search for the best ways to increase access to high-quality health care at an affordable expense, there are several other efforts underway to improve America's health care system. As you prepare for your role in health care, it's important to also be aware of these trends and issues.

THINK ABOUT IT

WHERE DO YOU STAND ON HEALTH CARE REFORM?

Where do you stand on the Affordable Care Act and efforts to reform the nation's health care system? Since you work in health care, people will assume that you know what's going on and will have thoughts to share.

- What role, if any, should the government play in the health insurance market?
- Should taxpayers and/or businesses help cover the cost of health insurance for people who can't afford it?
- Should people be required to have health insurance or pay a tax if they don't want the insurance, believe they don't need it, or can't afford it?
- Should employers with more than 50 employees have to provide health insurance for their employees or pay a penalty?
- What changes, if any, should be made to Medicare and Medicaid to adequately fund the programs while reducing costs to taxpayers?

Quality Improvement

Improving the quality of health care services to achieve better patient outcomes has always been a top priority in health care. But it's even more important today when the goal is to "do more, with less, and get better results." By closely monitoring patient outcomes, providers can make sure that quality doesn't drop as cost-cutting and health care reform efforts kick in.

One of the most important steps in improving quality is closely examining the **process** (a set of actions or steps that must be accomplished correctly and in the proper order) by which work gets done—looking at each action or step in the flow of work that must be accomplished correctly and in the proper order. Examining work processes is especially important when something goes wrong. In health care, this is called **continuous quality improvement** (CQI)—using methods and tools to identify, prevent, and reduce the impact of process failures. By studying the process, you can determine if there's a better way to do things. When something goes wrong, it's important to figure out what happened and implement a better process to prevent the occurrence from happening again. You must continually evaluate your processes and make the necessary adjustments. Also make sure that quality improvement efforts in your department don't result in a negative impact on other departments.

When doing QI projects, you must remain focused on what you're trying to do. Ask yourself these questions: (1) What are we trying to accomplish? (2) How will we know if we are successful? (3) What options do we have and which ones might work best?

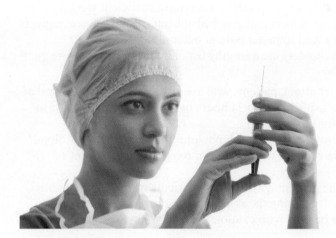

Figure 1-5 Surgical nurse double-checking the correct dosage (*India Picture/Shutterstock*)

Quality improvement goals include:

- Eliminating **adverse effects** (unfavorable or harmful outcomes) such as patient falls and bed sores
- Reducing waste and unnecessary expense, such as duplicating blood tests or keeping patients in the hospital longer than necessary
- Avoiding costly hospital **readmissions** (quick return to a hospital after discharge)
- Preventing undesirable patient outcomes such as hospital-acquired infections or medication overdoses

Of course, quality improvement is much more than just preventing things from going wrong. Hospitals and other health care providers use quality improvement approaches such as PDSA to figure out how to make things that are working well work even better.

Plan: creating a plan or a test to see how a different approach would work
Do: implementing the plan to see what happens
Study: reviewing the results to determine what was learned
Act: taking action based on what was learned

When using the PDSA approach, you might have to go through the four-step cycle several times before you get the results you're seeking. Using **metrics** (a set of measurements that quantify results) is the key. In most QI projects, you must be able to measure things to know if your approach was an improvement or not. You gather **baseline data** (information gathered before a change begins to form a basis for analyzing subsequent changes) before you start and compare those statistics with your **outcome data** (information gathered after a change has taken place to examine the impact or results of the change) after you have finished to see if there's been any change and, if so, how much.

There are many ways to improve quality in health care, not the least of which relates to **staffing levels** (the number of people with certain qualifications who are assigned to work at a given time). For example, studies have shown that having an adequate supply of registered nurses on a patient care unit is directly related to the quality of care those patients receive. When hospitals, clinics, and doctors' offices cut back on staff, there's a greater likelihood that quality and patient care will suffer. So it's important for health care providers to maintain sufficient staffing levels while monitoring their labor costs. Staffing models that give bedside nurses and other caregivers more responsibility for quality and safety lead to better patient outcomes.

Health care providers and other stakeholders use a lengthy list of indicators to measure quality. Here are just a few examples:

- *Aspirin at arrival*: The percent of heart attack patients who are given aspirin upon arrival at the hospital. (Patients should receive aspirin within 24 hours before or after they arrive at the hospital to reduce the potential for blood clots.)
- *Oxygenation assessment*: The percent of patients with pneumonia who have their blood/oxygen level measured. (Pneumonia reduces the amount of oxygen in the patient's blood.)
- *Surgical infection prevention care*: The percentage of surgery patients who receive an antibiotic within one hour before surgically cutting the skin. (Antibiotics reduce the risk of infection. However, antibiotics must be used with caution to avoid risks associated with multiresistant organisms.)

Hospitals are known for long waits in the emergency department, overuse of paperwork, duplicated tests and treatments, and other wasteful characteristics. Similar problems occur in clinics, physician practices, and other places where people access health care. **Lean Sigma** combines two quality improvement approaches: Lean and Six Sigma. Lean initiatives aim to streamline processes, reduce or eliminate waste, and increase speed and efficiency. Six Sigma initiatives, used successfully for many years in the manufacturing industry, aim to reduce variations and defects as a means of improving quality and reducing costs. When combined and applied in a health care organization, Lean Sigma concepts can improve work flow, productivity, timely delivery of services, and patient satisfaction while reducing waste, errors, and costs. Teams from different units or departments work together to examine each step in a process. When the process breaks down, they look for the **root cause** (the factor that led to the problem and that, when fixed, will solve the problem and prevent it from happening again) instead of just blaming someone. By openly sharing information across units or departments, Lean Sigma teams try to develop a perfect process where each step creates value for the patient. Organizations don't have to sacrifice quality to save money. They use strategies and tools to measure short-term improvements and then continue to track outcomes and data over time.

Approximately half of all health care organizations have incorporated Lean Sigma projects as part of their overall improvement efforts to reduce costs while increasing capacity and quality. Many of them report impressive results. Examples include:

- Reducing preparation time for chemotherapy treatments by 40% while eliminating most errors
- Reducing patient time spent in the emergency department by 20%
- Reducing the wait time for radiology oncology services from referral to treatment by 60%, down to six days
- Improving the pregnancy rate in an infertility clinic by 24%
- Reducing the number of steps that ER nurses take to get supplies by 78%
- Increasing patient satisfaction by 50%
- Cutting costs by 15% by redesigning a hospital's transplant unit
- Decreasing in-hospital mortality rates by almost 48%

Quality improvement projects are often closely aligned with efforts to improve patient safety. Let's take a closer look at the situation.

RECENT DEVELOPMENTS_____

A SINGLE DROP OF BLOOD

Researchers are discovering that a single drop of your blood may provide far more information about your current and future health than previously thought. The human body has about 1.5 gallons of blood circulating in its system. Thanks to new technology, blood tests will soon help doctors understand how sickness results from molecular abnormalities. Tests on just one drop of blood can detect a wide range of conditions including Alzheimer's disease, cancer, multiple sclerosis, and Down syndrome. Characteristics such as nut allergies, the sex of a fetus, fertility level, and the risks of suicide, heart attack, and death after surgery may also be uncovered. Breast cancer may be found more quickly through blood testing than through mammography, and Alzheimer's may be diagnosed before it severely affects the brain. Thousands of viruses can be detected from a drop of blood within seconds, including evidence of every virus a patient has ever had in the past.

Decoding the secrets of blood offers significant benefits for patients. Blood samples are easily obtained without having to undergo invasive procedures such tissue biopsies and surgeries. Instead of waiting to feel a lump on a breast, patients with an earlier diagnosis could begin cancer treatment much sooner. Blood tests are much less expensive than diagnostic imaging exams such as CT and MRI scans. The quick turnaround time for test results could allow coaches to determine if athletes with possible brain concussions are safe to return to the game. Only time will tell the extent to which a single drop of blood can greatly improve the diagnosis and effective treatment of many different conditions and diseases.

Patient Safety

Health care is one of the most, if not *the* most, complex industries on Earth. Hundreds of medical miracles occur every day as dedicated, hard-working health care professionals do their best to care for patients. But as you've already learned, the health care system is not perfect. Consider the following sober statistics:

- Death by preventable medical **mistakes** (to understand, interpret, or estimate incorrectly) is the third leading cause of death in the United States. Heart disease and cancer are the top two causes of death.
- Each day 1,000 people die as a result of medical errors at a cost of $1 trillion per year to the United States.
- Each day 200 people die from hospital-acquired infections, totaling more than 70,000 deaths per year.
- Although the U.S. spends the most money on health care among other developed nations, it scores more poorly than most on quality indicators.

Improving patient safety requires a heightened awareness of errors and mistakes and a culture that encourages nurses and other health care workers to speak up when they see mistakes about to occur. Nurses and other health professionals who interact frequently with their patients get to know their patients quite well. These caregivers must feel **empowered** (given authority, enabled, or permitted) to question things when they don't seem right. For example, a nurse might question the doctor's order to give the patient a certain drug if the nurse believes the drug might cause a complication with other drugs the patient is taking. Or a medical assistant might notice that a busy doctor forgot to properly wash his or her hands when moving from a patient with the flu to the next patient there for prenatal care.

Speaking up when you spot something that doesn't seem right may require some courage on your part, especially when questioning someone with more authority. But it's absolutely essential in protecting the patient's safety. Ask yourself this: If you were about to make a mistake that could potentially harm a patient, wouldn't you want someone to speak up, even if it might cause you some embarrassment? Health care professionals always put what is best for their patients ahead of what is best for them. Be on the lookout for potential mistakes and errors and never hesitate to speak up.

A primary goal of patient safety is preventing a **sentinel event**—an unexpected occurrence involving death or serious physical or psychological injury, or the risk thereof, with "serious injuries" including the loss of a limb or function. Each accredited hospital or health care organization is required to define a sentinel event for their purposes and to have a plan in place to identify, report, and manage these kinds of events. Once the event has been reported, the circumstances can be studied and processes can be put into place to prevent the occurrence from happening again.

Each year, National Patient Safety Goals from The Joint Commission provide a series of specific actions that accredited organizations are expected to implement to prevent medical errors. The goals for 2015 were:

- *Identify patients correctly.* Use at least two ways to identify patients. For example, use the patient's name and date of birth. This is done to make sure that each patient gets the correct medicine and treatment. Make sure that the correct patient gets the correct blood when they get a blood transfusion.
- *Improve staff communication.* Get important test results to the right staff person on time.
- *Use medicines safely.* Before a procedure, label medicines that are not labeled, for example, medicines in syringes, cups, and basins. Do this in the area where medicines and supplies are set up. Take extra care with patients who take medicines to thin their blood. Record and pass along correct information about a patient's medicines. Find out what medicines the patient is taking. Compare those medicines to new medicines given to the patient. Make sure the patient knows which medicines to take when they are at home. Tell the patient it is important to bring their up-to-date list of medicines every time they visit a doctor.
- *Use alarms safely.* Make improvements to ensure that alarms on medical equipment are heard and responded to on time.
- *Prevent infection.* Use the handwashing guidelines from the Centers for Disease Control and Prevention or the World Health Organization. Set goals for improving handwashing. Use the goals to improve handwashing. Use proven guidelines to prevent infections that are difficult to treat. Use proven guidelines to prevent infection of the blood from central lines. Use proven guidelines to prevent infection after surgery. Use proven guidelines to prevent infections of the urinary tract that are caused by catheters.
- *Identify patient safety risks.* Find out which patients are most likely to try to commit suicide.
- *Prevent mistakes in surgery.* Make sure that the correct surgery is done on the correct patient and at the correct place on the patient's body. Mark the correct place on the patient's body where the surgery is to be done. Pause before the surgery to make sure that a mistake is not being made. (*National Patient Safety Goals from 2015 Hospital National Patient Safety Goals. Copyright © 2015 by The Joint Commission.*)

As mentioned earlier, having an adequate supply of registered nurses and other health care providers on hand is crucial to ensuring quality care and patient safety. But shifting trends in the supply and demand of health care workers is causing serious concerns.

Workforce Supply and Demand

Much has already been said about the impact of the Baby Boomer population on the health care industry. But the Baby Boomers' increasing demand for health care services as patients is only part of the problem. Millions of Baby Boomers work in health care, serving as doctors, nurses, and other health care workers. As they age, they will retire from their health care jobs in large numbers. These rising retirement rates could lead to major labor shortages during the same period of time when Baby Boomers are increasing the demand for health care services.

Consider the following:

- About one-third of all registered nurses are currently 50 years of age or older.
- About 55% of RNs plan to retire in the next 10 years.
- By 2020 there will be a shortage of one million nurses in the United States.
- While 50% of nurses currently work in hospitals, the demand in other care settings is growing.
- The number of new RNs graduating from college is not sufficient to replace all of the retiring nurses.
- To meet the demand, new nursing graduates would have to increase by 90% a year.
- As the demand for RNs increases worldwide, there will be fewer foreign-trained nurses working in the United States.

Labor shortages are also predicted for other types of health care professionals, including doctors.

- About 40% of U.S. doctors are age 55 or older.
- By 2020, there will be at least 100,000 fewer doctors in the workplace than today.
- By 2025, the U.S. population will grow by 30 million people, yet there will be a shortage of about 65,000 doctors including both primary care and specialists.

The number of Americans over 65 years of age will almost double by 2025, requiring about 25,000 **geriatric** (elderly; a medical specialty or service for older adults) doctors to care for them. But with just 7,500 geriatricians currently in the United States, there's a major need to start educating more of them.

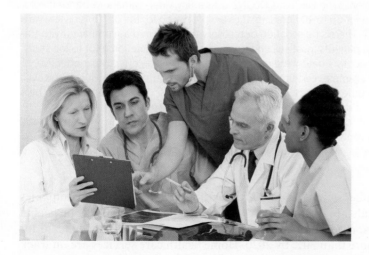

Figure 1-6 Doctor, nurse practitioners, and physician assistants discussing a patient (*Rido/Shutterstock*)

When you match these labor forecasts with the expected demands of the Baby Boomer population, you can easily understand some of the serious challenges facing the American health care system. One method of addressing the shortage of doctors is the rapidly increasing use of **advanced practice providers** (APPs). APPs include physician assistants, certified nurse practitioners, certified nurse midwives, clinical nurse specialists, and certified registered nurse anesthetists. With additional education, clinical experience, and certifications and licenses, these caregivers typically function under the direct supervision of a physician, although some states now allow certified nurse practitioners to function independently. Advanced practice nurses and PAs have been part of the health care workforce for many years but their numbers are growing. Between 1999 and 2013, the number of nurse practitioners increased from 60,000 to 171,000. The number of PAs increased from 83,466 in 2010 to 101,977 in 2015. Working in physician practices, clinics, hospitals, and other settings, APPs assist physicians with surgeries and complex medical procedures and perform a variety of tests and treatments including tissue biopsies, lumbar punctures, pelvic and breast exams, and replacing chest tubes. They serve as "first assistants" in the operating room, order and interpret lab and radiology tests, read electrocardiograms, and prescribe medications.

HOT TOPICS

NEW TOOLS IN DIAGNOSIS AND TREATMENT

Diabetic patients may soon have an alternative to frequent fingerpricks to obtain blood samples. Scientists are studying how light, fiber optics, and lasers can be used for diagnostic purposes. Since compounds such as glucose absorb wavelengths of infrared light, shining a laser beam on a patient's palm can identify glucose blood levels without the need for blood testing. Light is also being studied for use in treatments. Through photodynamic therapy, certain drugs that are activated by wavelengths of light can treat tumors on the skin or on the surface of organs. In other studies, tiny pieces of glass or fiber optics can provide data such as body temperature and the levels of oxygen and carbon dioxide in the blood. Before long, needles may become obsolete for some types of medical testing.

As an alternative to undergoing a traditional colonoscopy procedure, patients can now just swallow a pill to examine the inside of their colons. The PillCam COLON2 uses a tiny video camera to transmit color photos as it travels through the colon for up to 10 hours. Images are processed for the doctor's review via a belt worn around the patient's waist. There's no sedation or recovery time required as compared with traditional colonoscopy procedures, but patients must still undergo a cleansing preparation prior to the study.

Genetic DNA tests are helping doctors determine which medications will be effective, ineffective, or harmful for individual patients. For example, certain genes can identify which patients will respond well to specific antidepressants whereas other patients will suffer bad side effects. Genetic tests can also help determine the most effective doses of drugs, preventing serious and life-threatening overdoses.

These are just a few examples of some of the new tools designed to improve the diagnosis and treatment of diseases and other medical conditions.

As mentioned earlier, the number of jobs in outpatient settings and home health companies are growing while jobs in hospitals are declining. In fact, between 2012 and 2022, physician practices will add 1.2 million jobs, more than any other sector of health care. The demand for medical assistants will grow by more than 30% by 2020. Home health care services are on track to be the fastest-growing industry in the U.S. economy, with almost 60% job growth between 2012 and 2022. Hospitals will continue to provide ample job opportunities since about 39% of all health care jobs in 2013 were in hospitals, but the growth rate for new jobs in hospitals will decline sharply over the next decade.

Advancements in technology are improving patient care, quality, and safety in ways we couldn't even imagine just a few years ago, resulting in job growth in disciplines such as health information technology (HIT). Employment in HIT is expected to increase by 20% by 2018. This above-average employment outlook is based on the rise of the **electronic health record** or EHR (computerized health record) and the growing need to keep patient information secure and confidential. Health information technicians, also known as medical records technicians, assemble and organize patient records. They manage health information data to ensure accuracy and security and they communicate with other health care workers to clarify information and gather additional details. HIT professionals interact with software programs and computer systems and provide support for health information networks.

Health care workers who enter information in an EHR must be certified or licensed, leading to a new job title: medical scribe. Medical scribes are usually certified or registered medical assistants who enter information into the patient's EHR during the patient's conversation in the exam room with the doctor. Medical scribes enter this information in real time as the conversation is happening. This saves the doctor's time at the end of the day, reducing the need to dictate notes. Scribing also reduces errors since the doctor doesn't have to remember the details of what was said during the office visits with each and every patient.

Let's take a closer look at EHRs and how this new technology is improving patient care.

Electronic Health Records

Electronic health records are now common in hospitals, doctor's offices, and clinics where patient information needs to be shared quickly and frequently among providers at several different locations. But until just a few years ago, medical records were routinely kept on paper and stored in a patient's chart or file. When doctors and specialists needed to review a patient's paper medical records, the pages had to be copied, mailed, faxed, scanned and emailed, or hand-carried to other locations. This process consumed a lot of time and delayed the patient's tests and treatments, often posing serious problems in emergency situations. During the advent of computerized record-keeping, switching from paper records to electronic records was voluntary. Doctors, nurses, and other health care workers had to be trained to use EHRs. Mastering new skills and moving to a totally new format took time and led to backlogs in patient care until the staff was up to speed

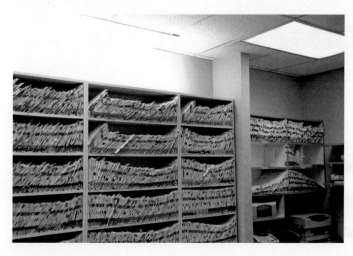

Figure 1-7 Medical records stored on paper (*Elena Elisseeva/Shutterstock*)

with the new technology. Some people, especially older workers and doctors, resisted having to learn new skills and undergo such a radical change.

But today, EHRs are the only acceptable way that health care facilities may keep records on their patients without facing financial penalties. When patients move among doctor's offices, specialists, clinics, and hospitals, their medical information needs to move with them. This can only be accomplished by using technology. When providers can access comprehensive, up-to-date information on each patient, the quality and continuity of care increases and the cost associated with unnecessary duplication of blood tests and radiographs, for example, decreases. EHRs offer several other advantages. They:

- *Save paper and space.* Instead of keeping paper files on patients, their medical records are kept in computer files, which save space and reduce the cost of paper.
- *Enhance coordination.* All members of the patient's health care team, regardless of their locations, have access to the same medical information. They can see what other team members are doing to care for the patient as they develop their own treatment plans.
- *Improve quality.* When patients are being seen by several specialists at the same time, there's a risk that one doctor might prescribe a drug that isn't compatible with the drugs prescribed by one of the patient's other doctors. With EHRs, each doctor can see what the other doctors are prescribing. This is just one example of quality improvement via EHRs.
- *Reduce delays.* When doctors use technology to gain immediate access to records, tests and treatments can begin much sooner.
- *Ensure **legibility*** (the ability of handwriting to be read and interpreted accurately by others). Handwritten doctors' orders and treatment notes can be difficult to read, sometimes leading to confusion or mistakes. When orders and treatment notes are typed into an electronic record, illegible handwriting is no longer a concern, but typos can still occur.

As with most technologic advancements, there are also some disadvantages to EHRs:

- *System incompatibility.* There is no universal EHR and the different systems won't interact with one another. This is one reason why health care providers are joining networks, so that all members within the network can use the same electronic systems.

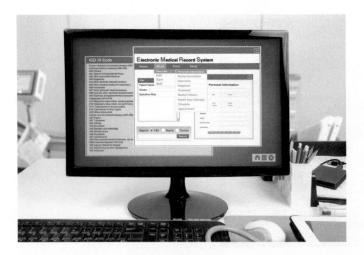

Figure 1-8 Medical records stored electronically (*pandpstock001/Shutterstock*)

- *Security concerns.* Having medical information stored on computers raises concerns about potential security issues and the accidental release of private information. When storing, transmitting, and transporting medical records electronically, strict security measures must be followed to avoid a **breach** (a break, failure, or interruption) in **confidentiality** (maintaining the privacy of certain matters).

Investing in information technology is very expensive but the future holds great promise. EHRs contain a great deal of valuable data. Once new tools and processes are in place to combine and analyze "big data" from thousands of individual patient records, major improvements in quality of care, patient safety, and cost-effectiveness will emerge. Data-driven medicine and evidence-based care will lead to benefits such as predictive care models, standard order sets, and the ability to identify and share best practices among health care providers. EHRs are still in the infancy stage and their long-term benefits will likely be worth the investment.

CASE STUDY

Carla started her medical assisting career working for a small medical practice owned by three family medicine doctors. When the doctors decided to join a large network and switch from paper medical records to an electronic format, Carla considered leaving the practice to work in a clinic across town that wasn't undergoing such extensive change. But she decided to stay and she's glad she did. Joining the network turned out to be a positive change for everyone, including the practice's patients. Switching to electronic health records wasn't easy, but Carla and the doctors and staff all survived the extra training and transition.

Once the practice joined the network, things started happening quickly. The practice's management plan was restructured and the network's policies and procedures were put into place. The practice's electronic health records were synched with the network's system to share patient information among the network's multiple locations. New diagnostic equipment was installed and additional medical procedures were implemented. The number and diversity of patients coming in for office visits increased, and Carla noticed that a large percentage of the new patients were older, disabled, and suffering from multiple chronic conditions. As the practice grew, the office expanded into vacant space next door. Three more doctors joined the staff along with three medical assistants and five new advanced practice providers (three nurse practitioners and two physician assistants). The practice's hours were expanded to accommodate the increased patient load.

Carla's practice had never been busier. When she thought about her town and other local health care providers, she realized that fewer patients were being hospitalized due to expanding outpatient care. When patients did have to be admitted to the hospital, they stayed a shorter period of time than in the past even though their medical conditions were still serious. There was no doubt about it, things were changing and changing rapidly.

Carla thought about her career and where it was headed. She loved working with patients but was also intrigued by the business side of health care. A few years ago she had served on a new interdisciplinary team to design and open a new clinic across town. The group got off to a rocky start, but Carla stepped up to help the group function more smoothly and was soon designated team leader of the new Patient Experience subcommittee. She learned a lot about patient satisfaction, customer service, and how to improve patients' interactions with their health care providers. In fact, she got so involved in researching best practices among health care networks around the country she started a **blog** (an online personal journal available to the public) to share what she had learned with colleagues in other states.

Having completed several prerequisite courses at a local community college, Carla decided to work toward a BS degree in Health Care Management and Supervision. She took advantage of workshops, seminars, and classes offered through her practice's network and through her state's medical assisting professional association. After attending several

(continued)

meetings and networking with colleagues, she became active in the organization and joined the annual meeting planning committee. Carla also volunteered for team assignments at work to hone her skills and studied Lean Sigma and Quality Improvement techniques. Things were going quite well for Carla careerwise.

One day Carla was asked to meet with her practice manager. A supervisor position had opened up and the manager encouraged Carla to apply for it. After several interviews with the doctors and network leaders, she was offered a promotion and readily accepted it. Her new duties included recruiting and selecting new office staff, coordinating work schedules and payroll, enforcing policies and procedures, conducting performance reviews, representing the practice on various network planning teams, and assisting her manager with budgeting and other business functions.

One of Carla's first assignments was to bring her staff up to speed on the Affordable Care Act and its implications for their facility and network. She had just become the newest member of the strategic planning team charged with transitioning the network into an accountable care organization and she suddenly realized she had a great deal to learn before she could explain things to other people.

What should Carla do to prepare for this first assignment? What would you do if you were in Carla's place?

Advancements in Technology

There are far too many examples of how technology is improving the health care industry to list them all. But here are a few more examples:

- Remember the IBM supercomputer called "Watson" that beat the experts at chess and Jeopardy matches? Researchers at a New York hospital are testing the computer to determine how it could help doctors improve their diagnostic and therapeutic skills.
- Asthma sufferers can send data to their doctors simply by blowing into their **smartphones** (cell phones that also function as hand-held computers).
- New mobile **apps** (applications; software programs that perform specific functions on smartphones and hand-held computer devices) and devices such as Fitbit and Lark are tracking sleep patterns, exercise activity, and eating habits to help people stay active and healthy.
- Omnifluent Health provides an app that instantly translates messages spoken into a smartphone into a different language. Since more than 40 million Americans lack English skills, the app helps doctors and other caregivers communicate directly with patients without the need for a translator.
- Sherpaa, based in New York City, saves trips to the emergency room by offering online and telephone medical consultations with some of the top medical practitioners in the area.
- Doximity, led by a cofounder of LinkedIn, provides a social networking site just for doctors throughout the United States to facilitate collaboration on complex medical cases.
- Telemedicine, also known as telehealth, allows patients to video-chat with a doctor and receive a full medical assessment without having to appear for an office visit. This technology is especially valuable in rural settings where patients don't have ready access to a local physician or specialist. Research shows that patients in intensive care units with telehealth equipment can be discharged up to 20% more quickly and with a 26% lower mortality rate when compared with ICUs without the technology.
- Portal technology allows patients to communicate with their doctors online, access test results and medical information, and schedule follow-up appointments. Patients become better educated and empowered to accept more responsibility for their health and health care.

- Self-service kiosks are reducing labor costs and speeding up the outpatient and hospital registration processes by collecting co-pays, verifying identification, and completing paperwork without the patient having to interact with a registration worker.
- Home monitoring systems are now used by about 3 million people worldwide to reduce visits to the doctor's office. Data from a patient's cardiac pacemaker, for example, can be sent to a remote location and monitored for any problems. On average, about 25% of heart disease patients have to be readmitted to the hospital for follow-up care. But the readmission rate at a hospital in Minnesota dropped to just 2% by using a home monitoring system.
- Sensors and wearable medical devices are on the rise. If a patient falls down, for example, or if a minor cut becomes infected, sensors can alert the patient's caregiver that something unusual has happened. "Smart helmets" send an alert when an athlete might have suffered a concussion. Patients can swallow a sensor powered by stomach fluids that sends data such as heart rates to a patch on their bodies. Bracelets can alert doctors if they haven't washed their hands properly.
- e-NABLE's three-dimensional (3D) printing process is revolutionizing medical prosthetics, producing low-cost limbs customized to each patient's needs. The organization aims to meet the demand for 1,000 free prosthetic hands for people throughout the world.
- The U.S. Food and Drug Administration (FDA) recently approved Spritam, the first prescription drug produced via 3D printing. This dissolvable tablet helps patients deal with some types of epileptic seizures.
- Before long, you'll be able to enter a booth at your local department or grocery store, have labs and diagnostics run, and participate in a personal visit with a health care provider via a remote feed. Pilot projects for this new technology are already underway.

What could be more exciting than watching new technology emerge in health care? You'll need to know what types of new technology are on the drawing board for your profession,

THE MORE YOU KNOW

ROBOTS IN MEDICINE

A good example of advancements in health care technology involves the use of robotics. Robots have been used in hospitals for years to deliver meals, clean linens, and supplies and to remove medical waste and trash. Pharmacy robots have automated the sorting, storing, delivery, and restocking of drugs and medications. But a major breakthrough occurred in 1985 with PUMA, the first medical robot to assist with brain biopsies and prostate surgery. In just a few years, the da Vinci Surgical Robot was developed to assist with prostate and heart surgeries. Surgeons use remote control to adjust the robot's arms while looking through a camera with a high-definition 3D view. Due to the less-invasive procedure, da Vinci robots help surgeons perform a wide variety of complex operations with less pain and blood loss for the patient, fewer infections and complications, reduced scarring, and a faster recovery period compared with normal surgeries.

Promising research is now underway in other countries such as Switzerland, where scientists are developing pills that, when swallowed, release tiny robots to conduct surgical procedures inside the human body. Micro-cameras shaped like pills study the gastrointestinal tract, but the devices are limited and can't take samples or administer drugs to the site. A project in Europe called ARES (Assembling Reconfigurable Endoluminal Surgical System) is creating miniature robots with remote-controlled limbs that move like insects, freely allowing the robots to move within the stomach. Research is exploring the use of devices such as ARES to gather biopsy samples without the need for a surgical incision.

and how that technology will affect your patients and your work. Most of the digital software, drugs, devices, and medical procedures that will be routine tomorrow haven't even been developed yet. Maybe you will play a role in discovering a medical breakthrough at some point in your career.

The Big Picture and Where You Fit In

Having taken a step back to look at the "big picture" of the health care industry and some of the major trends and issues, it should be obvious by now that you've chosen to work in an industry like no other, challenged by unprecedented and radical change. No one knows what the health care industry will look like 10 years from now. For some people, that's a scary prospect. For others, it's an exciting opportunity to get involved and help shape the future of an industry that impacts every single American.

For decades, the hospital has always been the center of health care, but that's quickly changing. As medical homes and ACOs grow, patients are becoming the new center of health care. As consumers, patients will seek out preventive and health care services that are convenient, friendly, high quality, and low cost. They'll want appointments right now, not next week. They'll choose to get their tests and treatments from their doctor's office, their local drug or department store, or a concierge service that offers highly personalized care, same-day appointments, 24/7 access to their physician, and shorter waits for ordering tests and getting results. Instead of waiting until an injury or disease sends a patient to the ER or a hospital, patients will benefit from an increased focus on wellness and disease and injury prevention. In effect, these current trends are transforming what has been a "sick care system" into an actual "health care system."

A major force in improving patient care and safety will be patient engagement. Patients must become more directly involved in making decisions about their health and health care. Motivating patients to change their behaviors won't be easy, but it's a critical part of improving the overall health of the nation. About 25% of ER visits are due to depression, anxiety, and other behavioral health issues, so social workers, psychologists, and other behavioral health workers are joining patient care teams in hospitals and physician offices. Having resources available such as these to help patients manage and cope with their chronic conditions will be key.

Another important trend will be redesigning the death and dying experience for Americans. While most everyone agrees that end-of-life decisions should be made by patients and their doctors and family members, the cost of caring for terminally ill people is significant. About 20% of America's overall health care expense per year goes to Medicare, and Medicare spends about 28% of that ($170B in 2011) on the last six months of patients' lives. Studies show that about a third of that expenditure has no direct benefit to the patients. Medicare now reimburses doctors for discussing aspects of death and dying with their patients, and efforts are underway to increase **palliative care** (care designed to reduce pain and suffering and to improve the quality of life) and **hospice services** (care provided for the terminally ill that focuses on comfort and quality of life instead of a cure) to provide the kinds of support that dying patients need.

It's absolutely critical that health care professionals stay current and understand how their industry is financed and regulated, and how it will change as consumers become more engaged. As a health care worker yourself, you must be able to view the health care industry from both the business side and the service side and try to keep both in balance. You'll wear at least three different hats—as a patient, a taxpayer, and a health care professional. Each time you change a hat, your **perspective** (the manner in which a person views something) will change along with it. Some of your perspectives might conflict with others. Here are a few examples:

- What's best for you as a patient might not be what's best for you as a taxpayer. As a patient, you want the very best health care that money can buy, no matter what the cost. But as a taxpayer, you know that resources to fund medical care are limited.
- What's best for you as a health care professional might not be what's best for you as a patient. As a health care professional, you want to leave work on time to get on with your busy personal life. But as a patient, you want your caregiver to stay as late as necessary to finish your procedure without handing you off to the next shift.
- What's best for you as a taxpayer might not be what's best for you as a health care professional. As a taxpayer, you want to reduce the cost of health care to avoid tax increases. But as a health care professional, you want the government to fund medical research to help develop new treatments and cures.

In order to make the best decisions, you must keep all of these perspectives in mind as you move through the day. Always try to see things through the eyes of your patients. When you're at work wearing your health care professional hat, your patients must always come first.

PROFESSIONALISM ONLINE

DIGITAL COMMUNICATION AND SOCIAL MEDIA

No discussion about professionalism in today's world would be complete without exploring the appropriate use of digital communication and social media. Let's start with some definitions.

Digital communication involves the use of computers, software, and networks to store and share information including data, video, and voice. Interactivity is an important feature of digital communication where messages can be sent and received quickly between two people or among larger numbers of people. Users can choose to participate in networks where they can easily create groups and instantly communicate about desired topics. Interactivity and group-forming are what make digital communication so unique and valuable. **Social media** is electronic communication that enables users to establish online communities for the purpose of sharing content, ideas, personal messages, and other information such as videos and photographs.

Examples of social media include Facebook, LinkedIn, Twitter, Instagram, Snapchat, Pinterest, and YouTube, to name just a few. Facebook is a social networking website where users can keep in touch with family and friends by creating personal profiles, posting photos and videos, and exchanging messages. Facebook users, called members, create lists of "friends" who then share comments among themselves about the content that members have posted. Members can allow anyone and everyone to view their Facebook information or they can restrict access to some or all of their content. Facebook, available in 37 different languages, provides a private messaging system similar to email and helps members organize events, tap into classified ads, and find people with whom to interact.

LinkedIn is a large social networking site for business people who already know one another through their jobs, schools, professional associations, etc. Members establish a professional identity online by creating a profile page listing their education, employment history, and professional affiliations and activities. They connect with other professionals to share information, ideas, and professional opportunities. If members move or change jobs, they can remain connected.

Twitter is a social networking site that allows users to broadcast short messages of 140 characters or less called tweets to a group of people called followers. Users can import their email addresses or use the Twitter search function to locate people and invite them to participate. Tweets can be made available to the public to anyone who wishes to view them, or users can restrict access to their

(continued)

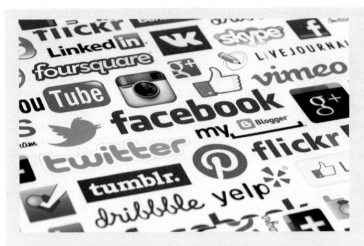

Figure 1-9 Social media websites (*Anatolii Babii/Alamy*)

followers. Tweets use hashtags, which are #prefixes that identify topics so they can be searched as a group (e.g., #healthcareprofessionals).

Instagram is an online video- and photo-sharing service. Users can upload photos, apply filters to enhance their appearance, and then share their pictures with other people via the Instagram website or through other social media sites such as Facebook or Twitter.

Snapchat is a videomessaging site that allows users to take photographs and record short videos. These "snaps" can then be sent to a specific group of recipients who have just seconds to view them before they are deleted from the recipient's device.

Facebook, LinkedIn, Twitter, Instagram, and Snapchat are just a few examples of the growing number and variety of social media sites. In today's world, digital communication and social media are used by almost everyone, and quite frequently. Facebook has 728 million users per day, with 1.5 billion monthly active users (people who have logged on in the past 30 days). LinkedIn has 364 million members in more than 200 countries. About 6,000 tweets are tweeted every second, adding up to about 200 billion tweets per year. About 75 million people use Instagram and 16 million people use Snapchat every day.

Digital communication is highly accessible via desktop computers, tablets, cell phones, and other devices. For many users, their cell phones are either already in their hands or just a reach away. A text message is an electronic communication from one cell phone to another. Texting uses typed words, often in an abbreviated form. This has led to a new language for digital communication, full of acronyms such as LOL for "laughing out loud," GR8 for "great," and BTW for "by the way." Users may also choose from hundreds of different **emoji** (pictures or characters representing facial expressions, objects, places, or other concepts) inserted in their messages. This new language can easily confuse people who aren't up to speed with digital communication.

There's no doubt that digital communication and social media are part of our everyday lives now. The benefits are obvious. We can find detailed information instantly about restaurant menus, store discounts, weather forecasts, traffic reports, and sports scores. We can get answers to our questions, locate old friends, research our ancestors, buy things online, and get directions. We can make and change reservations, search for the lowest prices, watch TV programs or videos, and organize family reunions and other events. The list goes on and on. Digital communication provides convenience, saves us money, and connects individuals and groups who otherwise might not get together.

But there's also a downside to digital communication and social media, including the potential for dishonesty, criminal acts, embarrassment, invasion of privacy, and the unintended release of personal and confidential information. Boundaries must be established and enforced to set limits and to draw the line between acceptable and unacceptable behavior. This becomes especially important in health care in order to protect the "social contract" between health care providers and their patients where maintaining trust and professional reputations are critical. These topics and how they relate to professionalism in health care are fully explored in the chapters that follow.

REALITY CHECK

It's time to get real and think about answering the questions, What role are you going to play? Are you looking for a job or a career? There's a big difference. Some people just pass through the health care industry, skipping from job to job and paycheck to paycheck. Others take time to think, plan, and build their careers one step at a time. Health care workers are like renters and owners. Renters have a short-term outlook. They don't feel a sense of ownership, so they avoid investing their time, money, and energy in making improvements. Owners, on the other hand, are in it for the long term. They not only invest in improvements, they take pride in the results.

Health care is a unique and rewarding career for people who like the work and enjoy serving others in a complex, team-oriented environment. Because of the criticality of the work, the industry needs workers who want more than a job. It needs professionals who are dedicated to the work they are doing and focused on performing to the best of their ability regardless of the job they hold.

Innovation is now the name of the game in health care. Strategic thinkers are needed at every level in health care organizations to solve problems and find new and better ways of doing business. This is the industry you've chosen and the future is now before you. What you make of it is up to you. If you're serious about a career in health care, and your goal is to be recognized as a health care professional, then keep reading. It's time to focus on what's going to be expected of you. The remainder of this book is your roadmap to success.

For More Information

The Health Care Industry
American Hospital Association
www.aha.org

Health Care Reform and the ACA
U.S. Department of Health and Human Services
www.hhs.gov/healthcare/facts/

The Baby Boomer Population
www.babyboomers.com

Health Care Labor Forecasts
Bureau of Labor Statistics, U.S. Department of Labor
www.bls.gov

National Patient Safety Goals
The Joint Commission
www.jointcommission.org/standards

Quality Improvement
Agency for Healthcare Research and Quality (AHRQ)
U.S. Department of Health and Human Services
www.ahrq.gov

Lean Six Sigma in Healthcare
iSixSigma
www.isixsigma.com

Electronic Health Records
www.healthit.gov

Social Media
www.socialmediatoday.com

KEY POINTS

- Remember that soft skills are just as important as hard skills in achieving success at work.
- Keep up-to-date with the business side of health care and where it appears to be headed.
- Monitor current trends and issues so you can discuss them intelligently with other people.
- Be on the lookout for new technology and how it might impact your patients and your work.
- Watch for opportunities to improve the quality of care and speak up when something doesn't seem right.
- Monitor National Patient Safety Goals and avoid making mistakes and errors.
- Learn as much as you can about caring for geriatric patients.
- Think about the different hats you wear and always put your patients first.
- Consider that boundaries must be established and enforced when digital communication and social media are used to connect and interact with other people.
- Think about what role *you* want to play in health care, and keep learning.

LEARNING ACTIVITIES

Using information from Chapter One:
- Answer the Chapter Review Questions
- Respond to the What If? Scenarios

Chapter Review Questions

Using information presented in Chapter One, answer each of the following questions.

1. List four benefits of working in the health care industry.

2. Explain the difference between *soft skills* and *hard skills*.

3. List two reasons why health care workers must be aware of current trends and issues in the health care industry.

4. List three reasons why health care is expensive and the costs continue to rise.

5. Identify two ways that the Baby Boomer population will impact the health care industry.

6. Describe two controversial issues associated with health care reform.

7. Define *continuous quality improvement*.

8. List two quality improvement goals.

9. Define *sentinel event*.

10. Explain the connection between sentinel events and patient safety.

11. Identify two trends in the supply and demand of health care workers.

12. List two advantages of electronic health records.

13. Define *social media*.

14. Give two examples of social media sites.

What If? Scenarios

Think about what you would do in the following situations and record your answers.

1. You're the leader of a team that includes a new employee. He has years of experience working in another hospital and knows more than the rest of the team about operating the new high-tech equipment just installed in your department. When you ask him to show his coworkers how to use the new equipment, he refuses by saying, "I wasn't hired to be a teacher." He mostly keeps to himself and doesn't get along very well with other team members. You're beginning to wonder which is more important: hard skills or soft skills?

2. You've been invited to participate on a conference panel next month to discuss the impact of health care reform on your profession. You really want to accept the invitation but you don't feel prepared. You've heard just enough about health care reform and the Affordable Care Act on TV to know they are controversial topics. You read a newspaper article stating that health insurance is changing and you overheard a heated conversation last week between your father and uncle arguing about taxes, Medicare, and something called an individual mandate.

3. Your neighbor has paid you a visit, very upset about the bill he just received for having some blood tests run at a local clinic. He said the cost this year was 25% higher than what he was charged for the same tests a year ago. Since you work in health care, he wants you to explain why the cost has gone up so much and what is being done to reduce the expense.

4. The outpatient surgery center where you work just experienced a sentinel event, resulting in serious harm to one of the patients. It was a complicated case and no one knows exactly what went wrong. The surgeons and staff are highly concerned that the same thing might happen again unless the cause can be identified and fixed.

5. A doctor on your unit just ordered a drug for one of your patients. You're pretty sure that the drug she ordered will cause a serious complication with another drug ordered by another doctor just yesterday. You are new on the unit and not sure if you should speak up or not.

6. You really need the day off tomorrow but forgot to take your name off the schedule. You could call in sick but your absence would cause the staffing level to drop below what's safe for the patients.

7. You have just moved across the country to a new town and left your family and friends behind. Now you're wondering what might be the best way to keep in touch with everyone and share news about your new home and job.

2 Your Work Ethic and Performance

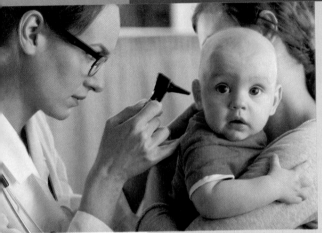

A pessimist sees the difficulty in every opportunity. An optimist sees the opportunity in every difficulty.

—Winston Churchill (1874–1965),
British prime minister

(Photographee.eu/Shutterstock)

CHAPTER OBJECTIVES

Having completed this chapter, you will be able to:

- Define *interdependence* as it relates to health care workers.
- Describe why health care workers need to have a systems perspective.
- Give one example of how failing to use common sense with social media can lead to a HIPAA violation.
- Explain why it's important to be "present in the moment" at work.
- Define *critical thinking*.
- List three things that critical thinkers do to make good decisions.
- List five factors that demonstrate a strong work ethic.
- Describe the attitudinal differences between optimists and pessimists.

- Explain why health care workers must function within the legal scope of practice for the state in which they are employed.
- Explain why it's important for health care workers to comply with federal, state, and local health laws and regulations as they relate to health care settings.
- Explain how HIPAA protects the confidentiality of medical information.
- List two things you should do when representing your employer.
- List three ways to prepare for a performance evaluation.
- Differentiate between objective and subjective evaluation criteria.

KEY TERMS

360-degree feedback	discretion	job description	reasoning
cloud	dismissal	mindfulness	reimbursement
common sense	fraud	objective	reliable
compliance	front-line workers	optimists	responsibility
conflict of interest	goals	organizational chart	sexual harassment
consent	hacked	peers	stagnant
constructive criticism	hostile workplace	performance-based pay	subjective
contingency plans	HIPAA	performance evaluation	subordinates
corporate mission	HITECH	pessimists	systematic
corporate values	impaired	probationary period	systems perspective
corrective action	insubordination	problem solving	unethical
critical thinking	intentional	punctual	up-code
diligent	interdependence	rational	whistleblower

Making a Commitment to Your Job

As previously mentioned, no job is insignificant and no worker is unimportant in health care. Most people are familiar with the critical roles that doctors, nurses, and pharmacists play in health care. But patients and the general public may not be as familiar with the roles of other caregivers such as medical assistants, nuclear medicine technologists, occupational therapists, electroneurodiagnostic (END) technologists, and sonographers, to name just a few. People who work behind the scenes may be even less known to patients and the public. This includes instrument technicians, biomedical engineers, research assistants, and medical coders whose roles are also vital. When you add chefs, security officers, lawyers, and maintenance workers, large urban hospitals and medical centers employ so many different types of workers they begin to resemble small towns. Depending on how you add them up, there are several hundred different jobs in health care organizations.

If your job involves direct patient care, it should be obvious that professionalism is important. The same holds true with jobs where workers interact with visitors, guests, and vendors or function in support roles behind the scenes. Examples include customer service agents, telephone operators, purchasing agents, billing clerks, insurance processors, and medical secretaries. Professionalism is important in all jobs.

- What if phlebotomists confuse blood samples and label them incorrectly?
- What if clerical workers misspell medical terms on patient records?
- What if housekeepers don't dispose of soiled linen properly?
- What if radiographers position patients incorrectly and have to repeat imaging exams?
- What if registered nurses give the wrong dose of a vaccination?
- What if pharmacy technicians fail to remove expired drugs from the stock room?
- What if medical assistants enter information in the wrong patient record?

It should be obvious that professionalism is vital in every job. Each job exists for a reason and performing the job well requires making a commitment to your job and taking a professional approach to your work.

Interdependence

As mentioned previously, no matter what your job may involve, you must be able to view the "big picture" and know where you fit in. Having examined the health care industry in general, let's focus more closely on your job and how it connects with the roles of other workers. This starts with developing a **systems perspective**—standing back, viewing the entire process of how a patient moves through your organization, and understanding how your role fits into that process. No one in health care works alone—everyone's work is interconnected. This need to rely on another is called **interdependence** and without it, the work flow breaks down.

Think about your role and responsibilities:

- How do your responsibilities connect with those of other workers?
- Which other workers do you have to depend on to get your work done?
- Which other workers have to depend on you to get their work done?
- Where do the patients fit into this picture?

Most companies have an **organizational chart**—an illustration of the components of a company and how they relate to each other. Typical organizational charts include the hierarchy of the company—people and work units arranged by rank. In other words, "who" reports "to whom." Large companies have detailed illustrations showing the flow of work processes within and across departments. Regardless of the size and structure of the company, there's always one common thread—all departments and employees must work together and depend on one another to get the work done and done well.

From a systems perspective, ask yourself what would happen if you:

- Don't show up for work on time and fail to notify someone?
- Get sloppy and make an error?
- Appear for work **impaired** (having a reduced ability to function properly) by alcohol or an illegal or prescription drug?

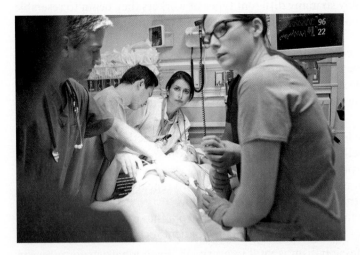

Figure 2-1 Working together to provide emergency care (*Monkey Business Images/Shutterstock*)

How would these behaviors affect other workers who are counting on you? If you fail to commit to your job, you won't be there for long. You may be able to hide incompetence, sloppiness, and indifference for a little while, but eventually poor performance will catch up with you. What's worse, someone could be harmed by your lack of commitment and professionalism in the meantime.

PROFESSIONALISM ONLINE

DIGITAL COMMUNICATION AND PRIVACY

Computers play a major role in health care. They store large amounts of data and process information with amazing speed, accuracy, and consistency. They guide doctors and other caregivers in making patient care decisions and assist with accounting, purchasing, and personnel functions. Computers maintain health records, schedule medical procedures, order supplies, create treatment plans, monitor patient conditions, perform diagnostic tests, and process medical bills, to list just a few of their functions. It's hard to imagine today's modern health care industry without such reliance on computers. But computers can be misused, either on purpose or by accident, and misuse can lead to serious problems. Health care workers must be fully aware of their employer's policies regarding passwords and computer security and comply with procedures detailing the appropriate use of company computers and the Internet.

The advent of digital communication and social media has greatly expanded the benefits of using computers and other digital devices in health care. But an increasing number of health care employers are now implementing new policies and procedures to address growing concerns about the inappropriate and **unethical** (violating standards of conduct and moral judgment) use of computers among their workforce. It's important to be aware of these concerns and to avoid the unprofessional behaviors that can prevent you from getting a job or keeping a job.

Let's start with **HIPAA** (Health Insurance Portability and Accountability Act of 1996). The law's goals are to make it easier for people to keep health insurance, protect the confidentiality and security of their health care information, and help to control health care administrative costs. When you take a photograph (or video) at work that includes a patient's image, identity, or medical information and then share it with someone else via social media, you could be violating the patient's privacy and confidentiality. With your cell phone just a reach away, it might be tempting to just "snap" a quick photo and send it to a friend via Snapchat thinking the photo will be deleted in a few seconds anyway. But stop and think—deleted Snapchat photos can still be viewed by the site's administrators after they've disappeared from your friend's device. If you post a patient's photo or his or her information on Facebook, the content can be altered and shared with other people without your knowledge. HIPAA violations can lead to serious repercussions when confidential or private information about patients is shared or posted online.

Once a photograph, video, message, or other content is posted on social media it becomes public. Anyone anywhere can view the information, alter it, and send it to other people without your knowledge or permission. The information is no longer private or confidential. It's "out there" permanently and it's easy to access and share. Someone can alter a photo of your face and paste it on another body, or place an image of you in a different setting or within a different group. Whether you posted it or not, once it's out there, it's out there forever and you have no control over it. Furthermore, if you have posted information that was protected by copyright or patent, you will have violated those protections and could be vulnerable to a lawsuit from the author or the legal owner of the material.

(continued)

You may think privacy settings on your social media pages prevent unauthorized people from viewing your postings, but is that really the case? The people who operate and maintain social media sites and the **cloud** (a network of remote servers on the Internet used to store, manage, and process data) behind the scenes have access to the content posted on those sites. Cell phones, tablets, and other digital devices can be **hacked** (being the victim of unauthorized access gained by a computer), lost, stolen, or accidently viewed by someone else such as your child or spouse. Even the firewalls on secure websites can be overcome.

Let's take a closer look at the concept of privacy and how social media could impact your employment. It's not at all unusual these days for employers to search Google, the Internet, blogs, and social media sites for information about their job applicants. If they don't like what they see, they may decide you aren't a good fit for the organization and deny you an interview. Your current employer may be tracking your online presence as well. You may mention the organization you work for in the "About" information on your Facebook or other social media site. In fact, Facebook and others encourage you to provide this information as part of your biography. However, if you post content or comments that undermine or damage the company's reputation from your employer's point of view, you could be suspended or fired from your job. You may think this is an invasion of your privacy. After all, what you post on your Facebook page should be *your private business*, correct? Digital communication and social media blur the lines between what's private and what's public. Information transmitted electronically is not confidential or private. You can post whatever content you desire, but if someone else believes they have been harmed by what you've posted, you may have to suffer the consequences.

Engaging in digital communication and social media calls for **common sense** (using good judgment and thinking and behaving in a reasonable way). The problem is—there's nothing common about common sense. Some of the lessons to be learned in using social media may have to be learned "the hard way." For example:

- Don't call in sick and then post photographs of yourself having fun out in public.
- Don't waste time checking your Twitter messages when you should be taking care of patients.
- Don't take photographs of patients.
- Don't send sexually oriented photographs or tweets.
- Don't post photos of yourself naked, drunk, or engaged in illegal activity.
- Don't send tweets to patients asking them to buy things such as Girl Scout cookies.
- Don't vent your anger about your boss or company online.
- Use privacy settings but don't count on them to ensure privacy.

The list of dos and don'ts and the lessons to be learned regarding social media go on and on. What's the bottom line? Use your common sense. Stop and think before you click.

Self-Awareness

One of the challenges of working in a busy environment is avoiding distractions and paying attention to what's going on around you. This requires a certain degree of understanding where you are, what you are doing, and why you are doing it, or **mindfulness**, and being "present in the moment." When you are "present in the moment" you can filter out distractions and concentrate on what's in front of you at any given time. This ability to focus is absolutely critical in emergency situations, in protecting patient safety, and in avoiding mistakes and errors. Always stop and think before you act. Everything that you say and do should be **intentional** (done on purpose). This means thinking things through instead of just quickly reacting to whatever situation occurs.

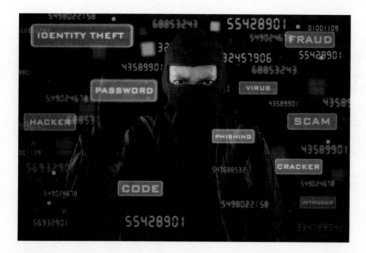

Figure 2-2 Computer hacking to steal private information (*Creativa Images/Shutterstock*)

When you are at work you need to filter out distractions from your personal life, which is easier said than done. Family conflicts, an argument with your spouse, bill collectors finding you at work, children left unsupervised, legal issues and court dates, and your own medical concerns are just a few examples of how your personal life can cause distractions at work. Let's face it—you're just one person and it's not easy to keep everything in balance. Concentrating on the task at hand when there's so much else going on in your life can be quite a challenge, but it's absolutely critical and something you must work hard to achieve.

One of the best ways to reduce distractions at work is to avoid becoming a distraction yourself. You aren't there to sell things, convince coworkers to adopt your political or religious beliefs, plan social gatherings, spread gossip, text friends, visit social networking sites, shop online, wager bets, or collect donations for your favorite charity. You are there to work, not to advance your personal agenda. Save distracting activities such as these for after work hours.

Working in health care is stressful. Each day that you come to work you'll be faced with a variety of decisions to make and problems to solve. The facts and data that you've learned in school will certainly help. But making good decisions and finding workable solutions requires the ability to fully understand, explore, question, and apply the information you've learned in the past.

Critical Thinking

When it comes to patient care, there isn't always just one right way to do things. You have to think through each situation, decide on a strategy, test it, observe the results, and adjust accordingly. This is where **critical thinking** (using reasoning and evidence to make an analysis or reach a decision) becomes a valuable skill. By using critical thinking skills and a step-by-step **systematic** (methodical) approach to decision making, you can reduce your stress and find effective solutions to most any problem. Critical thinkers use **reasoning** (forming conclusions based on logical thinking) and evidence to make decisions about what to do or what to believe without being influenced by emotions. When you think critically, you:

- Look at things from a **rational** (based on reason; logical) and practical perspective.
- Ask essential questions to get to the heart of the matter.
- Identify and analyze relevant information and evidence.
- Differentiate between facts, opinions, and personal feelings.
- Think with an open mind and question assumptions.
- Exercise caution in drawing conclusions.
- Test conclusions against relevant standards.

When faced with a problem, critical thinking skills can help you:

- Avoid jumping to conclusions.
- Identify and clarify the problem.
- Gather as much information as you can.
- Examine the evidence you've found.
- Identify options to solve the problem.
- Decide which option would work best.
- Implement your solution.
- Evaluate the results.

There's almost always a good solution to every problem, but you may have to invest some time and energy to find it.

Effective **problem solving** (a systematic process to find solutions to difficult issues and situations) and critical thinking skills are mandatory for a well-orchestrated personal and professional life. Interpreting the "small print" in credit card agreements, creating a budget for your family, comparing options for car insurance, and figuring out how to resolve an argument with a friend are just a few examples where critical-thinking skills can help you personally. Selecting the

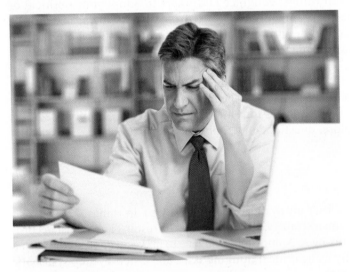

Figure 2-3 Using critical thinking skills to solve a difficult problem (*Kurhan/Shutterstock*)

CASE STUDY

Carla read everything she could find about health care reform, the Affordable Care Act (ACA), and affordable care organizations (ACOs). She studied relevant trends and issues, met with other leaders, and attended several workshops and conferences. Before long she had a working knowledge of the **goals** (aims, objectives, or ends that one strives to attain), concepts, metrics, and terminology associated with health care reform and she was ready to move forward. She developed printed handouts and held several in-service sessions with her staff to explain things. She invited the leader of the network's ACO team to participate in the sessions and she's glad she did. The staff asked far more questions than she had anticipated and it helped to have an expert in the room. People weren't just curious about how an ACO would affect the network, they were also concerned about how health care reform would affect their personal health insurance and medical care.

In addition to performing her supervisory duties, Carla continued to rotate through front and back office roles in the practice to maintain her medical assisting skills. Her attendance had always been exemplary, as Carla was reminded when her manager offered Carla her promotion. But now that she was a supervisor in charge of work schedules, her perspective had broadened as she saw the "big picture" of

what could happen when employees weren't in their assigned positions ready to work when the office opened for business each day. She soon noticed patterns of tardiness and poor attendance among three members of her staff. She monitored the situation, counseled the employees, put all three of them on probation, and documented her actions. Over the next 30 days, two of the employees did fine and were removed from probation but the third person failed to improve and had to be fired. The employee was a medical assisting colleague of Carla's who had worked at the practice for several years, and Carla was really sad to see her leave. But the patients' needs always came first in the practice, and everyone knew it.

Now Carla was dealing with another personnel issue. It seems a clerical worker, on the job for only one month, had accessed her husband's medical records to check for a history of sexually transmitted diseases (STDs). When the clerical worker confronted her husband about what she had found, her husband called his doctor to complain that his privacy had been violated. The doctor apologized to the patient and referred the matter to Carla, the employee's supervisor, for follow-up.

What should Carla do about the potential HIPAA violation? What would you do if you were in Carla's place?

appropriate equipment settings, revising a patient's treatment plan, interpreting blood test results, and deciding whether to apply for a promotion are just a few examples of how critical-thinking skills can help guide you in the right direction professionally. Developing critical-thinking and problem-solving skills is an important part of being, and being viewed as, a professional. Health care employers need problem solvers, not problem complainers. The more you use your critical-thinking and problem-solving skills, the more effective they will become.

Developing a Strong Work Ethic

Ask employers what characteristic is most important in a good employee and the majority will respond, "a strong work ethic." Positioning your job as a high priority in your life and making sound decisions about how you approach your work are critical to success in health care. Employees with a strong work ethic:

- Stay focused and leave their personal problems at home.
- Apply themselves to the task at hand.

- Get their work done right the first time.
- Exercise self-discipline and self-control.
- Know what management expects of them and they measure up.
- Don't wait to be told what to do.
- Demonstrate a positive attitude and enthusiasm for their work.

Employers today often complain about a perceived lack of work ethic among younger workers. Generational conflict may relate to the belief that young people may have chosen their professions for different reasons than their supervisors, they're more demanding of their work environment and employer, and they grasp and use technology much easier. These differences may create a divide between younger workers and their older supervisors because their shared experiences aren't the same. Regardless of your age, as a new health care professional you're going to encounter a wide variety of people and it's your job to demonstrate a strong work ethic. Here are some more examples:

- Come prepared to do your job.
- Work hard to complete your assignments.
- Offer to help others.
- Be tidy and neat.
- Be a good communicator and team member.
- Be positive and curious.
- Do what you say you will do.

If you have a few extra minutes, it's always a good idea to help out, even if it's not part of your job. Tidy a room, converse with patients and families, get the area ready for the next patient, and stock the supplies. People will notice that you've "gone the extra mile" to be of help.

Let's examine some additional factors that describe a strong work ethic.

Attendance and Punctuality

It's nearly impossible to demonstrate a commitment to your job without being there. Performing the duties of your job requires showing up for work every day and being **punctual** (arriving on time). Poor attendance usually results in other people having to cover for you when you aren't there yourself. How would you feel if your coworkers called in sick frequently, leaving you to do your work plus theirs? How would your coworkers feel if your attendance leaves a lot to be desired? Many health care organizations are already lean on staffing and can't afford to have people absent on a regular basis. When people are counting on you, it's important to be there and to arrive on time.

When you arrive late for work:

- The patient's diagnosis, treatment, surgery, or discharge from the hospital might be delayed
- Necessary supplies might not get delivered on time
- Paperwork might get filed too late to meet a deadline
- Other people might have to work late to catch up

Remember how the roles of health care workers are interconnected? You may think arriving late won't cause a problem for your work group, but what complications might you be causing other people?

Most everyone must miss work or arrive late on occasion. But when poor attendance or punctuality becomes a habit, it may result in a performance issue leading to **corrective action** (steps taken to overcome a problem) or **dismissal** (involuntary termination from a job).

What steps can you take to ensure good attendance and punctuality?

- Make a commitment to show up for work every day and arrive on time.
- When your shift starts, make sure you are in the area and ready to go.
- Have **contingency plans** (backup plans prepared in case original plans don't work) to cover situations when your children or spouse gets sick or when your transportation isn't **reliable** (can be counted upon; trustworthy).
- Protect your health and safety to keep from getting sick or injured.
- Eat well, get plenty of sleep, and consider getting a flu shot.

Allow some extra time at the end of your shift in case you get held over. Never leave a patient or coworker in the middle of a procedure by rushing out the door the minute your shift ends. Make sure there's a smooth transition between shifts and don't leave your work for other people to finish up. Remember interdependence? Other people are counting on you to arrive on time and get your part of the work done.

Reliability and Accountability

Being reliable and accountable for your actions are key factors in a strong work ethic. If reliable people have agreed to do something, their coworkers know they will follow through. Following through on commitments is a big part of the team effort. If you are there for other people when you say you will be, it's more likely they will be there for you when you need them.

People who are accountable accept **responsibility** (an obligation or a sense of duty binding someone to a course of action) for the consequences of their actions. They "own up" to what they've done and avoid blaming other people. If you make a mistake, admit it and accept full responsibility. Apologize to those who have been inconvenienced. But keep in mind that it's important to apologize for a mistake, but that doesn't erase the fact that a mistake was made. Learn from the experience and avoid making the same mistake twice. Your supervisor and coworkers will appreciate your "the buck stops here" attitude.

Follow through on all work assignments that you are qualified and prepared to perform. If you are given a work assignment that you are not qualified or prepared to perform, discuss the situation with your supervisor immediately. Refusal to do an assigned task or to follow established rules may be construed as **insubordination** and grounds for dismissal.

When serving the needs of patients, it's important to avoid passing judgment or projecting your own personal beliefs on others. If you object to an assignment because it conflicts with your religious beliefs or values, you must discuss these concerns with your supervisor. It's best to resolve issues like these when you first consider a job offer. If you wish to not participate in abortions, sex-change operations, end-of-life procedures, or other such activities, many employers will allow you to opt out. But this must be discussed ahead of time so that patient care isn't delayed or jeopardized.

BY THE NUMBERS

DISHONESTY AT WORK

Research shows that 70% of applicants overstate their qualifications on job applications. More than one-third lie about their experience and achievements and 12% fail to disclose criminal records. About a third of all job applicants admit to thinking about stealing from their employers.

What happens when these applicants become employees? About half of all new hires don't work out, often the result of dishonest behavior before and during employment. The result can be devastating to the

(continued)

companies that hire them. About 30% of all business failures in the United States are caused by employee theft. Employee theft is growing by 15% a year and as much as 75% of internal theft is never detected. In addition to theft, work-related violent crimes affect about 2 million people every year.

According to a recent study, as many as 80% of group practice physicians could be victimized by embezzlers during their careers, mostly involving office personnel who handle cash before and after office hours. The problem is sometimes detected when workers refuse to take time off for fear their dishonest acts will be discovered while they're away from the office. To reduce the potential for theft, doctors run periodic credit checks on employees who handle cash and they rotate assignments so that more than one person is responsible for overseeing the finances.

Attitude and Enthusiasm

How often have you witnessed another person's behavior and thought to yourself, "What a bad attitude!" For some people, negativity is a way of life. As **pessimists** (one who looks on the dark side of things)**,** they "see the glass as half empty." From their perspective, the situation is always bad and getting worse. They complain about everything and nothing seems to satisfy them. They rarely smile, appear happy, or convey enthusiasm about their work. They spread negativity to everyone around them and undermine morale, teamwork, and a spirit of cooperation.

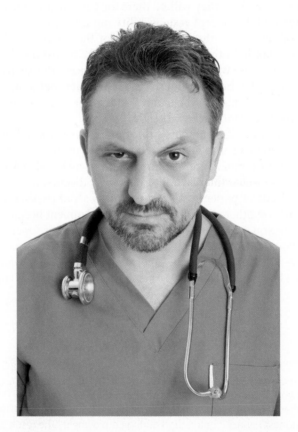

Figure 2-4 Displaying a negative attitude (*Pop Paul-Catalin/Shutterstock*)

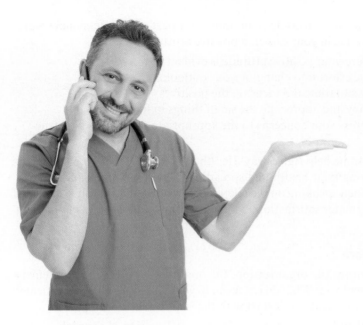

Figure 2-5 Displaying a positive attitude (*Pop Paul-Catalin/Shutterstock*)

Optimists (one who looks on the bright side of things), on the other hand, display a positive attitude most of the time. They "see the glass as half full" and approach life with enthusiasm. When they experience things they disagree with, they voice their complaints in a constructive manner. They look for reasons to feel happy and content and they appreciate the small things in life. They tend to smile a lot and convey a friendly and cooperative attitude.

Working in health care can really challenge your attitude. People who have worked in health care for several years may feel as if things are getting worse. They may be critical, resentful, and angry about some of the changes they've seen occur. Perhaps cutting staff to reduce costs has resulted in longer work hours, additional duties, and more holiday shifts to cover. Some of the benefits they enjoyed in the past may have been reduced or eliminated to save money. Their job titles and job duties might have been altered as part of a reorganization or merger of companies.

As mentioned earlier, health care is constantly changing. When workers feel like something of value has been taken away, their attitudes can suffer. It's important to look for the advantages that come with change and avoid focusing on the negatives.

People who are relatively new in their health careers may also face attitudinal challenges. Young workers may become impatient when job promotions and pay raises don't occur quickly enough. They might question long-standing policies and procedures that don't seem relevant anymore. Dress code requirements barring visible tattoos, facial piercings, and nontraditional hair colors and styles may cause discontent.

The bottom line is this: No job or place of employment will ever be perfect. Even though companies may work hard to enhance job satisfaction and be seen as an "employer of choice," people will still find things to complain about. That's just human nature. The key to maintaining a positive attitude is to always look for what's good in any situation and remain optimistic that things will get better.

Displaying enthusiasm and a positive attitude is an important part of a professional's work ethic. If you want to excel and advance in your career, a positive attitude is a must.

- If you are an optimist, make sure your positive attitude is evident at work.
- If you are a pessimist, put some effort into changing your outlook.
- Look for the bright side in any situation and focus on the positives.
- Seize opportunities to feel happy and appreciate the small things in life.
- When you must complain, express your concerns to the appropriate person in a constructive manner.

If you feel "stressed out," get some help right away. Health care workers who don't alleviate their stress run the risk of damaging their health and spreading their stress among coworkers. Smile every chance you get, even when speaking on the telephone. By adopting a positive attitude, you will experience more joy and greater satisfaction in life, and your optimism and enthusiasm will spread to those around you.

Competence and Quality of Work

No matter where your job falls within the organization, the quality of your work is extremely important. What does quality mean to you? What does it mean to your employer and your patients? How can you support quality improvement? Let's start with the importance of competency.

- Make sure you are well trained and competent to perform every function of your job.
- Never take a chance and just "wing it."
- Keep your knowledge up-to-date and your skills sharp.
- Learn about the latest procedures, techniques, and new equipment.
- Attend in-service sessions, register for continuing education workshops, and read professional publications in your field.
- Don't hesitate to ask questions or request help.

Keep in mind that your education won't end when you graduate from school. Nothing stays **stagnant** (without motion; dull, sluggish) in health care. As a professional, it's your responsibility to continue learning, strengthen your skills, and improve the quality of your work.

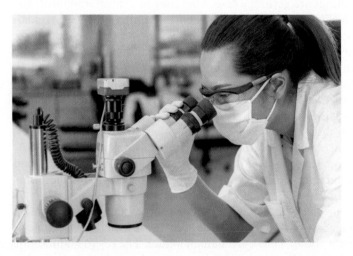

Figure 2-6 Checking a microscopic slide to ensure accuracy (*Bullstar/Shutterstock*)

Perhaps you've heard the saying, "Quality is in the details." This means paying attention to even the smallest things, because making a small mistake or overlooking a minor detail can have a big impact on quality. Stocking items on the wrong shelf, misfiling a document, losing a phone number, miscalculating a bill, or missing an important meeting can all negatively impact quality. Each day brings many opportunities for details to "fall through the cracks." Being **diligent** (careful and conscientious in one's work) about quality and careful in your work will help prevent these kinds of problems.

Contributing to quality improvement efforts companywide is an important aspect of your work ethic. No one has a better handle on how to improve work processes and quality outcomes than the people who do the work on a daily basis. Management can't improve the company's quality without the help of their **subordinates** (people at a lower rank or under someone's supervision).

- When you have a suggestion for quality improvement, submit it to your supervisor.
- When you spot a potential problem, report it.
- If your work unit receives periodic quality-related data, pay attention to the reports and do your best to support improvements.

Sometimes you may be asked to do things that don't fall within your **job description** (a list of the essential duties of and qualifications for a job). (Refer to Appendix A, Sample Job Description.) Responding to one of these requests by saying, "That's not my job!" isn't acceptable. Doing what's asked of you might not fall within your job duties, but one of two things needs to happen. Either you should go ahead and perform the task because you are capable and willing to do it, or you should refer the matter to the appropriate person and make sure he or she follows through.

No task is too menial when working in health care.

- If a patient or visitor becomes ill in the parking lot, offer assistance or send for help.
- If someone looks lost, provide directions; if necessary, guide them to their destination.
- If you notice a spill in a public area, don't wait for a housekeeper to discover it. Clean it up yourself (using safety precautions) or report it to the appropriate person and stay in the area until it's cleaned up to prevent possible injuries.
- If you observe a piece of equipment not working properly or spot a situation that could pose a health or safety hazard, take action. Don't just ignore things and go on about your business.

A commitment to quality requires paying attention to what's going on around you and addressing concerns before they escalate into serious problems.

TRENDS AND ISSUES

YOU CAN'T ALWAYS TRUST CAREGIVERS

Doctors are supposed to be open and honest in sharing information with patients about their medical conditions. Yet according to a recent survey, more than half of all doctors admitted to giving patients false hope. Ten percent of doctors reported telling their patients a lie within the past year. These findings emphasize why it's important for patients to make their wishes clearly known. If patients want the truth from their doctors, they need to speak up. Seriously ill patients who get accurate information can plan ahead and get their affairs in order. Yet many doctors are reluctant to convey bad news.

Almost 20% of the doctors surveyed failed to disclose mistakes they had made, based on the fear of being sued. Yet studies among patients indicate that when doctors admit up-front they've made a mistake

(continued)

and apologize for it, patients are less likely to sue. One third of the doctors included in the survey don't agree that mistakes should be divulged.

In very rare situations, caregivers cause intentional harm to their patients. A nurse anesthetist in Minnesota addicted to pain medications took most of a surgery patient's painkillers herself. As the patient screamed in pain on the surgery table, she told him to "man up" because he couldn't be given any more medication. Prior to surgery, the patient had been told that his kidney stone removal wouldn't be painful since patients are typically heavily sedated or asleep during the procedure. As the man told doctors he was in terrible pain, he heard staff members discuss putting him in restraints. The patient's medical records revealed that he had only been given one-third of the drug he should have received. After the incident, officials found empty syringes in the nurse's pocket. She refused to take a drug test and resigned.

There have been several cases where health care workers have killed one or more patients for various reasons. Fortunately, incidences involving such extreme and heinous conduct are very rare.

Compliance

Compliance (acting in accordance with laws and with a company's rules, policies, and procedures) is extremely important. Ignoring a rule, violating a policy, or breaking the law can compromise quality, hurt a patient or coworker, and get you fired from your job. What might happen if employees:

- Don't wear their identification badges at work?
- Share private business matters or confidential patient information?
- Make threats against other employees?
- Attempt to perform duties beyond their scope of practice?

Health care workers must always function within their scope of practice. Performing duties beyond what you're legally permitted to do is highly risky and illegal. Some jobs require a special license to practice. State agencies grant licenses only to people who have met preestablished qualifications, and only licensed workers may legally perform the job. Other jobs may require a special certification. State agencies and professional associations certify people who have met certain competency standards. Although noncertified people may legally perform the job, employers may prefer to hire only those workers who possess certification and who are eligible to use the professional title associated with that certification. When a license, certification, or some other special credential is required for your job, make sure you meet those requirements and maintain "active" status. In some professions this means completing annual continuing education requirements or periodic competency retesting.

Rules and policies are established for good reasons and everyone has the responsibility to comply with them. Health care companies usually have written policies and procedures plus employee handbooks to communicate their expectations. Know where to find these documents and, if you don't understand something, ask for clarification.

Complying with laws and policies has always been important in health care. But compliance is gaining even more attention these days because the government is stepping up its efforts to identify violators and prosecute them. Some companies have hotlines so employees can report compliance concerns anonymously with no fear of backlash.

Violating a law, regulation, or policy can get you and your employer in serious trouble. You could end up fired, prosecuted, fined, or incarcerated. Your employer could face stiff fines and exclusion from vital government programs such as Medicare or Medicaid. Complying with laws,

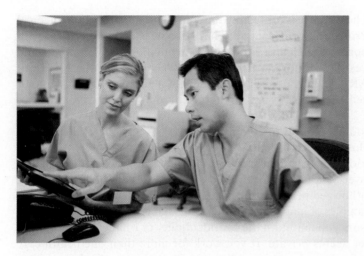

Figure 2-7 Discussing policies to comply with regulations (*Monkey Business Images/Shutterstock*)

regulations, and policies because you have to is important, but there's more to it than that. Professionals comply because *it's the right thing to do.*

- Make sure you're aware of and understand all of the federal, state, and local health laws and regulations pertaining to your profession, as well as the policies and procedures for your job.
- Become familiar with medical/legal issues specific to your profession.
- Comply with your company's Internet and computer security policies and procedures.
- Learn about security and fire safety procedures and how to protect your patients, coworkers, and company.
- Know what your company expects of you in practicing sound business practices.

If accused of an illegal activity, claiming that you weren't aware of the law isn't an acceptable legal defense. It's your job to know what laws, regulations, and policies apply to you and your job. If you're uncertain about compliance responsibilities, ask for clarification.

THINK ABOUT IT

THE RIGHT THING TO DO

Do you always follow the rules? Or do you "bend" or break the rules when you're sure you won't get caught? For example, do you:

- Exceed the speed limit in road construction zones when no police are present?
- Park in a handicapped spot when no one is looking?
- Borrow someone else's ID to get his or her discount on your purchase?
- Wear a piece of clothing and then return it to the store for a refund?
- Share copyrighted music or books with friends without paying for it?
- Return a mail-order item that your child broke, claiming it was damaged in shipment?

Professionals don't do the right thing because they're afraid of getting caught. They do the right thing because *it's the right thing to do.*

A major part of compliance in health care is protecting the confidentiality of patient medical records via HIPAA regulations. Protecting confidentiality has become even more critical with the advent of electronic health records. The Health Information Technology for Economic and Clinical Health (**HITECH**) Act was signed into law in February 2009 as part of the American Recovery and Reinvestment Act (ARRA). Portions of the HITECH Act address the confidentiality of health information transmitted electronically and strengthen the enforcement and penalties associated with HIPAA rules.

Become familiar with what you need to do to comply with HIPAA and the HITECH Act to prevent the inappropriate disclosure of confidential information and avoid potential fines against you and your employer. Violating a patient's right to privacy is a very serious offense, but sometimes workers forget or overlook actions that would constitute a violation. Discussing a patient's condition with an unauthorized person or releasing the name or address of a patient without permission are just two examples of inappropriate behavior that could result in a HIPAA violation and lawsuit. Also make sure you maintain the confidentiality of financial information and other materials your employer deems private. If you work for more than one health care company at the same time, or move from employer to employer, it's important to not share private information among employers.

HOT TOPICS

THE HEALTH INSURANCE PORTABILITY AND ACCOUNTABILITY ACT (HIPAA)

The confidentiality of a patient's medical information is protected by the Health Insurance Portability and Accountability Act (HIPAA). This law regulates the sharing of medical information. Regulations in the act help ensure that a patient's medical information is kept secure and confidential. All health care workers must be familiar with the HIPAA regulations that apply to their jobs.

Here are a few examples of the kinds of information protected by HIPAA:

- Information in medical records
- Conversations between health care providers about patient care or treatment
- Health insurance information
- Patient billing information
- Most other information about a patient's health

Confidential communications are protected under law against any disclosure (forced or voluntary) over the objection of the patient. If confidential information needs to be released to other people, the patient must give his or her written **consent** (permission given for something to happen). The rationale behind the rule is that a level of trust must exist between a doctor and the patient so that the doctor can properly treat the patient. If the patient were fearful of telling the truth to the doctor because he or she believed the doctor would report such behavior to others, then the treatment process could be far more difficult.

Certain types of information may be considered exempt from HIPAA regulations. This includes:

- Suspected **fraud** (intentional deceit through false information or misrepresentation)
- Births and deaths
- Injuries caused by violence, including child abuse

(continued)

- Drug abuse
- Communicable diseases
- Sexually transmitted diseases (STDs)

A medical facility, doctor, or health care worker can be fined, sued, or lose his or her job for sharing *any* confidential information about patients with other people, including the patient's family members. Violations of patient confidentiality must be reported.

Some other areas of risk that can result in compliance concerns include safety and environmental precautions, labor laws, retention of records, Medicare billing and **reimbursement** (paying back or compensation for money spent), licenses and credentials, and **conflict of interest** (an inappropriate relationship between personal interests and official responsibilities).

Examples of illegal or unethical behaviors include:

- Fraud such as billing for a test or treatment that wasn't performed
- Improperly changing or destroying records
- **Sexual harassment** (unwelcome sexual advances, requests for sexual favors, and other verbal and physical contact of a sexual nature)
- Creating a **hostile workplace** (an uncomfortable or unsafe workplace)
- Stealing property.

Issues related to sexual harassment can cause major problems at work. Avoid any suggestion of unwelcome sexually oriented advances or comments that could lead to sexual harassment charges being filed against you. Examples include verbal communication, visual and written materials, unwanted touching, sexually explicit texting or postings on social networking sites, or any other actions that have the potential to make another person uncomfortable. Even if you think your actions are harmless, the other person (or someone else present at the time) might see things differently.

If you are the victim of sexual harassment or intimidation, report the incident to your supervisor or another superior immediately. Keep written notes on what you've observed or experienced, including details such as the date, time, place, who was present, what exactly happened, and what you did to follow up. Information such as this will be very important should an investigation take place.

There are far too many examples of compliance issues to list them all. Here are some important things to keep in mind:

- Don't modify or destroy patient or financial records without proper authority.
- If your job involves preparing bills for patient procedures, make sure the codes you use to identify specific diagnoses or procedures are accurate; never **up-code** (modify the classification of a procedure to increase financial reimbursement) a procedure.
- Always work within your scope of practice.
- Don't accept pay for hours that you did not work.
- Avoid any suggestion of a conflict of interest.
- If your job involves awarding contracts to outside companies, don't accept gifts or free meals in exchange.

- Don't ask a vendor that your company does business with to give you a special discount on a personal purchase.
- Don't refer patients to one of your relatives who just happens to be in the health care business.

Inappropriate Behavior

Inappropriate behavior can result in serious compliance issues. As a professional, you would never knowingly engage in an illegal or unethical act yourself, but you might observe someone else doing something suspicious. Or you might feel that you are a victim of sexual harassment or a hostile work environment.

- You should never bring a weapon to work or create an environment where someone else could feel intimidated or unsafe. Verbal threats, nasty letters, or other forms of hostile behavior may lead to charges of intimidation.
- If you have a concern about something you see going on at work that might put you, your employer, coworkers, or patients at risk, let your supervisor know or report your concern via a hotline if one is available.
- If your supervisor is one of the people involved in the activity, report the matter to your supervisor's boss, a human resources representative, or someone in legal services.

Stay alert! If you find yourself in a situation where you aren't sure how to proceed, ask yourself some questions. Is what's going on legal and ethical? Is it in the best interests of my employer and patients? How would this look to others outside my organization? Then take action.

You've probably heard the term **whistleblower**, a person who exposes the illegal or unethical practices of another person or of an organization or company. "Blowing the whistle" can be a scary proposition for employees, but the law protects whistleblowers from retribution. In fact, whistleblowers might receive a portion of the fine the government collects when a health care provider is found guilty of Medicare fraud, for example.

- If you suspect someone of illegal or unethical behavior, it's your responsibility to report it.
- Try to resolve your concerns within your organization first. Avoid going to the government or the media unless repeated internal attempts have failed.
- If you've tried your best to report and stop illegal or unethical practices but have been unsuccessful, you might need to think about finding a job at another company.

CONSIDER THIS

REPORTING ILLEGAL BEHAVIOR

If you know someone is engaged in illegal behavior, it's your responsibility to report it. If you don't, you could get in trouble as well. In fact, even if you didn't know the illegal behavior was occurring but you should have known, you can be liable for legal action.

For example, if you observe someone stealing from a patient, report it immediately. If you don't report it and your supervisor finds out that you knew what was going on, you could be disciplined as well as the thief. If your job involves maintaining an inventory of supplies and a coworker gets fired for stealing some of them, you could get in trouble for not noticing the items were missing.

Although you might be tempted to say, "It's none of my business," reporting the illegal behavior of a coworker actually *is* your business.

Representing Your Employer

When you accept a job offer, show up for work, and receive a paycheck, you become a representative of the company. To patients, visitors, guests, and vendors, *you are the company you work for*. Everything you do and say can have an impact on the company's reputation. By accepting employment, you not only agree to follow your company's rules and policies but also agree to support its mission and values.

Get a copy of your company's **corporate mission** (the special duties, functions, or purposes of a company) and **corporate values** (beliefs held in high esteem by a company), review the documents, and think about what you should do to support your employer. Even though you don't own the company, it's important to take an active interest and get involved.

- Learn about the history and structure of your company.
- Read company newsletters and keep up with the latest news and events.
- Participate in your company's social events and sports teams.
- Volunteer to serve on committees and your local speaker's bureau.
- Substitute words such as "we" and "us" for "they" and "them." For example, instead of saying, "They told us they are going to open a new clinic next year," it would be better to say, "We are opening our new clinic next year."

Become familiar with your company's long- and short-term goals and its vision for the future. As you focus on the duties of your job, think about how your performance each and every day aligns with your employer's mission, vision, and values. Health care companies need people who are viewed as a "good fit" for the organization, so take some pride and ownership in the company for which you work.

Regardless of what job you have, your appearance, attitudes, and behaviors affect your company's image in the community. **Front-line workers** (employees who have the most frequent or direct contact with a company's customers) such as nurses, medical assistants, housekeepers, patient transporters, and cafeteria workers have some of the greatest influence on their company's

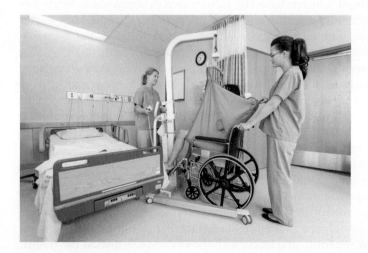

Figure 2-8 Front-line workers use a lift to move a patient from a wheelchair to her bed (*Tyler Olson/Shutterstock*)

reputation because they have the most frequent contact with patients, visitors, and guests. What might happen if you publicly criticize your employer, complain about a company policy, or question how a physician treated a patient? By damaging the reputation of your employer, you're hurting yourself and countless other employees who come to work every day to do a good job. If you take issue with something going on at work, speak with the appropriate person and communicate your concerns in a professional manner.

- Don't make negative remarks about your company or its employees in public or in a public forum such as Facebook.
- Use **discretion** (taking care and using good judgment about what one says or does).
- Give your employer and your coworkers the benefit of the doubt; assume that everyone is there to do his or her best.
- If you have serious doubts about your employer and the way your company does business, it's probably best to look for employment at another company.

Evaluating Your Performance

Now that you're familiar with what it takes to demonstrate a strong work ethic, let's examine how health care employers evaluate job performance. If you take your job seriously and apply everything you are learning in this book, you should have no problem when it comes time for your **performance evaluation** (a measurement of success in executing job duties). But if you lack the competence or the commitment required to perform your job effectively, your deficiencies will soon become apparent.

The process used to conduct performance evaluations varies from company to company. Sometimes it's called a "performance appraisal" or "performance management." The purpose of a performance evaluation is not to determine how well an employee "is liked" or how his or her supervisor "feels" about the employee, as this would involve **subjective** criteria (affected by one's state of mind or feelings). Instead, employers evaluate job performance using **objective** criteria (real or actual; not affected by feelings), which is based on factors such as competence, behaviors (customer service, teamwork, problem solving), and traits (attitude, appearance, initiative). Evaluating competence and behaviors using objective criteria is fairly straightforward. But assessing traits such as "appearance" and "attitude" without becoming subjective can be difficult.

It's not unusual for new employees to undergo a **probationary period** whereby their attendance and performance are closely monitored for the first few months to make sure they are a good fit for the organization and the position. New employees are evaluated at the end of their probationary period and the decision is made to retain the employees or not. Having successfully completed their probationary period, employees are then subject to regular performance evaluations from that point forward, typically done on an annual basis.

Small organizations may evaluate performance on an informal basis. The supervisor observes the employee's performance over a period of time and provides verbal feedback regarding strengths, weaknesses, and areas for improvement. Informal evaluations may or may not be documented in writing and kept in the employee's personnel file. Larger companies typically evaluate performance on a more formal basis. The supervisor observes the employee's performance during the year, completes a written performance evaluation form, and meets with the employee to discuss the results. The performance evaluation form and notes from the meeting are documented in writing and kept in the employee's personnel file. (Refer to Appendix B for a Sample Performance Evaluation.)

Some companies give their employees the opportunity to do a self-evaluation. This can be very helpful in preparing for your evaluation meeting with your supervisor.

RECENT DEVELOPMENTS

360-DEGREE FEEDBACK

Employers are now using **360-degree feedback** tools as part of performance evaluations. People who have worked with the employee are asked to provide input to the employee's evaluation. This could include **peers** (people at the same rank within a company or society), subordinates, team members, customers, people from other departments, and people outside the organization. Getting feedback from people in addition to the employee's supervisor helps reduce subjectivity and provides a broader view of the employee's performance. When employees work on teams, getting performance feedback from other team members helps evaluate the employee's team skills as well as his or her individual performance.

In addition to focusing on previous performance, the evaluation process also lays out plans for the coming year. Through discussions with supervisors, employees develop goals for the coming year to help them progress from where they are to where they eventually want to be. The goal-setting process helps employees overcome deficiencies, enhance skills, and work toward job promotions and career advancement.

Each company has its own rating scale. Typically, a few employees will receive an "outstanding" evaluation, most will receive an "average" evaluation, and a few may receive a "poor" evaluation. Performance evaluations may result in more than just feedback about how well you're doing on the job. Many companies now tie the amount of an individual's compensation or pay increase to the score on his or her performance evaluation. This is called **performance-based pay**, also known as merit-based pay or pay for performance. Employees who receive high scores on their performance evaluations receive higher pay raises than employees who receive lower scores. Employees with poor scores may not receive a pay raise at all. When pay is tied to performance, it's even more important to focus on objective criteria rather than subjective criteria in the evaluation process.

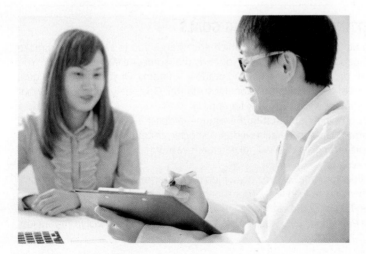

Figure 2-9 Discussing the results of a performance review (*Nonwarit/Shutterstock*)

Which behaviors result in outstanding evaluations? Keep reading because most everything you need to know to earn an outstanding evaluation is covered in these chapters. As you read, start evaluating your own strengths and weaknesses. Think about what you need to improve upon and what steps you will take.

Preparing throughout the year for your performance evaluation is a good idea.

- Review your job description once a month.
- If you have goals for the year, ask yourself: "Am I making progress on my goals? If not, why not? What should I do to improve?"
- Keep any thank-you notes or emails from doctors, coworkers, or patients in a file.
- Maintain a list of projects you've worked on and committee participation.
- Keep records of any workshops you have attended or classes you've taken.
- Track suggestions that you've submitted to improve quality, safety, and cost-effectiveness.
- Keep notes about other things you've done to make things better for your company and your patients.

When your performance review gets close:

- Review your job description again and make sure you're familiar with the essential duties of your position.
- If your company uses a performance evaluation form, ask for a copy. Make sure you understand the performance criteria and how performance is evaluated and scored.
- If your company's performance evaluation process is computerized, make sure you have the computer skills you need to complete your part of the process.
- Complete your self-evaluation and make a copy for your supervisor.
- Think about the goals you set for the past year. Did you accomplish them? Why or why not? Jot down your accomplishments and note what you would like to achieve in the coming year.
- Think about your performance and what you've accomplished. Prepare your notes and other materials that you've assembled during the year to share with your supervisor during the meeting.
- Make a list of questions you might want to ask your supervisor when you meet.

THE MORE YOU KNOW

SETTING AND ACHIEVING GOALS

Wanting or needing something can be a strong motivator, which encourages you to set goals and make decisions that will lead to success. Goals are aims, objectives, or ends that someone strives to attain. You might set a goal to obtain something specific, such as a passing grade in anatomy. Or you might set a goal to achieve a position, such as president of your local professional association. Goals help you focus on what is really important to you and what you are willing to work toward.

Long-term goals help you focus on what you want in the future—at least a year from now, or even five or 10 years from now. Short-term goals can be achieved in a shorter amount of time. For example, completing a first aid course is a short-term goal that will take just a few months. Becoming employed as a registered nurse will take years to achieve.

If your supervisor has identified areas for improvement in your job performance, it's important to not only establish some goals but to achieve them. More than likely, your supervisor will be watching you to make sure you're taking the situation seriously and doing your best to measure up to expectations. Failure to achieve the goals set forth through a performance evaluation could lead to a probationary period or dismissal from your job.

The night before your review, get plenty of sleep and try to relax. This is when being prepared really helps. During the meeting with your supervisor:

- Practice good listening skills, pay attention to everything your supervisor says, take notes, and ask for clarification when you don't understand something.
- If you disagree with something, state your reasons in an objective, respectful manner and avoid becoming defensive.

Keep in mind that some supervisors are more skilled and experienced than others in providing constructive feedback and coaching their subordinates for improvement. Performance evaluations can create some uncomfortable conflict. Employees aren't the only people who experience anxiety over these sessions—many supervisors do, too.

- Brace yourself for some negative feedback. If you've done your best all year long, you should also hear lots of positive comments.
- Accept **constructive criticism** (positive and negative comments and opinions offered to help another person improve) and learn from it.
- Compare the scores on your self-evaluation with the scores your supervisor gave you and discuss any differences.
- If you disagree with what's been said during your evaluation, state your opinions clearly and objectively, but don't expect your scores to change.
- If you're expected to make improvements during the coming year, make sure you know exactly what's expected of you and how improvements will be measured.
- At the end of the session, summarize important "next steps" and thank your supervisor for the time he or she spent with you.

Take your performance review seriously, but not as "an attack" on you personally. Remember, no one is perfect and everyone has more to learn. Many companies are moving from a hierarchical management structure, where employees have just one supervisor, to a matrix management structure, where employees have two or more supervisors. For example, registered nurses might be assigned to work on two separate patient care units each month, or medical assistants might work with three different doctors. Radiographers might rotate to work two different shifts, or audiologists might provide services for three area clinics. Matrix management can lead to some confusion regarding "Who is really my boss?" and "Who should I listen to?" In situations like this, you'll be challenged to meet the expectations of all of your supervisors. And most likely, all of them will have input to your performance evaluation.

Even if your company doesn't have a performance evaluation process, you can (and should) request periodic feedback. This can be as simple as asking, "How do you think I'm doing?" You don't have to wait until annual review time to ask. Solicit feedback from your supervisor and coworkers on a regular basis and then act upon what they've told you. If your performance becomes an issue, chances are your supervisor will let you know as soon as the problem becomes apparent. But don't subscribe to the "no news is good news" theory. Soliciting feedback from those most familiar with your performance is the best way to increase your value to the organization.

Understanding the elements of a strong work ethic and performing well on the job are vital in developing your reputation as a health care professional. The next step is examining your personal traits and how they impact your work.

REALITY CHECK

Perhaps you've already had one or more jobs where you've been held to certain performance standards and had to comply with company policies and procedures. If you appeared for work every day and on time, demonstrated competence and a commitment to your job, and proved to be a reliable and enthusiastic employee, then you probably earned a satisfactory performance evaluation and maybe a pay raise or job promotion. If so, this experience and what you learned from it will serve you well as you assume your new role in health care.

But as mentioned previously, working in health care presents some unique challenges. More than likely, you'll be working in a complex, stressful environment where everything that you say and do will make an impact on other people. It's like throwing a pebble in a pond and watching the ripple effect. You can see some of the ripples created because they happen right in front of you. But other ripples are off in the distance, too far away to observe.

Your attitude and behaviors at work cause ripples. Some ripples you will see, others you will not. When you smile and project a friendly attitude, you create positive ripples. When you complain and spread negativity, you create negative ripples. When you "go above and beyond the call of duty" to do something special for a patient or a coworker, you create positive ripples. When you get lazy and develop an "I don't care" attitude about your work, you create negative ripples. As with the pebble in the pond, you probably won't know just how much of an impact you've actually made, whether positive or negative. It all comes back to being intentional about everything you say and do. Stop and think before you act, because the ripples *you* create should only be the positive ones.

For More Information

Health Care Compliance
Health Care Compliance Association
www.hcca-info.org

HIPAA and HITECH Act
U.S. Department of Health and Human Services
www.hhs.gov/ocr/privacy/

Sexual Harassment
U.S. Department of State
www.state.gov/s/ocr/c14800.htm

Workplace Violence and Harassment
U.S. Department of Labor
Occupational Safety and Health Administration
https://www.osha.gov/SLTC/healthcarefacilities/violence.html

KEY POINTS

- Commit to your job and make it a high priority in your life.
- From a systems perspective, know where your role fits in.
- Remember the concept of common sense when using digital communication and social media.
- Be mindful, aware of what you're doing, and present in the moment.
- Stop and think before you act; everything you say and do should be intentional.
- Develop effective critical thinking skills to help solve problems.
- Report for work when scheduled and arrive on time.
- Adopt an optimistic attitude and display enthusiasm at work.
- Maintain your competency and always work within your scope of practice.
- Pay attention to quality and submit suggestions to improve it.
- Comply with all policies, laws, and rules that apply to your job.
- Avoid illegal, unethical, and inappropriate behavior.
- Represent your employer in a professional manner.
- Ask for feedback about your job performance and make improvements as needed.

LEARNING ACTIVITIES

Using information from Chapter Two:
- Answer the Chapter Review Questions
- Respond to the What If? Scenarios

Chapter Review Questions

Using information from Chapter Two, answer each of the following questions:

1. Define *interdependence* as it relates to health care workers.

2. Describe why health care workers need to have a systems perspective.

3. Give one example of how failing to use common sense with social media can lead to a HIPAA violation.

4. Explain why it's important to be "present in the moment" at work.

5. Define *critical thinking*.

6. List three things that critical thinkers do to make good decisions.

7. List five factors that demonstrate a strong work ethic.

8. Describe the attitudinal differences between optimists and pessimists.

9. Explain why health care workers must function within the legal scope of practice for the state in which they are employed.

10. Explain why it's important for health care workers to comply with federal, state, and local health laws and regulations as they relate to health care settings.

11. Discuss how HIPAA protects the confidentiality of medical information.

12. List two things you should do when representing your employer.

13. List three ways to prepare for a performance evaluation.

14. Differentiate between objective and subjective evaluation criteria.

What If? Scenarios

Think about what you would do in the following situations and record your answers.

1. You were out with friends until very late last night and had to report for work this morning at 7:00 A.M. You know your coworkers won't arrive for another half an hour. You've got just enough time for a quick run to the corner coffee shop before your coworkers arrive.

2. You promised your coworkers you'd work the day shift on Thanksgiving so they could be home with their families. Then two days before the holiday, an old friend from out of town calls to say he'd like you to be his guest for lunch on Thanksgiving Day.

3. Your shift ends in 30 minutes and you've got about 30 minutes of work left to do, but you haven't gotten to take your afternoon break yet.

4. Your niece needs to sell 10 more packs of popcorn to earn a fundraising prize at school. You're pretty sure your coworkers would buy some.

5. Your supervisor has asked you out on a date twice. Both times you declined saying you'd prefer to not date people from work. Now he's asking again and reminds you that your performance review is coming up next month.

6. The office manager tells you to enter a code on an insurance form that she knows is not correct. If you enter the incorrect code as she has told you to do, the clinic will receive more money from the insurance company than it would if you enter the correct code.

7. One of your neighbors is admitted to the unit where you work. A relative of yours calls to tell you he's heard a rumor that the neighbor has a communicable disease. Because you work on the unit and have access to records, your relative asks you to find out if the rumor is true.

8. A coworker invites you to a party. When you arrive, you notice three people that you work with complaining about low wages and telling a group of strangers that one of the surgeons at your hospital made a mistake last week and lied to the patient's family to cover it up.

9. A doctor mistakes you for a registered nurse and tells you to prepare a medication for him to administer to a patient. Even though you prepared medications in your previous job, it's not within the scope of practice for your current job.

10. A coworker left for her lunch break and returned 90 minutes later. When you asked why she was gone so long, she said she had an appointment to get her hair cut.

11. You notice that a radiographer with whom you work routinely overexposes his patients and then uses digital settings to correct the images.

12. A coworker took a photograph of a patient at the clinic and posted it on his Facebook page.

3

Personal Traits of the Health Care Professional

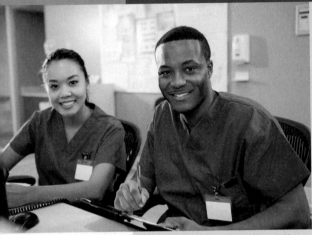

The ultimate measure of a man is not where he stands in moments of comfort and convenience, but where he stands at times of challenge and controversy.

—Martin Luther King, Jr. (1929–1968), civil rights leader

(Monkey Business Images/Shutterstock)

CHAPTER OBJECTIVES

Having completed this chapter, you will be able to:

- Describe how your character affects your reputation as a professional.
- List four examples of the lack of character in the workplace.
- Explain how your character traits and personal values affect your behavior and attitude.
- Give three examples of dishonest behaviors.
- Define *ethics*.
- List three important questions to ask yourself when making difficult ethical decisions.
- Define *morals*.
- Explain the importance of protecting your professional reputation on social media sites.
- Give three examples of fraud in health care.

- Name and define two examples of criminal law terms.
- Name and define two examples of civil law terms.
- Explain why it's important to comply with the code of ethics for your profession.
- Differentiate between personal ethics and professional ethics.
- Explain the connection between negligence and malpractice.
- Describe why some types of health care workers need personal liability insurance.
- Explain why it's important to follow protocol if you suspect a reportable incident.
- List three examples of complex ethical, moral, and legal dilemmas in health care.

KEY TERMS

abuse	ethics	libel	protocol
assault	false imprisonment	loyalty	prudent
battery	felony	malpractice	reasonable care
callous	gross misconduct	moral convictions	reportable conditions
character	harassment	morale	reportable incident
cheating	inconsistent	morals	résumé
clone	integrity	negligence	slander
code of ethics	invasion of privacy	opioid	standards of care
conduct	judgment	personal values	torts
conscience	liable	priorities	trustworthiness
duty to act			

Character and Personal Values

Professionalism brings together who you are as a person and how you contribute those traits in the workplace. Before you can achieve success "doing" something, you have to "be" something and being a health care professional depends greatly on who you are as a person. It takes a long time to develop a good reputation and only a split second to lose it. Much of this comes down to your **character** and **personal values**.

- *Character:* a person's moral behavior and qualities
- *Personal values:* things of great worth and importance to a person
- *Reputation:* a person's character, values, and behavior as viewed by others

Employers are becoming increasingly concerned about a lack of character and positive personal values in the workplace. Each year in businesses throughout the country, employees are responsible for a variety of dishonest, illegal, and unethical behaviors and this includes people working for health care companies.

- Hidden video cameras in hospitals reveal employees stealing computers, office supplies, syringes, medications, and patients' personal possessions.
- Job applicants falsify information on employment applications and overstate their education and work records.
- Countless numbers of fraudulent workers' compensation claims are filed each year.
- Employees bring weapons to work and arguments, fistfights, workplace violence, and **harassment** (any verbal or physical abuse of a person because of race, religion, age, gender, or disability) are becoming more commonplace.

This is one reason why health care employers increasingly run criminal history background checks, credit checks, and drug screens on job candidates before they start work. Employers are also placing more emphasis on the character of their employees to help reduce theft, absenteeism, dishonesty, workplace violence, substance abuse, safety infractions, **negligence** (failure to perform or give care in a reasonably careful and cautious manner), and low productivity. Increasingly, employers are hiring for character, praising for character, and promoting for character. Character reflects a person's **morals** and influences their **integrity** and **trustworthiness**, two key factors in professionalism.

- *Morals:* standards of behavior or belief based on differentiating between right and wrong
- *Integrity:* the quality of being honest and of sound moral principle

- *Trustworthiness:* the quality of deserving others' confidence in one's honesty, integrity, and reliability

How do personal values, reputation, morals, integrity, and trustworthiness apply to you as a person? How do they affect the way you approach your work? Do you know the difference between right and wrong? Are you honest? Can you be trusted? If you make a bad decision, can you overcome it and get back on track?

THE MORE YOU KNOW_____

PERSONAL VALUES AND ETHICAL CONDUCT

Recognition as a health care professional requires meeting your ethical responsibilities as well as your legal responsibilities. **Ethics** (standards of conduct and moral judgment) is a system of moral principles—the standard of *right* versus *wrong*. Knowing how to comply with laws is fairly straightforward. Laws appear in writing and, if you violate a law, you know what the penalties could involve. Living up to ethical responsibilities, on the other hand, is more challenging. Moral **conduct** (behavior or standard of behavior) is subject to interpretation, and not everyone is held to the same penalties for unethical behavior.

A person's perspective on right versus wrong is influenced by his or her family, friends, teachers, coworkers, religion, and society in general. If you associate with people who lie and cheat, at some point you may decide there's nothing wrong with lying and **cheating** (deceiving by trickery). If your supervisor gets personal gifts from a vendor in exchange for giving the vendor your organization's business, you may decide the practice is acceptable. If your mother uses someone else's membership card to qualify for a discount, you may think it is okay to be dishonest.

People are subjected to many different influences every day, from television and magazine advertisements, to political and religious perspectives. All of these messages can influence your morals and your sense of right and wrong. But when it comes down to behavior, ethical conduct is up to the individual. This is where professionalism plays such an important role.

Health care professionals meet high standards for ethical conduct. They reveal their character traits in everything that they say and do.

Character Traits

Character traits lead to a person's behavior, thoughts, and emotions. Here are a couple of examples:

- "Amiable" (good humored and friendly) versus "ill-natured" (unpleasant disposition)
  Would you like to work with an amiable person, one who is good humored, friendly, and able to establish positive relationships with patients and coworkers? Or would you rather work with a grumpy person who doesn't seem to like being around other people?
- "Ambitious" (strong desire to achieve) versus "shiftless" (lacking ambition and initiative)
  Would you prefer to have an ambitious coworker, one who strives to exceed expectations? Or would you prefer a shiftless coworker, one who fails to take initiative and doesn't seem to care?

If you were choosing a new team member, which of these character traits would you look for?

Depending on the reference, you can find lengthy lists of character traits. Here are several examples to consider, identifying both the positive and negative aspects of each type of trait. Think about each trait. Which of these describe you? How might each trait affect customer service, relationships, and **morale** (the general mood or spirit of a person or group) in the workplace?

CHARACTER TRAITS

Appreciative/Ungrateful
- Feeling or expressing gratitude
- Not thankful or appreciative

Caring/Callous
- Feeling of concern and interest
- Insensitive and emotionally hardened

Cheerful/Grumpy
- In good spirits
- Ill-tempered

Conscientious/Careless
- Taking extreme care and attention to details
- Lack of attention and forethought

Courteous/Impolite
- Polite, uses good manners
- Failure to demonstrate good manners

Dependable/Undependable
- Worthy of trust, can be counted on
- Unworthy of trust, cannot be counted on

Diligent/Neglectful
- Careful in one's work
- Failure to show care or attention

Generous/Selfish
- Willing to give and share with others
- Concerned with one's self to the detriment of others

Honest/Deceitful
- Marked by truth
- Deliberately false and fraudulent

Humble/Boastful
- Marked by modesty and a lack of arrogance
- Exhibiting self-importance

Honorable/Immoral
- Of sound moral principle; having integrity
- Failure to differentiate between right and wrong

(continued)

Loyal/Disloyal
- Faithful to people that one is under obligation to defend or support
- Deserting people that one is under obligation to defend or support

Reliable/Unreliable
- Can be counted upon, trustworthy
- Not worthy of reliance or trust

Respectful/Disrespectful
- Feeling or showing honor or esteem
- Failure to feel or show respect, rude and discourteous

Sincere/Hypocritical
- Open and genuine, not deceitful
- Pretending to be, or feel, something that is not real

Self-disciplined/Indulgent
- Ability to control one's impulses, avoids temptations
- Inability to control one's impulses, gives in to temptations

Tolerant/Intolerant
- Showing respect for the rights, opinions, and practices of others
- Narrow-minded, unwilling to show respect for the rights, opinions, and practices of others

Truthful/Untruthful
- Conforming to the truth, does not lie
- Intentionally lies and spreads false information

Reputation

No single factor is more important in being recognized as a professional than your reputation. How do people view *your* character, values, and behavior? As mentioned earlier, it takes a long time to develop a good reputation and only a split second to lose it. After years of being an honest, law-abiding individual, all it takes is one dishonest act or a single incident of unprofessional behavior to shake people's confidence in you and lose their trust. This is why professionals must work hard each and every day to do what's right and to maintain the trust and respect of others.

If a person has developed a pattern of behavior over the years based on lying, cheating, stealing, and taking advantage of other people, then changing those traits would be quite a challenge, but it's possible. Our sense of acceptable behavior starts at a very young age when our parents and other influential people teach us the difference between right and wrong. As children, we experiment with different kinds of behavior to see what reactions we get. If those who raised a child believed in guidance and discipline, that child probably soon learned the consequences of "doing something bad." As children, most of us were taught to get along with others, share our toys, wash our hands before we eat, and treat older people with respect. Unacceptable behavior may have resulted in "getting grounded" or losing privileges like playing with friends or watching television.

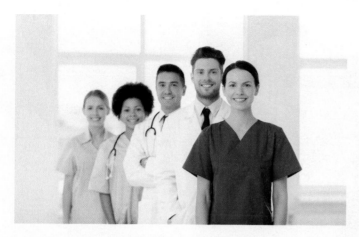

Figure 3-1 A team of health care professionals (*Syda Productions/Shutterstock*)

Over the years, we learned to make calls based on good **judgment** (ability to make considered decisions and choices and reach reasonable conclusions). We learned the concept of self-control and the importance of avoiding temptation. Through relationships with other people, we learned about fairness, respect, ethics, and **loyalty** (demonstrating allegiance to people that one is under obligation to defend or support). We learned to care, to give, and to appreciate. And before long, our character, values, and **priorities** (things having precedence in time, order, or importance) began to define who we are as people and how we conduct our lives.

HOT TOPICS

FROM PRESCRIPTION PAINKILLERS TO HEROIN

About 100 million Americans suffer chronic pain from broken bones, surgical procedures, chronic diseases such as arthritis and lupus, or other conditions. Such severe or long-term pain impacts the quality of life. In the past, people would take over-the-counter drugs such as aspirin or acetaminophen to help relieve their pain. Only patients dealing with terminal diseases such as cancer would be given heavy-duty **opioid** (a narcotic with an opium-like effect but not derived from opium) painkillers such as codeine or morphine. But by the late 1980s, researchers thought that patients might be suffering needlessly and that the risk of becoming dependent on opioids was very low for people with no history of addiction. Drug companies started testing and by 1994 new prescription drugs such as OxyContin, Vicodin, and Percocet were available on the market.

Over the next two decades, more than 20 new drugs were approved by the U.S. Food and Drug Administration (FDA) to help patients with pain. States passed laws supporting opioid drugs, making it easier for doctors to prescribe them more frequently. Caregivers assessed pain levels like vital signs such as body temperature and blood pressure. People began believing that opioids were safe and effective. By 2011, prescriptions for opioid drugs had tripled to more than 200 million per year.

By 2014, one study showed that up to 20% of the populations of some small rural towns in the South were taking the drugs for extended periods of time. Usage was spreading nationwide and the addiction rate was growing. After becoming resistant to the drugs due to long-term use, patients started taking higher

(*continued*)

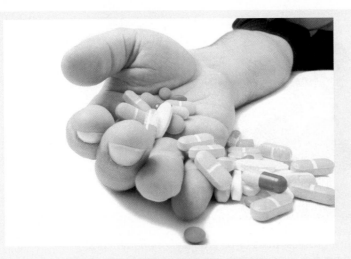

Figure 3-2 Overprescribed painkilling drugs (*Pop Paul-Catalin/Shutterstock*)

doses to get the same effect. By 2011, drug addiction had reached epidemic levels and 17,000 people per year were dying of prescription drug overdoses. Doctors backed off in prescribing the drugs for long-term use and some doctors stopped prescribing the drugs completely. Having been cut off, patients who were addicted then turned "to the street" to find the painkillers they needed. Patients began crushing the pills to snort or inject them and many people became heroin users. By 2014, 75% of heroin addicts said their drug use had started with prescription painkillers. Heroin is typically less expensive and easier to find than prescription narcotics. An OxyContin pill, for example, costs about $80 on the street. To get the same effect, people can buy heroin for just $10.

In years past, heroin addicts were associated with impoverished males living in urban areas. But by 2014, more than half of new heroin users were women, 90% were Caucasian, and the average age of users was less than 23 years. Reusing and sharing dirty needles from heroin injections has triggered another major public health emergency—the increasing rates of HIV and hepatitis C infections. A growing number of states and communities have begun approving needle-exchange programs to try to slow down the rising rates of these diseases.

Prescribing opioid drugs remains controversial. In 2015, the FDA approved a reformulated version of OxyContin for children as young as 11 years of age. Prescriptions are limited to short-term use for children who suffer pain from cancer, major surgery, or end-of-life medical conditions and who have no other options.

Judgment

As adults, we're faced with multiple decisions every day—what to do, why or why not to do it, how to do it, when to do it, where to do it, with whom to do it, and so on. Some of the decisions we have to make are small ones. But other decisions, especially those involving relationships with other people, require more thought and carry significant consequences—how to resolve a disagreement, when to say "no," and when to ask for help.

Several questions need to be considered when using judgment to make decisions:

- What are my choices?
- How do the options compare with one another?
- What might happen?

- Who might be affected?
- How would it make me feel?
- How would my decision be viewed by other people?

When the decisions you face involve your job, more questions arise:

- What would my supervisor think?
- How would my coworkers feel?
- How would this affect our patients?
- Could I lose my job?

PROFESSIONALISM ONLINE

YOUR REPUTATION ONLINE

Before the rise of digital communication and social media, people could expect some degree of separation between their personal lives and their professional lives. That's no longer the case because your personal life is no longer private. Anyone can Google you and find details about your past and present life. Grocery stores and online companies can track where you shop, what you purchase, and how much you spend. People can find and view your home online and in some cases, they can see pictures of the inside of your house. Your current location can be identified and monitored at any point in time without your knowledge. All of that happens without any action on your part. When you add social media, even more details of your personal life become evident. Some social media users tend to put everything out there for people to see details and photographs relating to their spouse, children, hobbies, sports, religion, political leanings, and thoughts and feelings. People send messages and post photos and videos of themselves while traveling and away from home. Like it or not, your personal life has become more public. Failure to limit access and protect the security of your personal information can lead to all sorts of problems including burglaries, stalking, bullying, harassment, physical attacks, identity theft, and computer hacking, to name a few.

Then there's your professional life and your professional reputation to consider. Now, no matter where you go, all it takes is one person with a cell phone to damage or ruin your reputation. Photos of you that you didn't even know were taken can be posted, altered, and shared without your knowledge or permission. Once they're public, there's not much you can do about it. If you have very private photos of yourself strictly meant for your spouse or boyfriend or girlfriend, for example, your device can be hacked and the photos shared with anyone and everyone.

Stop and think before you post anything on social media sites, and use good judgment. Protecting your reputation online is critical. If someone hasn't met you in person, their first impression of you will be based on what they see online. Don't post photographs, videos, comments, or other content that could lead a potential employer, or your current employer, to question your professionalism. Even if you intend to limit who can see the information, remember that nothing is totally private online. The audience who may receive, view, and share your content can grow instantaneously and without control. Speak with your family and friends to make sure they know that any content they post about you can affect your reputation at work. Ask them to never post anything about you without your permission. Someone may think that photos of you in an embarrassing situation are just humorous, without realizing that other people, such as your employer, might see things differently.

It's important to routinely monitor online material about yourself to find out what other people are seeing. If someone is posting negative or false information about you, it can be very difficult to have it changed or deleted. Due to free speech, people can voice their opinions openly. But if they're stating something as a fact rather than an opinion, and you can prove this caused you harm, you may have the basis for a defamation lawsuit. Remember—this also applies to things *you* say about other people. The best way to overcome negative online content is to make sure that more positive information gets posted.

Curriculum Knowledge Center (*continued*)
CEHHS
University of Michigan-Dearborn

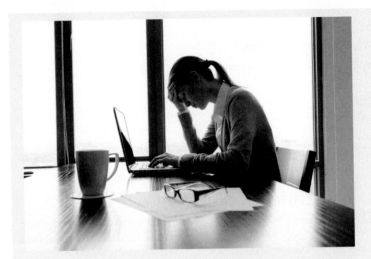

Figure 3-3 Discovering a violation of privacy online (*KieferPix/Shutterstock*)

In today's world, it's not unusual for patients to Google their doctors. And some of them might Google you, too. If you blog about patients or complain about them online without mentioning their names, they might find your content and identify themselves by what you've said about them. This could be considered a HIPAA violation. If you express negative comments about a patient, doctor, supervisor, or coworker and think that "free speech" will protect you, think again. The law protects people who can prove their reputation has been harmed by false information. For example, if you state, "Dr. Smith's incompetence lead to the death of three patients last month" you can probably expect a lawsuit. If you complain about your employer online and someone believes the comments are damaging to the company's reputation, you can be fired from your job.

Digital communication has created a host of identity concerns, making it easier for people to pretend to be someone else online. You would never want to do this yourself because it's unethical and, depending on the situation, it could also be illegal. Someone could impersonate you. They could use your name in a variety of embarrassing ways, or they could hack into your email and send messages from you to your list of contacts without your knowledge.

Here's the bottom line: Protect your reputation. Don't put yourself in a compromising situation online and do your best to prevent other people from doing so.

Conscience

Most people have a **conscience** (moral judgment that prohibits or opposes the violation of a previously recognized ethical principle). Your conscience is that little voice that gnaws away at you, keeps you from sleeping at night, and constantly says, "You *know* this *isn't* the right thing to do!" Your conscience can be quite reliable in reminding you of the difference between right and wrong. When you're facing some really difficult situations involving right versus wrong, more questions need to be answered:

- How would this look if it appeared in the newspaper?
- How would my children feel?

- Would my family support me?
- Could I look myself in the mirror?
- Would I be able to sleep at night?

The problem is that some people either have no conscience or have learned to ignore their conscience. It starts with something minor, like telling a little lie or stealing something small. And then it grows and grows until it becomes a way of life. Eventually dishonest and unethical behavior will become obvious, but in the meantime countless people including yourself could be affected.

The good news is that the majority of Americans are honest, law-abiding people with good character and sound moral values who sincerely want to do what's right in their lives.

- They face temptations but summon up the courage to say, "No!"
- They avoid engaging in dishonest behavior just because "everyone else does."
- When they become angry with someone, they forgive and move on.
- They look out for themselves but treat other people with fairness and respect.
- They exercise good judgment and make the right decisions for the right reasons.

In the health care workplace, personal traits such as character, values, morals, ethics, integrity, and trustworthiness are absolutely vital. If you were sick or injured, what kind of people would you want caring for you? If you owned a health care business, what kind of people would you want working for you?

RECENT DEVELOPMENTS

MISDIAGNOSING FOR PROFIT

A Michigan doctor was sentenced to 45 years in prison for misdiagnosing and treating patients for cancer who, in reality, were cancer-free. The hematologist oncologist who was "world renowned" according to his webpage, pleaded guilty to telling patients they had terminal cancer, giving them medically unnecessary infusions or injections, and then collecting more than $16 million in payments from Medicare and private insurance companies for the "care" he provided.

More than 550 patients were involved. People were subjected to years of painful chemotherapy and other treatments they didn't need, and some had organs surgically removed for no reason. Some of the doctor's patients did have cancer, but were intentionally misdiagnosed and given the wrong treatment. Many of the doctor's patients will have to live the rest of their lives dealing with the aftermath. One patient reported he had lost all of his teeth and his jaw changed its shape. Another man said he was grossly overtreated and found out he had a testicle removed for no reason. A woman said her husband had been "tortured" until his final breath. Another patient was still undergoing unnecessary and expensive blood plasma treatments when she saw her doctor on television being arrested.

Another doctor, a neurologist in Florida, was investigated for misdiagnosing his patients with multiple sclerosis (MS) in order to bill for treatments they didn't need. Concerns about the doctor's practice came to light after he was put on administrative leave following an affair with one of his patients. As hospital officials scheduled his patients for reevaluation, they investigated his records and found that he had misdiagnosed MS 65% of the time and made errors in diagnosing 90% of other neurological conditions. The doctor wrote more prescriptions (each costing $25,000) for a gel to treat MS than any other area neurologist and racked up consulting fees from the pharmaceutical companies that produced some of the expensive drugs he was prescribing.

(continued)

Having been diagnosed with an incurable disease that can lead to brain malfunction and paralysis, some of the doctor's patients made life-changing decisions. One woman quit her job and spent $50,000 to make her home wheelchair accessible. Another suffered welts all over her body and a burning in her throat as a result of the $5,000/month injections she was given needlessly. Another woman had her breast implants removed because she thought they were negatively impacting her health. Some patients, determined to spare their families the expense and difficulty of a painful death, were planning their suicides. After the doctor diagnosed his patients with MS, some just by looking in their eyes, he gave them Botox, steroid treatments, and spinal taps in order to bill for services rendered.

Trust

Part of developing a professional reputation is convincing people that they can trust you and the quality of the decisions you make. In today's society, we've become increasingly suspicious of other people. "Don't trust anyone!" is common advice. Unfortunately, that perspective gets reinforced each time we set ourselves up to believe in someone or depend on someone, only to end up disappointed or let down. The previous chapter discussed the importance of reliability and following through when someone is counting on you. When your word is "as good as gold," your supervisor and coworkers know they can trust you to keep your promises and meet your obligations.

- If you promised to give a coworker a ride to work, don't forget to pick him up.
- If you received training on a new procedure and your supervisor trusts you to perform it properly, make sure you apply what you learned.
- If you tell a patient you'll relay a message to her nurse, follow through.

If you want people to view you as a professional, make sure you can be trusted.

Honesty

Earning respect relies greatly on being viewed as an honest person. As mentioned earlier, dishonesty has become highly visible in the health care workplace. The cost of health care is high enough without employers having to pay for extra supplies, food, and equipment stolen by its employees. Most health care workers would deny that they steal from their employers or patients. But theft goes well beyond stealing a computer or a patient's wallet. Here are some examples of theft that you might not think of:

- Manipulating your time report to get paid for more hours than you worked
- Sleeping on the job, taking unauthorized breaks, or leaving your work area without permission
- Taking food off of a dietary cart delivered for someone else's lunch meeting
- Taking supplies off of a patient's bedside table to use at home

Anytime you take *anything* that doesn't belong to you without proper authorization, it can be construed as theft. Is a free sandwich or box of cotton swabs worth losing your job? What about an extra hour of pay that you didn't really deserve? This is where both honesty and good judgment enter the picture. Even if taking something that doesn't belong to you appears harmless, what might be the consequences?

BY THE NUMBERS

MEDICARE SCAMS AND FRAUD

There's so much money involved in Medicare that some people just can't avoid the temptation to try to take some of it for themselves. Estimates suggest that between 10 and 30% of Medicare's annual expenditures can be traced to scams and fraud, adding up to at least $60 billion per year. The culprits are often dishonest doctors working with scammers in pharmaceutical and medical supply companies. The doctors prescribe the drugs, products, or services and make the referrals. The companies bill Medicare, make lots of money, and everyone involved shares the profits. When scammers are uncovered in one part of the country, they move their operations to another locale. According to some fraud-detecting experts, the only people more creative than Medicare scammers are computer hackers.

Here are just a few examples:

- A state-of-the art, high-tech arthritis kit promises to relieve chronic joint pain at a cost to Medicare of $3,000 each. The kit actually contains Velcro braces and ankle and knee wraps.
- Doctors prescribe a topical pain-reducing cream to Medicare patients at a cost of $260 per tube. The cream isn't really needed and a cheaper product may be substituted for the real thing.
- People are pressured to sign up for professional home health services, which are then billed to Medicare. Patients actually receive low-end care or no services at all.
- Phony mental health centers provide fake psychological counseling services and collaborate with ambulance companies to provide unnecessary rides to the appointments, all of which are billed to Medicare.
- Pharmacists fill phony prescriptions and bill Medicare for expensive drugs that were never dispensed.
- Doctors order expensive diagnostic tests that patients don't need and Medicare covers the expense.
- Podiatrists perform toenail clippings and bill Medicare for the more expensive toenail removals.
- Physical therapists bill Medicare for expensive therapeutic treatments and give patients little more than backrubs.
- Medical supply companies bill Medicare for high-end, motorized wheelchairs and then deliver less expensive, nonmotorized models as substitutes.

Bribery is also a problem. In a recent scheme in New Jersey, 24 doctors and 37 people in total pleaded guilty to receiving more than $100 million in payments from Medicare and private insurance companies for accepting cash bribes for referring patients to a certain laboratory for blood tests. The lab received more than $400,000 in extra business due to the referrals.

When employees spend time on the clock doing something other than assigned job duties, they aren't just wasting time, they're stealing from their company by collecting pay for nonproductive time. Examples include texting friends, visiting social networking sites, accessing pornographic websites, gambling, checking sports scores, shopping online, and using company computers for other inappropriate activities. Employees may also be caught sleeping, watching television, and engaging in sexual activity while on the job.

Lying and cheating are two more dishonest behaviors that can get you in big trouble. Little, seemingly harmless "white lies" usually snowball into big, complicated lies that can become difficult to manage. Lies are eventually uncovered and, before long, people will wonder if they can believe *anything* you say. Being truthful is always the best approach.

Cheating is an example of dishonest behavior that results from giving in to temptation. Maybe you have to pass a written test to prove your competency for a job promotion but didn't have time to prepare. Dozens of people will be taking the test at the same time and no one would notice if you sneaked some notes into the room with you. After all, you could actually learn the material later on, after passing the test. If your supervisor finds out that you've cheated on the test, you'll be in big trouble. Forget the job promotion because your main concern will be keeping the job you've got. If you think your coworkers who are competing for the same job promotion will stand by quietly and let you get away with cheating on the test, think again. They prepared for the test and you didn't. If you get the job promotion as a result of cheating, your lack of competence may quickly become obvious and other people may suffer. Your professional reputation will be seriously damaged, perhaps beyond repair. Can you cheat just a little and get away with it? Ask your conscience.

A serious example of dishonest behavior is falsifying information, also known as fraud. As mentioned in the previous chapter, fraud is not only dishonest, it's illegal. A few examples of fraud include:

- Misrepresenting your education, credentials, or work experience on a job application, **résumé** (document summarizing one's qualifications for a job), or other document
- Billing an insurance company for a patient procedure that never occurred
- Back-dating a legal document, entering incorrect data on equipment maintenance records, or changing the results of a research study

As with stealing and cheating, there may be more to fraud than you realize. Fraud includes:

- Signing someone else's name without his or her permission
- Turning in a time card that you know is inaccurate
- Telling your supervisor that you passed a competency assessment when you really didn't

Since fraud is illegal, a fraud conviction cannot only cost you your job, it can also cost you your freedom.

CASE STUDY

Before Carla met with the employee who had viewed her husband's medical records without authorization to check for a history of STDs, she reviewed the employee's work record thus far. The clerical worker had been on the job for just six weeks and had already been warned three times about excessive use of her cell phone during working hours. She would disappear several times during her shift and, when located, was usually found text messaging on her phone. An MA had reported that two patients had been kept waiting at check-in while the employee fiddled with her phone, and a doctor complained that her patients weren't ready to be seen in a reasonable amount of time due to clerical delays. Carla checked attendance records and noticed that the employee had already called in sick two days and was tardy twice during her first six

weeks of employment. It was clear to Carla that the clerical worker wasn't taking her job seriously. She had already developed a poor attendance record and evidently cared more about texting her friends than performing her duties. Then there was the inexcusable violation of her husband's medical records. According to network policies, new employees are on probation for the first six months and can be readily fired for poor performance.

Carla met with the employee and discussed her performance issues including the most recent incident. The clerical worker said she knew she shouldn't have looked at her husband's records but needed to know if he had a transmittable disease. She expressed regret in having created the situation and said it would never happen again. But based on her poor judgment and other performance issues,

Carla decided the employee was not a good fit for the practice and terminated her employment. At the next in-service session, the entire staff was reminded about cell phone use, attendance policies, and the potential for HIPAA violations.

Firing people was the least favorite part of Carla's job as a supervisor. She wondered why people failed to use common sense when performing their jobs. She remembered someone saying, "There's nothing common about common sense" and believed it. Hopefully the clerical worker had learned a valuable lesson and would do better in her next job. The woman was still young and had her whole career in front of her. But there was no way she would get a positive employment reference from Carla's practice when she applied for her next job.

As Carla was thinking about her staff and the situations she had to deal with, a major scandal broke out in a nearby town. According to the news, a well-known doctor who ran a pain management clinic was under investigation for overprescribing prescription painkillers. Several of his patients had become addicted to the narcotics. When they could no longer obtain the prescriptions they needed, they turned to buying illegal painkillers on the street or, worse yet, using heroin as the alternative. Carla had heard about the rise in HIV and hepatitis C cases and knew that many had been traced back to people sharing needles after injecting drugs. The doctor's negligence came to light after three of his patients died of drug overdoses. Carla was shocked that something like this could be going on so close to home. Her concern escalated even more when the phone rang and she and her manager were asked to meet with an attorney in the network's risk management department. Evidently one of the practice's nurses had been a patient in the doctor's pain clinic and could possibly become implicated in the scandal. If the nurse was found guilty of taking illegal prescription drugs or using heroin she would likely be fired and lose her license. This was Carla's first really serious legal issue.

What should Carla do to prepare for her meeting with risk management? What would you do if you were in Carla's place?

Ethics

Another personal trait that factors into your reputation as a professional is ethics—standards of conduct and moral judgment. Would you:

- Inform your company's cafeteria cashier that she gave you too much change?
- Look in a confidential file that lists your supervisor's salary?
- Sign out for a friend who wants to leave work early?

If it seems like unethical behaviors overlap with lying, cheating, stealing, and other dishonest acts discussed earlier in this chapter, your observations are correct. It's hard to separate one type of unprofessional behavior from another. Consider the following:

- Failing to return extra change in the company cafeteria isn't just unethical, it's theft.
- Looking in a confidential file isn't just unethical, it's a breach of confidentiality.
- Signing out for a friend isn't just unethical, it's fraud.

The point is that every decision you make and every action you take can have a huge impact. One bad judgment call can erode someone's trust in you. One unethical decision can destroy your reputation. One illegal act can cause you to be fired from your job—or worse.

If you find yourself in a difficult situation weighing one option against another, and you're not quite sure which course of action to pursue, consider the following questions:

- Is it honest?
- Is it ethical?

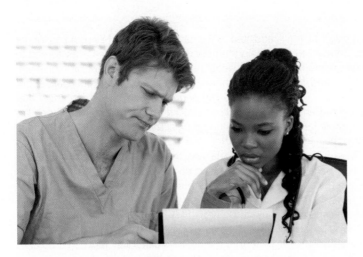

Figure 3-4 Considering a difficult ethical issue (*Wavebreakmedia/Shutterstock*)

- Does it reflect good character?
- Is it based on sound moral values?
- How would it affect my reputation?
- Would it damage the trust others have in me?
- What impact would my actions have on others?
- Would I be respected for my decision?
- What does my conscience tell me to do?
- What would a professional do?

CONSIDER THIS

FREE SHOES AND FRAUD

Eight companies, nine doctors, and 14 other health care workers in New York City (including nurse practitioners, cardiologists, pain management specialists, podiatrists, psychiatrists, physician assistants, office staff, managers, and a surgeon) were charged with submitting almost $7 million worth of Medicare and Medicaid fraudulent claims between 2012 and 2014. Poor people who could produce a Medicaid card were recruited from area homeless shelters and welfare offices and promised a free pair of sneakers in exchange for agreeing to unnecessary medical tests and medical equipment.

    Participants were subjected to physical therapy, cardiograms, vascular tests, and pain management evaluations so the health care companies and providers could submit medical bills and receive reimbursement for the participants' procedures. One of the female victims reported her concerns to authorities when she was taken to a clinic to be seen by a podiatrist and then given a knee brace that she didn't need along with her new free shoes. The two primary defendants in the case who orchestrated the corruption owned a durable medical equipment company.

Legal Issues and Implications

Criminal and Civil Law

As a health care worker, you have a legal responsibility to provide excellent care. Understanding legal responsibilities ensures a safe work environment, prevents lawsuits, and protects patients, workers, and health care facilities. Policies are in place to ensure that everyone practices and monitors sound legal behavior. A failure to provide the best care can result in lawsuits. Lawsuits are determined by the legal system based on the facts of the case. Avoiding illegal and unethical behavior promotes good patient care and helps avoid legal trouble.

Health care workers must perform to the best of their abilities or risk legal repercussions. These repercussions can fall under criminal or civil law.

- *Criminal law* is the type of law involved in punishing people for committing crimes against the state. Crimes against the state include many types of infractions of the law, such as stealing controlled substances from the hospital or stealing a patient's belongings.
- *Civil law* covers **torts**—wrongful acts that result in physical injury, property damages, or damages to a person's reputation for which the injured person is entitled to compensation. Tort law usually provides people with rights to compensation for the damages done. Torts may be categorized in two ways: intentional torts and unintentional (negligent) torts.

As a health care worker, you need to understand the law as it applies to medical negligence. Medical **malpractice** (failure to meet the standard of care or conduct prescribed by a profession), one type of tort, can result from any mistake in medical treatment. An example of malpractice would be when a health care worker mislabels a tissue sample and the patient has a breast removed via surgery based on a misdiagnosis of breast cancer.

Professional Standards of Care, Scope of Practice, and Professional Ethics

"Professional **standards of care**" (care that would be expected to be given to a patient by a similarly trained person under similar circumstances) are established on the basis of the standard that would be used by a reasonably **prudent** (careful and cautious) professional in that line of work. Professional standards of care are specific to professions. For example, a medical assistant is not held to the same standard of care as a doctor. Health care workers must always remember, however, that their actions have legal consequences. To that end, there are laws that authorize the scope of practice—or scope of care—under which health care workers function. For example, there are tasks that are within the scope of practice for a registered nurse, such as administering medications, and there are tasks that are *not* with the registered nurse's scope of practice, such as prescribing medications.

Each health care profession also has a **code of ethics** (standards by which a group decides the difference between right and wrong; behavioral expectations for people who practice in a given profession). Health care workers must not only display appropriate personal ethics as discussed earlier in this chapter, they must also be aware of and comply with the professional ethics established by their professional organizations.

In emergency situations, health care professionals have legal responsibilities. The first responsibility is a **duty to act** (the obligation to care for a patient who requires it) within the scope of practice for your profession. In an emergency, health care workers are accountable to themselves, their employers, and the public for actions that are in keeping with their health care training. The second responsibility is to stay constantly ready for emergencies by complying with your

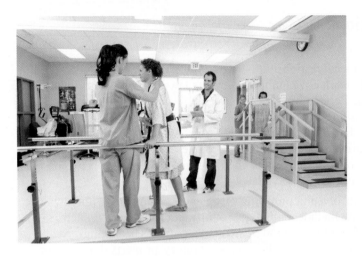

Figure 3-5 Working within a professional scope of practice (*Tyler Olson/Shutterstock*)

employer's policies and staying current with procedures and equipment. Everyone who works in a health care setting must do everything possible to prevent emergencies.

Medical Liability

As a health care worker, you are obliged to do everything you can to offer high-quality care and take steps to reduce errors. If you do anything less than provide the best quality care, you may have committed medical malpractice. Malpractice means *bad practice*—care that leads to faulty practice or neglect. Malpractice is a commonly heard term, but actually refers to one type of unintentional tort. For example, suppose a patient falls on a nail and the doctor does not order a tetanus shot or check to see when the patient last had one. Then, the patient develops tetanus or lockjaw. The failure to order a tetanus shot, or to check when the patient last had one, would be considered malpractice. The doctor could be held **liable** (legally responsible) for his or her actions. Be sure to check with your employer to find out whether or not you should purchase personal liability insurance.

Medical malpractice is a legal term. The legal system examines the facts of each case and determines whether or not the health care professional is guilty of malpractice. The specific facts are very important. Two very similar cases can be decided differently because of one small, but significant, difference.

What kinds of errors lead to medical malpractice lawsuits? Here are some examples:

- Medical errors and mistakes. Any serious error or mistake by a caregiver may result in a lawsuit.
- Inaccurate diagnosis. If a medical professional makes a mistake in diagnosing a patient's condition, that mistake may result in a lawsuit.
- Failure to diagnose a condition. If a medical professional fails to diagnose a patient's condition, that mistake may result in a lawsuit.
- Lack of informed consent. If a medical professional does not properly explain to a patient his or her treatment or the likely results of that treatment, that mistake may result in a lawsuit.

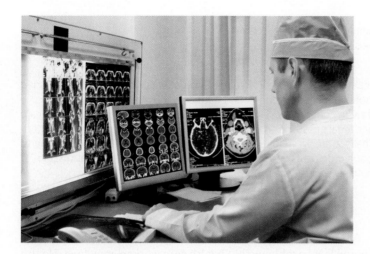

Figure 3-6 Double-checking to ensure a correct diagnosis (*Beerkoff/Shutterstock*)

- Mistakes during surgery. Any mistake during surgery may result in a lawsuit.
- Medical instruments left inside patients during surgery. If any instruments or equipment used during surgery remain inside a patient after the surgery is completed, that mistake may result in a lawsuit.

Just because a mistake was made and a lawsuit was filed, the professional who made the mistake has not necessarily committed medical malpractice. All the facts are presented to the legal system, and the decision is made there. Avoiding these mistakes in the first place, of course, ensures good care and helps avoid legal problems.

TRENDS AND ISSUES

IS THIS PROCEDURE REALLY NECESSARY?

Several groups of physicians are recommending ways to reduce wasteful spending without harming patients. This involves curtailing the use of certain medical tests and treatments that the physicians believe are overused, don't benefit patients, and are ordered largely to prevent possible lawsuits. If adopted, this approach would also help protect patients since some of the medical procedures involve risks and exposure to radiation. According to the doctors, reducing unnecessary expense would make more resources available for procedures that truly benefit patients. This movement aligns with current efforts to reform the health care industry and health insurance in order to cover more patients and provide better care. Instead of rewarding doctors for the volume of services they provide, the plan is to base payments on positive results and more highly coordinated care.

The doctors recommend no longer automatically ordering the following procedures:

- Repeat colonoscopies within 10 years of the first test
- Early imaging for most back pain

(*continued*)

- Brain scans for patients who fainted but didn't have seizures
- Antibiotics for mild to moderate sinus distress
- Cardiac stress tests for patients without coronary symptoms

They also suggest that cancer doctors stop treating tumors in end-stage patients who have not responded to multiple therapies and who are not eligible for experimental treatments.

These discussions, which are likely to continue as stakeholders search for ways to provide better care at lower costs, raise several ethical and legal questions. What could happen when some doctors decide not to order tests and treatments they believe are wasteful and unnecessary while other doctors continue to use these interventions? Should doctors order tests and treatments primarily to avoid potential lawsuits? If so, should health insurance plans routinely cover these procedures without question?

Other Legal Issues

Medical malpractice is just one of many legal problems that health care workers may face. Health care workers need to be aware of the whole range of possible medical-legal problems that can affect them. The following terms explain some of the other ways in which a health care worker can have a legal problem under criminal or civil law.

Criminal Law Terms

- **Assault** is a threat or an attempt to injure another person. *Example*: A health care worker threatens to hit a patient or coworker.
- **Battery** is the unlawful touching of another person without his or her consent, with or without an injury. Assault and battery are often charged together because of the successful attempt to injure. Both assault and battery are violations of criminal law, but they may also be subject to a civil lawsuit filed by a patient to recoup damages. *Example*: A health care worker hits a patient or coworker, or a doctor operates on a patient without obtaining a signed consent form.

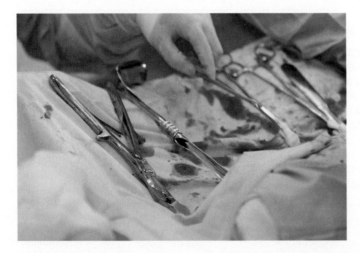

Figure 3-7 Counting surgical instruments to make sure none were left inside the patient (*Vz maze/Shutterstock*)

- **Felony** is a serious criminal offense that carries a penalty of imprisonment for more than one year and possibly the death penalty. *Example*: A health care worker withholds treatment for a terminally ill patient, which causes the patient's premature death.
- **Harassment** is any verbal or physical abuse of a person because of race, religion, age, gender, or disability. Any conduct that creates significant anguish for another person is harassment. Both state and federal criminal laws apply to harassment, but a civil lawsuit for harassment may also be filed. *Example:* A health care worker makes a joke about the religion of a patient.

Civil Law Terms

- **Libel** is a written false statement that damages a person's good reputation. Libel is a violation that pertains to civil law. *Example*: A newspaper writes damaging information about a local surgeon. The information is false and the paper is charged with libel. What you write in a patient record could be libel if you make a statement such as, "Mr. Smith is hoarding painkillers," when in reality Mr. Smith is only requesting, and taking, the medication that has been prescribed.
- **Slander** is a spoken statement of false charges that damages another person's good reputation. Slander is also a violation pertaining to civil law. *Example*: A health care worker tells friends that a famous person was treated for a drug overdose when in fact he or she was treated for a serious medical problem.
- **False imprisonment** is a civil tort in which a person is held or retained against his or her will. *Example*: A doctor or a health care worker refuses to allow a patient to leave the hospital.
- **Invasion of privacy** is a civil tort that unlawfully makes public knowledge of any private or personal information without the consent of the wronged person. *Example*: A health care worker gives personal information to a newspaper about a patient or coworker, or a health care worker leaves the door open while bathing a patient.
- **Reportable conditions** are situations where health care workers are required to file a confidential report to the county health department when they suspect child or adult **abuse** (improper, cruel, or violent treatment) or when certain diseases are diagnosed. Abuse is an intentional tort. There are three types of abuse: physical, verbal, and sexual. Reportable diseases include measles, tuberculosis, whooping cough, and other diagnoses that are important to public health. It's important to check your facility's policy and procedures manuals for a current listing of reportable diseases and the procedure for reporting abuse. *Example:* A child is at the doctor for a checkup and the doctor sees bruises and burns and suspects child abuse. Or, a health care worker intentionally pinches an older adult in a nursing home.
- **Negligence** is the failure to perform in a reasonably prudent manner. The legal definition of negligence can offer more clarification of this unintentional tort: Negligence occurs when a person "does not do what a reasonable and careful person would do, or does what a reasonable and careful person would not do." *Example*: A health care worker forgets to lock the brakes on a wheelchair, and the patient is injured.
- **Reasonable care** (use of the degree of caution and concern while providing care that a prudent and rational person would use in similar circumstances) is a legal requirement of health care workers. They must perform according to the standards of practice expected in their community for comparable workers. *Example*: Drawing blood takes training and skill. If a laboratory aide draws blood from a patient after watching the procedure several times but without proper training in the procedure, then reasonable care was not exercised.
- Sexual harassment is defined by federal regulations as "unwelcome sexual advances, requests for sexual favors, and other verbal and physical contact of a sexual nature." Innocent remarks, inappropriate pictures, and written material can be perceived as sexual. You can

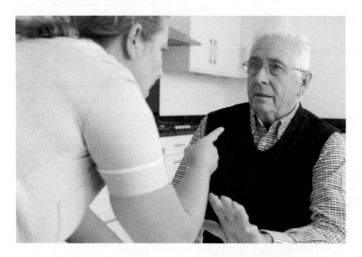

Figure 3-8 Verbally abusing an older patient (*SpeedKingz/Shutterstock*)

guard against harassment accusations by not making personal remarks or sexual gestures and by not participating in sexually explicit discussions around coworkers. *Example:* A coworker gets really close and frequently touches another person when talking. The closeness and physical touch could be interpreted as sexual harassment, even if it is innocent.

These definitions and examples provide the knowledge you need to help avoid medical-legal problems.

When you violate a policy, regulation, or law, you put yourself and your employer in legal jeopardy. Health care employers have enormous expenses to cover and they react very quickly when the illegal behavior of an employee results in extra legal fees, fines, or penalties. You can be one of the best-educated, most highly skilled professionals in your organization, but if you fail to meet your legal responsibilities, you won't have a job for long.

Violating patient confidentiality, divulging private business information, abusing a patient, or slandering a doctor or coworker is a sure way to get fired. Stealing from a patient, assaulting a coworker, or performing a procedure outside your scope of practice are examples of **gross misconduct** (unacceptable behavior of a serious nature often leading to dismissal from a job). Your employer may be sued and banned from participating in certain programs, and you may end up in jail.

Then there are the patients, the people who put their trust in you and your facility during some of the most vulnerable times in their lives. They're counting on their caregivers to put the needs of their patients first. The last thing a patient needs is a health care worker who makes mistakes and errors, abuses other people, or fails to live up to their legal obligations.

Policies, regulations, and laws are put into place to protect patients, employees, and health care employers. Every health care worker, regardless of job title or specific occupation, has the responsibility to comply with these rules. You also have a responsibility to report illegal activity if you are aware of it or suspect it. Check with your supervisor or a legal representative to make sure you follow the appropriate **protocol** (a prescribed policy or procedure) for dealing with a **reportable incident** (any event that can have an adverse effect on the health, safety, or welfare of people in the facility or organization).

THINK ABOUT IT_____

DOCTORS WHO CARE

So much of what is written today about health care fraud, scams, bribery, and other criminal behavior is depressing, disgusting, and heart-wrenching. You don't have to look far to find information about doctors who:

- Lie to patients, telling them they have a serious or terminal disease when they really don't
- Accept cash bribes for referring their business to certain companies
- Write phony prescriptions and submit fake Medicare bills
- Order expensive medical tests and treatments that patients don't need and shouldn't have

So much negative publicity might lead you to think that most doctors are greedy and unscrupulous. But nothing could be further from the truth. The vast majority of doctors are compassionate, honest, law-abiding people who strive to provide the best care possible for their patients. They study for years to become licensed physicians and may go deep into debt to pay for their education. They work long hours and make personal sacrifices to achieve their goals. The vast majority of doctors don't go into medicine to become wealthy by taking advantage of people and government programs. They choose a career in medicine because they have a calling to serve others, and a sincere desire to help relieve pain and suffering. You can find dishonest, **callous** (insensitive and emotionally hardened) people in every profession. But when doctors and health care workers get arrested, it makes front-page news.

Doctors, nurses, and other caregivers volunteer thousands of hours every year, sometimes at their own personal risk, to care for sick and injured people who would otherwise go untreated. They care for people in underserved areas of the United States and travel all over the world, serving in underdeveloped nations suffering from life-threatening crises such as natural disasters, wars, and disease epidemics.

Doctors Without Borders (Médecins Sans Frontières, or MSF) is a good example. For 40 years, MSF has been seeking out people who need medical care but wouldn't get it without their help. They've served millions of people in over 60 countries around the world where quality health care is lacking. The places where they work are often hard to get to and have limited resources such as electricity and safe drinking water. Some of the countries are war-torn, posing security and personal safety concerns. Even under the most severe and difficult conditions, MSF doctors strive to deliver the best medical care possible.

Here are just a few examples. MSF:

- Establishes hospitals in war-ravaged Syria to care for Sudanese refugees
- Operates a burn unit in a hospital in Port-au-Prince, Haiti
- Provides maternity services in Sierra Leone and Burundi
- Expands access to medical care for HIV/AIDS patients and for people infected with tuberculosis

In addition to directly caring for patients, MSF advocates for changes in policies and procedures that would benefit even more people, and they lobby for more funding to tackle global health problems. MSF was on the front lines of the recent Ebola epidemic in West Africa. They received about $93 million in private donations and $20 million in public funds in 2014 alone from people and organizations throughout the world. By the end of the year, they had spent about $80 million of those funds in Liberia, Sierra Leone, and Guinea, the three most highly affected countries.

Doctors Without Borders is just one example of doctors and other health care providers who go well beyond the call of duty in caring for people who need it the most.

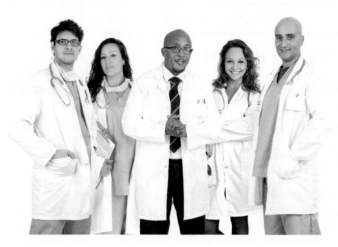

Figure 3-9 Doctors who care (*Luis Louro/Shutterstock*)

Ethical, Moral, and Legal Dilemmas

The information presented so far in this chapter relates to who you are as a person, how your character traits and values affect your work and your reputation as a professional, and what you need to know and do to avoid legal problems. People who work in the health care industry, as well as other stakeholders, also face a multitude of complex ethical, moral, and legal dilemmas that stretch well beyond how just one person thinks or behaves. Depending on the profession you have chosen, you may become directly involved in some of these issues yourself.

Here are some examples of the difficult and controversial questions that people are grappling with:

- *Abortion:* Should abortion remain legal? Should an abortion to save the mother's life or in cases of rape be legal? Should late-term abortions be legal? Should tax dollars be used to pay for abortions?
- *Genetic testing:* When prenatal genetic testing uncovers serious medical problems, is aborting the fetus acceptable?
- *Embryonic stem cell research:* Should embryonic stem cells be used for medical research when considering that the embryos must be destroyed as part of the process?
- *Rationing:* Should health care be rationed to reduce costs and reserve limited resources for those patients who would benefit the most?
- *Cloning:* Should scientists be permitted to **clone** (a group of cells that is genetically identical to the unit from which it was derived) human beings to produce organs for use in transplants and other medical procedures?
- *Medical marijuana:* Should patients who could benefit from using marijuana to reduce pain and the symptoms of chronic diseases be permitted to use the drug in states where marijuana is illegal?
- *End-of-life care:* Should life-sustaining treatments such as feeding tubes or ventilators be withdrawn to facilitate the death of terminally ill patients?
- *Euthanasia:* Is assisting someone with suicide ever justifiable and, if so, under what conditions?

- *Organ transplants:* When several patients are awaiting an organ for transplantation, which patients should get priority? Should age be a factor? Should an older patient who abuses alcohol about to die from liver disease be eligible for a transplant?
- *Refusing treatment:* Should parents be allowed to refuse treatment for a sick child based on their religious beliefs?

These are just a few of the complex ethical, moral, and legal issues associated with health care. How might you, your patients, or your employer become directly involved in some of these controversial issues? Based on your own personal values, morals, and ethics, how would you answer these questions? What would you say to someone whose opinions are different from yours? Is it possible to decide who is right and who is wrong?

As a health care worker, you may have strong personal opinions about some, or all, of these issues. You might be called upon to participate in patient procedures that you find to be **inconsistent** (at variance with one's principles; not staying the same throughout) with your personal values, morals, and beliefs. When choosing the right health career for you, it's important to think about these issues ahead of time. If you don't want to participate in abortions or sex-change operations, for example, no one will force you to compromise your principles. But you need to make your **moral convictions** (strong and absolute beliefs about what is right or wrong) known so that patient care won't be interrupted.

Having taken a closer look at your personal traits and how they affect your behavior, attitudes, and opinions, let's move on to examine what it takes to form and maintain effective interpersonal relationships at work.

REALITY CHECK

This chapter could provide a lot more examples of how your character and personal values affect who you are as a person and how you perform at work. But you already know what kind of person you are and you know the difference between right and wrong. You also know what's expected of health care professionals when it comes to ethics, honesty, morals, and legal requirements. You can either choose to live up to those high standards or you can try to slide by with less. No one can make that decision for you. If you've made some poor decisions in the past and failed to live up to professional standards, it's time to make some changes and get your life on track.

For More Information

Medical Ethics
The American Academy of Medical Ethics
www.ethicalhealthcare.org

Medicare Fraud and Abuse
www.medicare.gov/fraudabuse
Office of the Inspector General
U.S. Department of Health and Human Services
http://oig.hhs.gov/fraud/report-fraud/index.asp

Health Care Laws and Regulations
U.S. Department of Health and Human Services
www.hhs.gov/regulations/

Doctors Without Borders
www.doctorswithoutborders.org

KEY POINTS

- Keep in mind that it takes a long time to develop a professional reputation but only a split second to lose it.
- Review the list of positive character traits and decide which ones you need to improve upon.
- Use good judgment in making decisions.
- Listen to your conscience and avoid temptations to do the wrong thing.
- Make sure that your word is "as good as gold" and follow through on your commitments.
- Don't take anything that doesn't belong to you without proper authorization.
- Don't lie, cheat, steal, commit fraud, or engage in any other illegal or unethical acts.
- Be aware of the laws, standards of care, code of ethics, and the scope of practice that relate to your profession and abide by them.
- Report any concerns about improper patient care or illegal activity to the appropriate authorities.
- Keep up to date with the ethical, moral, and legal dilemmas that might affect your patients, your employer, and your work.
- Protect your professional reputation by stopping and thinking before posting information and photographs online.

LEARNING ACTIVITIES

Using information from Chapter Three:
- Answer the Chapter Review Questions
- Respond to the What If? Scenarios

Chapter Review Questions

Using information from Chapter Three, answer each of the following questions:
1. Describe how your character affects your reputation as a professional.

2. List four examples of the lack of character in the workplace.

3. Explain how your character traits and personal values affect your behavior and attitude.

4. Give three examples of dishonest behaviors.

5. Define *ethics*.

6. List three important questions to ask yourself when making difficult ethical decisions.

7. Define *morals*.

8. Explain the importance of protecting your professional reputation on social media sites.

9. Give three examples of fraud in health care.

10. Name and define two examples of criminal law terms.

11. Name and define two examples of civil law terms.

12. Explain why it's important to comply with the code of ethics for your profession.

13. Differentiate between personal ethics and professional ethics.

14. Explain the connection between negligence and malpractice.

15. Describe why some types of health care workers need personal liability insurance.

16. Explain why it's important to follow protocol if you suspect a reportable incident.

17. List three examples of complex ethical, moral, and legal dilemmas in health care.

What If? Scenarios

Think about what you would do in the following situations and record your answers.

1. You witness a coworker taking money from the petty cash box in your department. She says she needs to borrow the money to get her car fixed and she'll pay it back when she gets her next paycheck. She reminds you that she did you a big favor when you first started your job and asks that you not report her to the supervisor.

2. You have one more paper to turn in for a course you're taking that's required for your job. You keep the weekend open to write it, but a dear friend calls and says he'll be in town for the weekend and would like to spend it with you. You have a copy of a paper that someone else wrote for the class two years ago that earned a grade of B. The instructor is new and would never know that you didn't write the paper yourself.

3. A patient on your unit gets discharged. While cleaning the room for the next patient, you find an expensive watch in the drawer in the bedside table. It's a woman's watch and the former patient was a man.

4. When you open up your paycheck, you realize that you got paid for a day that you didn't work.

5. As a research assistant, your salary is funded by a federal grant. If the research gets positive results, the grant and your job will get renewed for another year. The research director tells you to change some of the data to indicate better results.

6. When it's time for your competency evaluation, your supervisor announces that you and your coworkers will be checking each other off. Your coworkers get together and decide just to give each other a satisfactory evaluation without actually checking each person's competency level.

7. Your sons are returning to school tomorrow after summer break. You haven't had time to shop for school supplies and are short on cash. Your company is overstocked with office supplies and no one would miss a few pencils, pens, and tablets of paper.

8. Your best friend, who works in the same department you do, asks you to clock her out at 3:00 PM so that she can leave work at 2:00 PM to attend her daughter's dance recital.

9. A new supervisor schedules you to perform a procedure using new technology that was just installed but you don't feel competent to do so.

10. While working in a nursing home you notice a staff member who doesn't close the door when helping a resident use the bathroom.

11. You read a coworker's blog and discover that she's making up false stories about one of the nurses who work in your practice.

12. You suspect that your manager may be changing payroll information to increase the paycheck of one of her friends who works in the same department.

Relationships, Teamwork, and Communication Skills

4

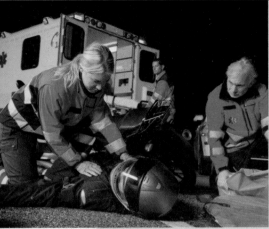

Think enthusiastically about everything, but especially about your job. If you do so, you'll put a touch of glory in your life. If you love your job with enthusiasm, you'll shake it to pieces.

—Normal Vincent Peale (1898–1993), clergyman and champion of positive thinking

(CandyBox Images/Shutterstock)

CHAPTER OBJECTIVES

Having completed this chapter, you will be able to:

- Explain the concept of interdependence among health care workers.
- List three ways to strengthen relationships at work.
- List two ways to demonstrate loyalty to your coworkers.
- Explain the role of courtesy, etiquette, and manners in the workplace.
- List three examples of netiquette when using digital communication.
- Give examples of two types of health care teams.
- Describe how group norms can help facilitate meetings.
- Explain why consensus is important but difficult to achieve.
- List the four essential elements for communication to take place.
- Describe how illiteracy impacts patient care.

- Explain two of the factors that may influence your communication with other people.
- Explain why labeling is a barrier to communication.
- Describe the role that body language plays in communication.
- Explain why conflict resolution is important in the workplace.
- Name the four styles of communication.
- Describe each of the four styles of communication including the likely outcome of each style.
- Identify the importance of assertive communication.
- List three types of communication technologies.
- List three problems that may occur when communicating electronically.
- Explain why it's important for health care professionals to develop their public speaking and presentation skills.

KEY TERMS

aggressive	consensus	hoard	personal space
assertive	cooperation	inclusive	plagiarize
attachment	courtesy	inferior	Platinum Rule
biased	de-escalate	interpersonal relationships	polite
body language	dialect	labeling	prejudiced
civility	diversity	literacy	selfie
cliques	emoticons	manners	slang
colleagues	etiquette	netiquette	synergy
conflict resolution	Golden Rule	passive	workplace bullies
confrontation	group norms	passive-aggressive	

Interpersonal Relationships

Now that we've examined character traits and how they're applied in the workplace, it's time to discuss how health care professionals work with other people. Your interactions with other people and the relationships you form with coworkers are the basis for success in the workplace. Interdependence is essential. No one person can do it all. Only groups of people working together can get the job done and done well.

Relationships, teamwork, and communication skills are some of the most important factors organizations are seeking in new health care workers. These skills directly impact quality of care, patient safety, the patients' experience, and the functioning of the care team. For example, about 85% of all medical errors are caused by poor communication and teamwork. Employers notice when effective communication is lacking. They want people who can collaborate with others to care for the patient and get the work done. They also want people who are positive and uplift the entire team. They want employees who can **de-escalate** (to reduce intensity or difficulty) and deal with conflict effectively. Finally, they want employees who can influence others while maintaining respect and the morale of the team.

Professionals devote a lot of energy to establishing positive **interpersonal relationships** (connections between or among people) and treating each other in a caring, respectful manner. Your ability to work well with coworkers contributes greatly to your reputation as a professional. Let's take a closer look at the need to work well with other people.

Coworkers as Customers

If you're employed on a full-time basis, you probably spend as much time with your coworkers as you do with your family and friends. People want to feel good about coming to work so it's important to create a positive, enjoyable work environment. Nothing can make your job more pleasant or miserable than your relationships with coworkers. Think about the relationships you've had in the past. Why did those relationships work well or not work well? Effective relationships are based on many of the factors already discussed in this text: trust, honesty, ethics, and morals. But several other traits and skills are also necessary.

You already know that patients, visitors, and guests are the customers of the health care company for which you work. But have you realized that coworkers are your customers as well? That

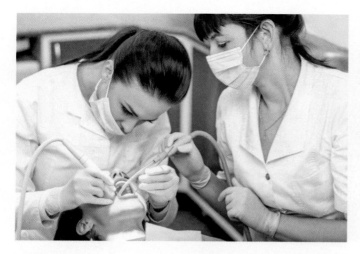

Figure 4-1 Working as a team (*RossHelen/Shutterstock*)

might seem strange, but your coworkers are your "internal" customers and they deserve to be treated with the same respect and compassion that you would give your patients and other customers.

As mentioned earlier, your attitude at work is important. Displaying a friendly, positive attitude, saying hello to people you pass in the hallway, and smiling every chance you get goes a long way in creating a pleasant environment at work. Always look for the best in people, give them the benefit of the doubt, and assume that everyone is there to do their best.

Professionals need to be viewed as team players. It's best to cooperate with your coworkers and avoid whining, complaining, and questioning authority. Complainers "poison" the workplace and stir up discontent. If you get labeled as a complainer or troublemaker, your opportunities for advancement could be limited.

Inclusion and Friendliness

In order to form effective relationships with coworkers, it's best to be **inclusive** (a tendency to include everyone). Instead of excluding people and participating in **cliques** (small, exclusive circles of people), invite your coworkers to join you for lunch and make them feel welcome. Don't leave people "out of the group." Excluding people can hurt their feelings and undermine their self-esteem. Self-esteem results, at least in part, from the feedback that people get from other people. So how you treat coworkers can have a direct impact on how they feel about themselves. If you want your coworkers to feel confident and good about themselves, then include them in your activities at work, reinforce their strengths and abilities, and help support their growth and advancement.

Because health care workers must depend on one another to get their work done, they must be willing to openly share information. Unfortunately, some people **hoard** (to resist giving something up) information because it gives them a sense of power. They know something that you don't know and that makes them feel important. But an attitude like this is counterproductive to relationships and teamwork. It's also important to share space, equipment, and supplies. After

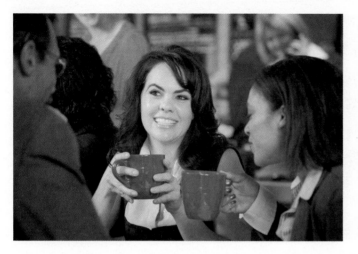

Figure 4-2 Strengthening relationships with coworkers (*Creatista/Shutterstock*)

all, you're all there for the same purpose—to serve patients and other customers, so there's no need for competition.

Laugh at yourself, be a good sport, and maintain your sense of humor. Avoid arrogance and don't be a snob. When you accomplish a goal, take pride but don't brag. Never look down on your coworkers or treat people in a demeaning way because they have less education, income, or status than you. There will always be people above and below you in the hierarchy of your organization and every person plays a critical role in accomplishing the company's mission. Remember the **Golden Rule** (a rule, held in most religions, that you should treat other people the way you would like to be treated; one familiar form of the Golden Rule is "Do unto others as you would have them do unto you.") In today's world, the **Platinum Rule** works best (a rule that you should treat other people the way *they* want to be treated, in contrast to the Golden Rule that you should treat other people the way *you* would like to be treated).

Building effective relationships doesn't happen overnight. It is hard work and you have to hang in there. Be patient and forgiving with yourself and your coworkers. No one is perfect—not even you! Get to know people better. You may discover a whole different side of someone's personality. Let your coworkers get to know you better, too. The better your relationships, the more likely your coworkers will be there for you when you need them, and vice versa.

Loyalty

Showing loyalty to the people who have helped you goes a long way in developing a professional reputation. One way to demonstrate loyalty to your coworkers is to be there for them when situations become stressful. Everyone who works in health care needs some encouragement and support from time to time. Getting the kind of emotional support that you need from people who don't work in health care themselves can be difficult. Even though family and friends may want to be helpful, it's hard to relate to the stress of working in health care unless you've experienced it yourself. This is especially true for employees who work on burn units and with critically ill children and patients facing death. Professionals need to "be there" for one another, to lend a helping hand or a shoulder to cry on. Let your coworkers know they can count on you. Protect their privacy. Don't talk about your coworkers' problems or situations at work with other people. When someone you work with needs support, be ready to help. Most of the time it means just listening—and understanding.

The concept of loyalty also relates to your relationship with your employer. Remember the statement, "*You* are the company you work for"? Stop and think about it. You don't actually work for a company, you work for the *people* who own and manage the company. Companies are just legal entities that own assets such as buildings, property, and equipment. You don't work for a building, you work for people! Professionals are able to make that distinction, and they feel a sense of loyalty to the people they *work for* as well as to the people they *work with*. You may not agree with management's policies, but don't forget that it's the people who manage your company that are providing you with a job and an opportunity to earn a living. When you disagree with a decision being made, you will need to trust leaders to do what's necessary to preserve and sustain the organization to fulfill its mission. If you support the mission, vision, and values of your company, you must remain loyal and positive even when you would have done things differently yourself. If you are unable or unwilling to do this, you might need to consider finding another place to work.

How can you demonstrate loyalty to your employer?

- Let management know you appreciate them and are proud to be part of the organization. Managers are people too, and they appreciate being appreciated.
- Give management the benefit of the doubt. Until you've walked in their shoes, you can't fully appreciate the challenges they face every day.
- If your employer invests in your education and training, help pay back their investment by continuing to work there for a reasonable length of time. If a local competitor offers you extra pay to switch companies, remember who invested in your education and show your loyalty. Someday you may need a recommendation from your current employer. If management views you as a loyal employee, it can only help.
- Represent your employer in a professional manner. Always speak highly of management when in public and do your best to enhance your company's reputation.

Cooperation

Cooperation (acting or working together for a common purpose) is essential in maintaining effective relationships at work. Offer to help your coworkers even if they haven't asked for assistance. When you've got a tough job to do or you're running late, isn't it a welcome relief to hear someone say, "Need a hand?" Offer to rotate shifts and holiday coverage—your coworkers will appreciate the consideration. Make personal sacrifices, such as coming in early or staying late, to help a coworker. Sensitivity and kindness are rewarded many times over. Learn to rely on one another, especially in emergencies and other stressful situations. Gain an appreciation for the strengths, abilities, and personal traits that each coworker contributes. Volunteer to serve on committees and sign up for employer-sponsored recreational activities to meet people and establish more relationships. Join people during your lunch break and widen your circle of **colleagues** (fellow workers in the same profession). You'll find there's **synergy** (people working together in a cooperative action to produce an effect greater than their separate efforts) in working with other people. After all, a group can accomplish so much more than individuals working on their own.

CASE STUDY

Prior to the meeting with risk management, Carla had researched the issues surrounding overprescribing prescription painkillers both nationally and within her state. She now had a better understanding of how the use of prescription painkillers could lead to heroin addiction, hepatitis C, drug overdoses, and death. Carla and her manager had reviewed the work records of the nurse in question and were prepared to discuss the employee's performance with network leaders. The nurse had worked for the practice for more than 10 years and had an impressive record. She had been involved in a car accident the year before and undergone surgery and several months of physical therapy. When she returned to work, her attendance and job performance were exemplary and there had been no complaints or incidents reported that would negatively affect her professional reputation.

When Carla and her manager met with staff from the risk management department they learned a great deal more about the pain management clinic, the doctor now under investigation, and the rising crisis facing their community. They were informed that a total of four employees within the network had been patients at the clinic, with just one of them working in Carla's practice. They learned that an internal investigation was underway and that network leaders were cooperating with local law enforcement on the next steps.

Within just a few days, Carla's nurse was released from the investigation. Although she had been seen twice at the pain clinic, she had never returned due to concerns about things she had witnessed there. When the case went to court several months later and the doctor was formally indicted, network leaders learned that the nurse had actually been the anonymous whistleblower who had notified law enforcement officials of potential wrongdoing at the site. Not only was the practice's nurse found innocent, she had taken the courageous step of revealing what was going on at the clinic and had probably saved several lives. Carla was relieved, and so proud of her colleague.

Carla's supervisory duties included coordinating several different types of teams. As groups got together from within the practice or with representatives from other parts of the network, effective communication skills became paramount. Establishing some **group norms** (expectations or guidelines for group behavior) helped, but disagreements often occurred and Carla spent considerable time helping to resolve interpersonal conflicts. She knew that staff members were committed to quality care and efficient business practices, but sometimes the stressful environment took its toll and people lashed out at one another. All too often, the issues involved behavioral concerns. Carla put topics like these on the agenda for the monthly meetings she held with her own staff. She raised topics, asked questions, and made sure that everyone had an opportunity to be heard. Group norms ensured that each staff member and his or her opinions were treated with dignity and respect.

One of the things Carla enjoyed most was guest lecturing at the local community college where she had earned her associate's degree. These lectures, which were more like informal discussions, helped Carla hone her public speaking and presentation skills. Next month she was scheduled to lead a discussion on social media **netiquette** (standards for appropriate conduct on the Internet). Since she and her staff had tackled several issues related to social media within the practice, she decided to ask her colleagues for input.

When Carla introduced the topic at the staff meeting just prior to her lecture date, the group erupted. Everyone wanted to speak at once! "Don't bring your cell phone to the dinner table!" "Get off the phone and get back to work!" "When you're speaking with someone in person, don't fiddle with your phone!" "People can't even use the restroom without talking on their phone!" "Stop texting while driving!" "Unplug at night and get some sleep!" "Quit texting risqué photos of yourself!" "Look up from your phone and watch where you're walking!" "You're on vacation, stop checking your messages!" "Lay that phone down once in a while and get a life!"

Carla was overwhelmed with the response and couldn't take notes fast enough. It was clear that social media was causing lots of frustration, both at work and at home. No one appeared exempt from the complaints as they cut across genders and all age groups. When people started relating stories about friends and family members who had suffered the consequences of poor judgment and posting inappropriate material on sites such as Facebook, Carla had to end the meeting because they were running out of time. She had plenty of feedback on social media netiquette. Stories about people who had become victimized would have to wait for a future discussion.

Carla reflected on what she had heard and thought about some of the issues related to social media that had occurred within the practice. She had already fired one employee who took and shared a **selfie** (a photograph of a person taken by him- or herself using a smartphone) that revealed confidential patient information. And while attending network meetings, she heard that several other employees had been put on probation or fired because of incidents involving social media. She began wondering if some new policies might be in order.

What should Carla do about the need for new policies related to social media? What would you do if you were in Carla's place?

Etiquette and Manners

A growing number of people, especially employers, are expressing concerns about the erosion of **civility** (politeness and consideration) in our society. People just aren't as **polite** (having good manners) and considerate of other people's needs as they should be. This concern is especially problematic in health care where people must work together, often under stressful conditions, to meet customer needs. So employers are increasingly emphasizing the roles that **courtesy**, **etiquette**, and **manners** play in forming and maintaining effective relationships.

- *Courtesy:* polite behavior, gestures, and remarks
- *Etiquette:* acceptable standards of behavior in polite society
- *Manners:* standards of behavior based on thoughtfulness and consideration of other people

Greetings, gestures, and other behaviors related to courtesy, etiquette, and manners may vary among different cultures of people. **Personal space** (the amount of space a person requires between him- or herself and another person in order to feel comfortable) and touching are described as *close contact* and *distant contact*. People comfortable with close contact may be more likely to touch an arm or shoulder of the other person, hold hands, and kiss one another on both cheeks. Distant contact people, however, prefer more space and may greet one another with a handshake or a hug if the other person is a close friend or family member.

It's important to use caution when touching another person because a touch can be misunderstood. Some Southeast Asian cultures believe that a person's spirit is on the head, so touching the head is often considered an insult. Making eye contact is another consideration. For Anglo-Americans, making direct eye contact with someone is important as it indicates interest, honesty, and listening. But in some American Indian and Asian cultures, for example, making direct eye contact is disrespectful or even hostile. If your job involves working with people from other cultures, learn about these differences and respect them in displaying appropriate courtesy, etiquette, and manners.

If it seems like the definitions of courtesy, etiquette, and manners overlap with one another, that's okay. What's important is the role that polite behavior plays at work, at home, and in all aspects of your life. Consider the following examples.

Courtesy

- Ask others before changing the room temperature, adjusting window blinds, turning on the TV, or playing music.
- Respect other people's possessions; return borrowed items quickly and, if you break something, repair it or replace it at your expense.

- Don't expect other people to clean up after you; keep your work area neat and orderly so it doesn't become an eyesore for others.
- Don't display risqué calendars, posters, or other personal items that might offend someone else.
- Listen while other people are talking and don't interrupt them.
- When riding on an elevator with a patient on a cart or in a wheelchair, protect their privacy and don't stare at them.

Personal Etiquette

- RSVP to invitations in plenty of time to let the host know if you'll be attending.
- Don't bring children or other guests with you to an event unless they've been invited.
- Acknowledge gifts by sending the giver a written thank-you note within two weeks.
- When seated for a meal, don't start eating your food until everyone at your table has been served; don't leave the table until everyone has finished eating.
- When walking down the street or up/down the stairs, stay to the right.
- When giving directions, don't point the way. Instead, use an open palm and gesture in an open manner when directing people. Better yet, escort the person to his or her destination.

Professional/Business Etiquette

- Shake hands with a firm grip when you meet someone. But be aware that some people will resist a handshake due to an injury, concern about spreading germs, or a cultural preference for distant contact.
- Refer to an older person or a superior (such as your boss's boss) by his or her last name (Mr. Smith, rather than Bill).
- Respect other people's time and don't make them wait on you.
- When you put people on hold on the telephone, check back every few minutes to let them know you haven't forgotten about them.
- When people arrive for a meeting, if possible, offer them a beverage.
- Maintain eye contact when speaking with people; when speaking to a group, make eye contact with everyone, not just one person. Keep in mind that some cultures refrain from any direct eye contact.
- When invited as a guest to eat with your supervisor or a coworker, don't order expensive menu items.
- When going through a buffet line, leave enough food for those in line behind you.

PROFESSIONALISM ONLINE

DIGITAL COMMUNICATION AND ETIQUETTE ONLINE

When it comes to the connections between "digital communication" and "relationships, teamwork, and communication skills," there are several issues to address. Let's start with some good news for digital communication.

Until recently, conventional wisdom taught us that leaving someone a voicemail message is more meaningful and conveys more emotion than sending someone an email message. This was thought to be especially true when expressing romantic feelings. But a doctoral student found just the opposite while conducting research for his dissertation. By using sensors on the face and feet of study participants, the student discovered that when people wrote romantic email messages they got sweatier feet than when they left voicemail messages. Sweaty feet indicated a higher level of excitement as people took more time to choose their words and edit their email messages carefully. Conversely, when study participants left voicemail messages, they only had one chance to get it right. Younger generations are growing up with texting and emails as a routine form of communication, so perhaps digital communication shouldn't be underestimated after all when it comes to expressing romantic thoughts and emotions.

You still need to keep in mind that digital communication is nonverbal. Without eye contact, facial expressions, and gestures, digital messages can be easily misunderstood. You might think you're sending a funny message while your recipient might think otherwise. Avoid expressing strong negative emotions via digital media. Stop and think about which form of communication would work best in conveying your thoughts. Sometimes that might require a face-to-face conversation.

Just as harassing, bullying, and stalking other people are unacceptable behaviors, so are cyberharassing, cyberbullying, and cyberstalking. Never use digital communication or social media to intimidate or threaten another person. If you are the target of such behavior yourself, collect evidence and report the situation to the proper authorities.

When it comes to written communication, never **plagiarize** (to use another person's work and claim credit for it) content that you find online. Plagiarizing is unethical and unprofessional. New software makes online plagiarizing easier to detect.

Let's state this one more time: Information that's sent electronically is not private or confidential. It's easy for someone to alter and forward your messages (email, voicemail, text, tweet, etc.) to other people without your knowledge, permission, or control. Don't put anything in a digital message that you wouldn't want to appear in the newspaper or on your employer's computer screen. Use security measures and privacy settings but don't count on them to protect you.

Keep in mind that it's easy to make mistakes when using electronic devices. You may be in a hurry and are probably using abbreviations, symbols, and a small-sized keyboard. Take a few extra seconds to reread your messages before you send them. Protect your cell phone and other mobile devices from unauthorized or accidental breaches. If your child is using your tablet, for example, make sure the content to which they have access is appropriate. Keep track of your devices and prevent them from being lost or stolen.

Let's move on to the subject of netiquette. Ask just about anyone and he or she will have a list of dos and don'ts related to courtesy, politeness, and manners when using digital devices. In fact, you probably have a list of your own. Here are some common netiquette tips:

- Don't text or talk on your cell phone during meals, meetings, or in other situations where you're with people who expect to have your full attention. If you're expecting a call and must take it, set your phone on vibration and lay it out of view.
- Don't disturb other people with your ringtones or personal conversations. If you must speak on the phone, move to a private area or lower your voice to avoid annoying the people around you. Don't speak on the phone in restrooms or in elevators, or when standing in line to order or pay in restaurants and stores. Don't make other people listen to your personal conversations.
- Use earbuds or headphones on airplanes, in waiting rooms, and in other places where your music or the noise made by your devices might not be welcome by people seated around you.
- Don't text or talk on the phone while crossing the street or walking through crowded areas.
- Don't use digital devices in dark places such as movie theatres or auditoriums where screen light will distract other people.
- Don't check or send messages or use digital devices when you're supposed to be sleeping. The light from electronic screens interrupts sleep patterns.
- Keep in mind that some people don't text or use social media or digital communication at all. Now and then it's a good idea to just pick up the phone and call someone. Or better yet, pay them a visit.
- Unplug once in awhile. Lay your phone down, turn it off, and put it away. Life will go on.

Here's *the* most important thing to remember: **Don't Text While Driving!** It would be better to miss a text than to miss the rest of your life or cause someone else to miss theirs.

Manners

- When you notice someone carrying a heavy or cumbersome package, offer to help.
- When in a crowded area, offer your seat to an elderly or handicapped person, a pregnant woman, or anyone else who needs the seat more than you do.
- Hold doors open for people who are entering or leaving the building right before or after you.
- If an elevator is crowded, step back and wait for the next one.
- When encountering a disfigured or handicapped person, don't stare or ignore the person; make eye contact and acknowledge their presence in a friendly manner.
- Always say "please" and "thank you" and acknowledge the kindness of other people.
- Cover your mouth and nose when you sneeze; wash your hands frequently during flu season to reduce the spread of germs. When you're sick, stay home.
- Acknowledge people when they walk into the room and make them feel welcome.

There are far too many examples of polite behavior to list them all here. If you feel you need to learn more about courtesy, etiquette, and manners there are many good books available on the subject.

TRENDS AND ISSUES

SOCIAL COMPETENCE AT WORK

Creating a positive and enjoyable work environment can be quite a challenge, especially if your job involves interacting with a diverse group of people in a high-stress setting. Keep this in mind—there's a difference between relationships with coworkers and relationships with friends. You and your coworkers don't need to be friends outside of work. Relationships with coworkers can enrich your professional life, but friendship is not the goal of your relationships at work. In fact, you might not even like some of the people with whom you must work. But you need to find ways to get along with them and respect the knowledge, skills, and talents they bring to the workplace.

According to a recent study, efforts to develop social competence skills should begin early in life. A 20-year study that followed 750 people through the age of 25 found that children in kindergarten who displayed strong emotional and social skills were more likely to graduate on time from high school, earn a degree, and secure full-time employment. Children who made friends and were cooperative and able to deal with conflict, showed interest in other kids' perspectives, and offered suggestions to classmates without being bossy achieved more success later in life as adults than their counterparts. When young children with weaker emotional and social skills became adults, they were more likely to be unemployed, arrested, substance abusers, and dependent on public assistance.

More than likely, the results of this study weren't at all surprising to Robert Fulghum. The information in his 1990 book, *All I Really Need to Know I Learned in Kindergarten*, provides helpful tips for getting along with other people: "Share everything. Play fair. Don't hit people. Put things back where you found them. Clean up your own mess. Don't take things that aren't yours. Say you're sorry when you hurt somebody. Wash your hands before you eat. Flush. Be aware of wonder. When you go out into the world, watch out for traffic, hold hands, and stick together" (Fulghum, Robert. *All I Really Need to Know I Learned in Kindergarten: Uncommon Thoughts on Common Things*. New York: Villard Books, 1988. Print.).

Teams and Teamwork

Your relationships with coworkers become even more important when working on teams, and teamwork is "the name of the game" in health care. In fact, many health care providers now rely on "high performance work teams" to care for patients and complete other assignments. Depending on your profession and where you work, you'll probably participate on many teams during your career.

Types of Teams

There are at least six different kinds of teams in health care. Some are based on disciplines that relate to different kinds of occupations and workers, such as radiographers, medical technologists, or unit secretaries. Some teams are composed of people from within the same department (*intra* means "within") while other teams are composed of people from different departments (*inter* means "across").

Intradisciplinary Teams

- People from the same discipline (radiography, for example) with similar educational backgrounds, job duties, and scopes of practice who work in the same department or different departments (main radiology, emergency department, outpatient radiology, etc.)
- A team of radiographers might work together to select some new diagnostic imaging equipment and prepare for installation and staff training

Interdisciplinary Teams

- People from different disciplines, with different educational backgrounds, job duties, and scopes of practice and who work in the same department or different departments
- A team of medical technologists, phlebotomists, and nurses might work together to coordinate the collecting and processing of patient blood samples

Intradepartmental Teams

- People from the same department or work unit, but with different educational backgrounds, job duties, and scopes of practice
- Surgical nurses, surgical technologists, and instrument technicians, for example, might form a team to improve instrument sterilization and packaging

Interdepartmental Teams

- People from different departments, with different educational backgrounds, job duties, and scopes of practice
- Representatives from the information technology, admitting, and patient registration departments might meet to streamline patient registration processes

There are at least two other types of teams in health care:

Work teams meet on an ongoing basis as part of their jobs. A group of paramedics, for example, might meet weekly to monitor patient transport and quality outcome data.

Project teams meet for a specified period of time and disband when their project has been completed. Some projects are short term (creating a new electronic form for patient billing) whereas others are more long term (creating a new computerized database to track patient discharges).

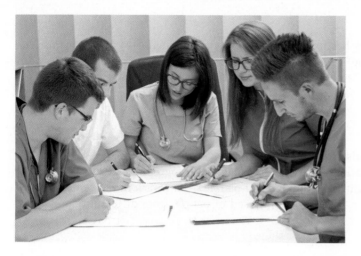

Figure 4-3 An intradepartmental team meeting (*Ocskay Mark/Shutterstock*)

Naming the teams you're on isn't necessary, but it's important to participate as an effective team member. High-performance work teams often work independently with little direct supervision. Management creates the team, identifies the members, arranges meeting times, communicates expectations, and clarifies the team's assignment. Then the team takes over:

- Arranging their own work schedules and holiday coverage
- Selecting new equipment and medical supplies
- Monitoring and improving quality outcomes
- Resolving budgetary and staffing issues
- Interviewing and selecting new team members

With 360-degree feedback performance evaluations, team members evaluate the performance of their teammates. With responsibilities such as these, you can see why effective communication skills are so important. Team members can also benefit from extra training in group dynamics, negotiation, delegation, resolving conflicts, and **diversity** (differences, dissimilarities, variations).

Regardless of what types of teams on which you serve, you will need to become skilled at both leading and following. You'll probably find yourself in both roles from time to time, even within the same team. "Shared leadership" is becoming more common. Members rotate the leadership role over time, or each team member takes the lead when the task to be completed falls within his or her area of expertise or interest.

Leading team members is not the same thing as supervising team members. In many situations team members are peers, so no one on the team reports to another person on the team. If one team member fails to complete his or her responsibilities, the whole team may suffer. In many health care settings, team performance is just as important (or more important) as individual performance. When the team performs well, each member is held in high regard. When the team fails, each member is held accountable.

Group Norms

It should be clear that, when working on teams, your success as an individual depends on the success of your team. Think about some of the teams on which you've participated. Which teams worked well together and which ones didn't? Establishing group norms might help. Group norms are guidelines that team members agree to follow to help the team function smoothly over time. For example, team members may be expected to:

- Attend all meetings, arrive on time, and stay until the end
- Speak up, play an active role, and participate in decision making
- Respect the ideas and opinions of others
- Follow through on obligations and complete assignments on time
- Carry their share of the workload
- Share information openly
- Cooperate and provide assistance when asked
- Focus on solutions instead of problems
- Serve as both leader and follower as needed

It's not unusual for employees who work in teams to cross-train with one another. As multi-skilled workers, these employees are capable of performing multiple functions, often in more than one discipline. For example:

- A housekeeper might be cross-trained to perform basic maintenance and repair duties
- A nursing assistant might learn to draw blood and prepare specimens for laboratory analysis
- A unit secretary might learn basic nursing assistant skills
- A maintenance worker might acquire carpentry skills

Multiskilled workers who participate on teams tend to be highly productive. They enhance convenience for patients and staff, add versatility and flexibility to the staffing plan, and save the company money in labor costs. Cross-training has become routine among health care employers so it's likely you will encounter this concept at some point during your career.

RECENT DEVELOPMENTS

VIRTUAL HEALTH CARE MEETINGS

Depending on your job and where you work, chances are you'll be spending a fair amount of time attending meetings. In settings where patient care requires teamwork, meetings are an efficient way for team members to communicate with one another. There are different types of meetings: a team meeting for coworkers to communicate about job duties; a staff meeting for supervisors to communicate about policies and schedules; a status meeting for team members to report on how patients are doing; and so forth.

Most of your meetings may be held in your facility or in a centralized location convenient to participants. Some meetings may be held via *conference calls* where participants "call in" and communicate as a group via telephone. A growing trend is to hold virtual meetings where participants use technology to "meet" with people spread out in various locations, sometimes in other states or even in other countries. Virtual meetings eliminate travel time and expense and allow people to communicate via online meeting services.

(continued)

Effective meetings require leadership to make sure that goals are achieved without wasting people's valuable time. If you are put in charge of leading a meeting, here are some things to think about:

- *Set goals.* Goals should be based on the topics that need to be covered. Envision what you hope to accomplish by the end of the session.
- *Issue invitations.* Identify who should attend the meeting based on the goals.
- *Schedule.* Set a time and location for the meeting. If participants need to call in or log on, provide them with details.
- *Confirm attendance.* Make sure that key participants plan to attend.
- *Prepare an agenda.* Develop a timeline for the session and share the agenda before, or at the start of, the meeting.
- *Maintain control.* Begin and end on time. Assign a note-taker or ask for a volunteer. Introduce each topic, guiding the team to focus and make decisions. If something cannot be resolved, set a time to address the issue after the meeting. At the end of the meeting, make sure all participants are aware of the next steps.
- *Follow up.* After the meeting, send a brief written summary. List action steps and a timeline for the team to achieve required follow-up activities. Thank participants for their time and attention.

Formal meetings require *parliamentary procedure*, typically following *Robert's Rules of Order.* Parliamentary procedure is used by professional organizations, government legislative bodies, and fraternal groups when debate and decision making must be done through a highly detailed, well-established, structured process. The first edition of *Robert's Rules of Order* was published in 1876; the most recent revision (11th edition) was released in 2011.

Consensus

Regardless of the types of teams that you serve on, one of your biggest challenges will involve achieving **consensus** (a decision accepted by all participants in a group) when decisions need to be made. Consensus is more than just voting on different options and declaring, "Majority rules." With majority rules, there are winners and losers—the majority wins and the minority loses. The

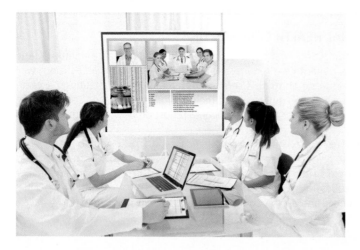

Figure 4-4 Participating in a virtual meeting (*Ndrey_Popov/Shutterstock*)

objective of consensus, however, is to arrive at a win–win solution where no one feels like a loser. Through group discussion, team members try to find an option that everyone can support. As you might imagine, achieving consensus is much more difficult than just taking a vote. But operating by consensus to find win–win solutions is the foundation of good teamwork.

Developing effective team skills takes time, especially when you're working with diverse groups of people from other cultures and with different personalities, values, and communication styles. But serving on a smooth-running, high-performing work team can be one of the most satisfying experiences you'll have as a health care professional. Let's examine how honing your communication skills can help.

Communication Skills

Unfortunately, treating your coworkers as customers and applying good etiquette and manners at work won't guarantee that you'll get along with everyone. In fact, you can pretty much count on some interpersonal conflict among the people with whom you work. Everyone is working in a stressful environment. When you're under pressure or feeling rushed, you don't always practice your best communication skills. Because of the diverse array of people you encounter, you can't help but experience some difficulty getting along with everyone. As mentioned earlier, you don't have to be friends with your coworkers, and it is okay if you don't like everyone with whom you work. But you can't choose your coworkers and you can't change them either, so you have to find ways to get along with everyone. Good communication skills can be a big help. Let's take a close look at communication and what it takes to be an effective communicator.

Elements of Communication

For communication to take place, there are four essential elements:

- *A message.* There must be something that you want to convey to another person. Perhaps the purpose of the message is to give information or to acquire information. Perhaps there is something you want another person to do.
- *A sender.* Unless there is someone who wants to send a message, there cannot be communication.
- *A receiver.* Even if there is a message and a sender, there must be a receiver. If there is no one to receive the message, communication is incomplete.
- *Feedback.* Capturing feedback is of critical importance. If you are not seen to be listening and acting on what you are told, why would people tell you anything?

Interference with any of these elements can disrupt communication. Remember that in order to ensure clear communication:

- The message must be clear.
- The sender must deliver the message in a clear and concise manner.
- The receiver must be able to hear and receive the message.
- The receiver must be able to understand the message.
- Interruptions or distractions must be avoided.

How can we ensure clear communication? We have to remember that communication is a two-way street. You must listen to others to make sure they listen to you. If you're interested in what the other person has to say, that person will more likely be interested in you. Remember to smile and maintain eye contact, so that the other person knows that you are interested in him or her. Use your voice, facial expressions, and gestures to show your enthusiasm.

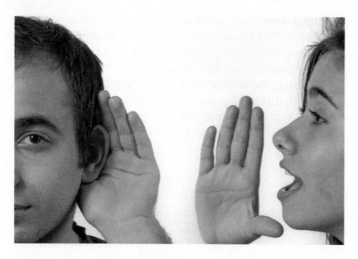

Figure 4-5 Practicing speaking and listening skills *(Sezer66/Shutterstock)*

There are many elements that can disrupt communication. Don't be competitive or make it seem as if what you have to say is more important than what the other person is saying. Watch your **body language** (nonverbal messages communicated by posture, hand gestures, facial expressions, and so forth). You don't want to appear bored or disinterested. Don't hunch your shoulders, fidget, tap your toes, or fiddle with your hair. Don't be too forceful or pushy in your conversation.

Listening is a very important element in all communication. If you do not receive the message that is being sent, communication has not taken place. Your understanding of how to be a good listener makes you a better health care worker. Here are some helpful tips:

- *Show interest.* It is important for you to show interest in the person who is sending you a message. If you follow all of the other rules of being a good listener but tune out the message because you are not interested, communication will not take place.
- *Hear the message.* People often think that they understand what is being said to them when they really do not. It is important to repeat what you believe you heard to be certain you heard correctly. It is not necessary to repeat exactly what was said, but check to see that you have understood the general message. Watch the speaker closely to observe actions that may contradict what the person is saying. Evaluate how well you listen and if you are using all of the above skills during and after each conversation.
- *Do not interrupt.* Have you ever tried to send a message and been frustrated by the receiver interrupting you? Allow the sender to give you the entire message without interruptions. If you need to ask a question to clarify the meaning, be patient and wait until the sender is finished. She or he may give you the information you need without your questions.
- *Pay attention.* This is critical. Eliminate distractions by moving to a quiet area for the conversations. Avoid thinking about how you are going to respond. Try to see the other person's point of view.
- *Maintain a positive attitude.* Keep your temper under control, even if you become irritated.

BY THE NUMBERS

ILLITERACY AND HEALTH LITERACY

Even though health care professionals focus on their communication skills to provide quality care, a large percentage of their patients may not be getting the full benefit. The problem is that a significant number of adult patients don't have the **literacy** (the ability to read and write) skills required to communicate effectively with their caregivers and understand the medical instructions and information they are given.

The term *health literacy* is gaining importance as efforts to improve the health and wellness of Americans continue to evolve. According to the U.S. Department of Health and Human Services, health literacy is defined as "the degree to which individuals have the capacity to obtain, process, and understand basic health information and services needed to make appropriate health decisions to prevent or treat illness." The National Literacy Act of 1991 defines *literacy* as "an individual's ability to read, write, and speak in English, and compute and solve problems at levels of proficiency necessary to function on the job and in society, to achieve one's goals, and develop one's knowledge and potential" *(Quick Guide to Health Literacy, U.S. Department of Health and Human Services)*. Based on a 2015 survey, 14% of U.S. adults (32 million people) can't read. About 19% of high school graduates haven't learned to read, and 21% of U.S. adults read below the fifth-grade level. The situation really hasn't improved over the past 10 years. Low literacy occurs most often among older adults, minority, poor, and medically underserved populations.

Many health care workers either aren't aware of the problem or don't have the skills required to overcome literacy-related communication issues. Patient education materials are available mostly in print and written at a 10th-grade or higher reading level. This means that millions of Americans struggle to understand the information they're given and apply it correctly.

Patients have a limited knowledge of medicine and health care to begin with, and medical language can be especially confusing. Problems occur when patients must read and follow medication instructions, share their medical histories, prepare for exams and treatments, manage chronic conditions, and provide follow-up self-care in a safe and effective manner. Concerns arise when patients must complete medical applications, sign consent forms, review insurance claims, and show up prepared for doctors' appointments. To make the situation more challenging, patients who are illiterate often hide their deficiencies from family members, friends, and health care providers out of shame or embarrassment.

It's not surprising that low literacy can result in less-than-optimum outcomes for patients. In fact, research shows that illiterate patients have higher rates of hospitalization than literate patients. To improve patient–provider communication, health care workers should:

- Watch for signs of low literacy and take extra steps to make sure that patients understand the information they're given.
- Reduce the reading level of printed information and include illustrations to add clarity; provide video- and audiotapes for patients who can't read.
- Communicate verbally with patients; ask follow-up questions to make sure they comprehend instructions and know how to follow them.
- Demonstrate self-care techniques (such as using an inhaler or checking blood pressure) and then have patients demonstrate the technique themselves to make sure things are done correctly.
- Speak slowly, explain things carefully, and use terms that patients can understand.
- Ask for assistance from a coworker, or from a patient's family member or friend, when English isn't the patient's primary language; provide print, video, and audio materials in languages other than English when possible.

Factors That Influence Your Communication with Other People

Prejudices

Everyone forms opinions and becomes **biased** (favoring one thing, person, or way over another based on some prior experience) and **prejudiced** (having judged or formed an opinion before the facts are known) as they grow up. These biases and prejudices affect how you feel about other people and how you relate to them. You may have very strong feelings about the backgrounds or the values of some of your coworkers or patients, and your feelings may affect how you communicate with them. For example, if you believe that certain people are lazy, overly emotional, or **inferior** (lower or less worthy), you need to think about your biases and prejudices. When you recognize and understand these feelings, you are better prepared to overcome them.

Frustrations

When you care for and work with other people, you may experience impatience, annoyance, and possibly anger. Perhaps other people do not understand your directions, or they move too slowly to suit you. This may cause you to feel frustrated or irritated. These feelings can interfere with your ability to communicate. Take time to understand why you feel frustrated or irritable. Evaluate the situation, and then try to correct it. It is your responsibility to control your behavior and to understand that coworkers, patients, and families have issues and problems of their own that influence their behavior.

How you act toward other people and how they act toward you affect the quality of communication. If you are disinterested or bored, if you are in a bad mood, or if you wish you were someplace else, communication can break down. However if you show interest and concern for others, your job will become easier and your communication more effective.

Life Experiences

People have new experiences every day. These experiences help us know what to expect in day-to-day living and how to act in certain situations. The most effective communication is based on shared experiences. These may be experiences you and other people went through together or experiences that you and others went through individually. Perhaps you grew up in the same community, went to the same school, or share the same language. It may be as simple as liking the same type of movies, music, or books. You will usually have more effective communication with someone who has shared some of your experiences. Of course, the reverse is true as well. Less shared experiences can cause communication to be more difficult and frustrating. This is especially true when communication involves **slang** (the informal language of a particular group) and **dialect** (language that is distinct to a culture).

To be a more effective communicator, look for things that you have in common with the other person. You can do this by listening to what they say and how they say it, looking for something familiar, and then focusing a bit more on that shared experience. As you find more and more areas in common, your communication with that person will become more effective.

Aging and Communication

What happens when a younger health care professional interacts with an older patient, or vice versa? There are, of course, possible physical issues that make communication with older adults more difficult, such as hearing or vision problems. There may be mental or emotional issues, such as older people who are afraid of losing the ability to think, reason, or explain themselves. Finally, there may be certain cultural issues, such as believing the doctor is always right or being afraid to complain about aches and pains. There are also fewer shared experiences between younger and older individuals, so it becomes even more important to work on finding some common ground that you may share.

HOT TOPICS

HEARING LOSS

The ability to hear plays a key role in interpersonal communication. The gradual hearing loss that occurs as you age (presbycusis) is a common condition. About 50% of people age 75 and older have hearing problems that affect their daily lives. Over recent years, the number of people experiencing hearing loss at younger ages has gradually increased. About 15% of adults age 18 and older (37.5 million people) in the United States have some degree of hearing loss.

Each day you're surrounded by a variety of sounds in your environment. Most sounds occur at safe levels that do not affect hearing. However, sounds that are too loud or last for a long time can damage sensitive structures called hair cells in the inner ear. The result is noise-induced hearing loss (NIHL).

Hair cells convert sound energy into electrical signals that travel to the brain. Once damaged, hair cells cannot grow back. Scientists once believed that the force of vibrations from loud sounds caused the damage to hair cells. Recent studies, however, have shown that exposure to harmful noise triggers the formation of molecules that can damage or kill hair cells.

NIHL can be caused by a single exposure to a quick, intense sound such as an explosion, or by long-term exposure to loud sounds over an extended period of time, such as noise generated in a woodworking shop. The loudness of sound is measured in decibels. Sources of noise that can cause NIHL range from 120 to 150 decibels. Examples include motorcycles, firecrackers, and small firearms.

Long or repeated exposure to sounds at or above 85 decibels can also cause hearing loss. The louder the sound, the shorter the time period before NIHL can occur. Sounds of less than 75 decibels, even after long exposure, are unlikely to cause hearing loss.

The good news is that NIHL is 100% preventable. In order to protect yourself, you must understand the hazards of noise and how to practice good hearing health in everyday life. To protect your hearing:

- Know which noises can cause damage.
- Wear earplugs or other hearing protective devices when involved in a loud activity.
- Be alert to hazardous noise in the environment.
- Protect the ears of children who are too young to protect their own.
- Make family, friends, and colleagues aware of the hazards of noise.

Exercise care when using headphones, earphones, and earbuds. Listening to loud music will have less of an impact on your hearing when you limit the amount of time and use higher-quality earphones that block out background noise as compared with the stock earbuds/earphones that come with iPods and MP3 players.

If you suspect hearing loss, have a medical examination by an otolaryngologist, a physician who specializes in diseases of the ears, nose, throat, head, and neck. You may also have a hearing test by an audiologist, a health professional trained to measure and help individuals deal with hearing loss.

Barriers to Communication

Recognizing barriers to communication can help you become an understanding health care professional. The following are four major communication barriers:

- *Labeling* (describing a person with a word that limits him or her, such as "lazy" or "mean"). Deciding the other person is mean, lazy, a complainer, or difficult causes a breakdown in communication. When labeling, you do not pay attention to the message being sent. If you listen, you might find out the reason for the behavior.
- *Sensory impairment.* Deafness or blindness can be a communication barrier. Always assess the people you are communicating with to determine if they have a sensory impairment.

- *Talking too fast.* It is especially important when you are working with older adults to speak slowly. Communication can break down when the message is delivered too rapidly.
- *Cognitive impairment.* Cognitive impairment includes memory, perception, problem solving, emotional reaction, and idea formulation. These types of impairments might result from autism, brain injury, Parkinson's, Alzheimer's, or old age. Be careful to make sure your patient understands what you are saying. You may want them to tell you, in their own words, what you have just explained to them. Or, you may write down suggestions for them.

When communicating verbally, here are some things to think about when you are the sender of a message:

- Be clear and concise so that your listener can easily understand.
- Use words and terms that your listener is familiar with.
- Give examples as further explanation.
- Avoid frustration when the other person just doesn't seem to "get it." Restate your message using different words.
- If the conversation seems to be going nowhere, ask a third person for help.

Effective listening skills are critical:

- Learn to listen carefully and concentrate on the message so that you fully understand the other person's point of view.
- Repeat what the person has said in your own words to make sure you received the message accurately.
- Don't "half-listen" to the other person while you're thinking about how to respond; you may miss part of the message.
- Ask the other person for clarification when you don't fully understand what he or she is saying. Or ask the person to state the message again using different words.
- Observe the person's body language to gather important information.

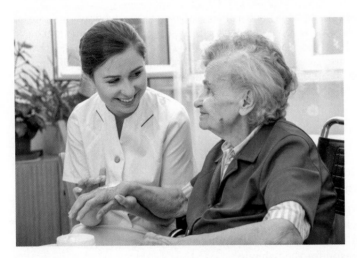

Figure 4-6 Using effective communication skills to give patient information
(*Alexander Raths/Shutterstock*)

Up to 90% of communication is nonverbal. About 55% of communication is through body language, 38% is through your tone of voice, and just 7% is based on the actual words you use. This means that most of the messages you send out are communicated nonverbally through your body language. This includes facial expressions, gestures, eye contact, "rolling" of the eyes, posture, body movements, tone and loudness of the voice, and so forth. Body language often communicates more information, and a greater accuracy of information, than the words people use. You can convey your anger, disappointment, or frustration with someone without even saying a word. Similarly, you can allow yourself to be taken advantage of slumping in your chair, cowering in the corner, or avoiding eye contact with the person with whom you are communicating.

Developing effective communication skills will help you become a more successful health care worker. Always be courteous and understanding. Take time to evaluate body language, gestures, facial expressions, and tone of voice to fully understand what is really being said. You may feel frustrated, angry, or irritated, but as a health care professional it's up to you to attempt to understand and to listen.

THINK ABOUT IT

COMMUNICATION DIFFERENCES BETWEEN MEN AND WOMEN

Studies have shown that men and women vary in the way they use nonverbal communication. Differences between men and women are found in their body movements, eye contact, and use of space.

Women tend to use facial expressions to express more emotion than men. They are more likely to smile and more likely to use facial and body expressions to show friendliness. In contrast, a man does not smile as much and is more likely to interrupt a person who is smiling. While women may show some friendly nonverbal cues, their posture tends to be more tense than men's posture. Men are more relaxed and more likely to use gestures.

While women do not often stare, men use staring to challenge power. This nonverbal cue for power is also seen when observing the behavior of a man during an initial gaze. Men will wait for the other person to turn away, while women are more likely to avert their eyes on initial gaze. Men also use staring to signal interest. Instead of staring, women signal interest by maintaining eye contact.

Men and women also differ in their use of personal space. Women tend to approach others more closely, while men want more personal space. However, men are more likely to invade another's personal space if necessary. These differences between men and women add to the complexity of communication.

Communication Styles and Conflict Resolution

You've no doubt heard the phrase "dealing with difficult people." Responding to **confrontation**, (facing boldly and defiantly), confronting people yourself, and resolving interpersonal conflict all require some special communication skills in **conflict resolution** (overcoming disagreements among two or more people).

When you confront someone or respond to someone who has confronted you, the goal is to communicate your point of view in an open, honest, direct manner. This means you are "open" to sharing your opinion, you are "honest" in stating your opinion, and you state your opinion in a "direct" manner to make sure the other person gets your point. Let's see how well these goals are met when using each of the four different styles of communication:

- **Aggressive** (likely to confront or attack)
- **Passive** (accepting without resistance)
- **Passive-aggressive** (acting in an aggressive manner while appearing to be passive)
- **Assertive** (confident and self-assured)

Here's the scenario. You and a coworker both want Christmas off. Both of you have relatives arriving in town and wish to spend time with them. After discussing the holiday schedule, it becomes obvious that one of you must work, so you start the conversation.

Aggressive Style

In a loud, angry tone of voice you say, "I've worked here longer than you, so I get the day off! Besides, my kids are coming and they live farther away than your kids!"

Your coworker replies, "You got Thanksgiving off and I had to work! So I deserve Christmas off more than you! And besides, you don't have grandchildren and I do!"

You reply, "Why do you always have to insist on getting your own way? Every time we do the schedule, you complain!"

"I complain?" your coworker responds. "You're the one who always refuses to work overtime!"

You can imagine where the "conversation" goes from here. With aggressive communication, the conflict usually gets worse. You've expressed your opinion in an open, honest, direct manner. So why didn't the aggressive style of communication work? You failed to show respect or consideration for your coworker, so he became defensive and fought back. Before long, anger took over, other issues entered the conversation, and the conflict escalated into an argument. Situations involving aggressive communication can turn violent and shouting or fistfights might result. The conversation might be overheard by other people including supervisors and patients. Did anyone "win" in this situation? Was the conflict resolved? It's clear the answer is "no." Let's try a different approach.

Passive Style

In a meek, quiet tone of voice you say, "Well, I guess if you want Christmas off, I'll have to work. Maybe my kids can come back for Easter."

That was a pretty short conversation. Using passive communication, you failed to express your opinion in an open, honest, direct manner. You turned into a floor mat to be walked on. Your coworker won, he got his needs met. But you lost, and came off looking (and feeling) weak and pitiful. Was the conflict resolved? Yes. But in the long run you'll resent your coworker and feel disappointed in yourself for not standing up for something that was important to you. Let's try again.

Passive-Aggressive Style

You say, "Well, I guess if you want Christmas off, I'll just go ahead and work. Maybe my kids can come back for Easter." And then as soon as you get the chance, you do something sneaky to "get even" with him. You send your supervisor an anonymous note saying your coworker takes longer breaks than he's supposed to. You spread malicious gossip about him behind his back. Or you call in sick on a busy day when the two of you are assigned to work together. After all, there are lots of ways to get even. Maybe getting even will make you feel better or maybe not. Using passive-aggressive communication, you still failed to express your opinion in an open, honest, direct manner. And to make matters worse, you did something sneaky and dishonest. Was the conflict resolved? No. Let's try one more time.

Assertive Style

In a normal tone of voice you say, "Well, we both want Christmas off. I'm sure you'd like to spend Christmas with your grandchildren. After all, you had to work Thanksgiving, didn't you? On the other hand, I've worked here twice as long as you so I have seniority. And my children are really looking forward to spending the day together as a family. So let's figure out a way to work this out so we can both get our needs met."

Maybe you could split the holiday shift. Maybe you could arrange a long weekend off to make up for one of you having to work the holiday itself. Maybe you could work together to find a third person who's willing to cover the holiday in exchange for a different day off. There is usually a workable solution to any problem. But if you're arguing with the other person, your energy is spent on the conflict, not the solution. Using assertive communication, you stated your opinion in an open, honest, direct manner and you did so in a way that showed respect and consideration for your coworker. Did it solve the problem? Maybe, maybe not. But assertive communication presents the best opportunity for you to work together, compromise, and come up with a solution that's acceptable to both of you. It's a win-win solution, which is the goal of conflict resolution.

It should be obvious that assertive communication is the only acceptable communication style at work. You must have enough self-respect to state your needs openly and honestly. You must not allow yourself to be "walked on," pitied, or tempted to do something underhanded and sneaky to get even. Professionals look out for themselves but do it in a way that shows respect for the needs and desires of their coworkers.

Assertive communication doesn't come easy—it takes practice. Maybe you're not used to standing up for yourself when someone confronts you or disagrees with you. Maybe aggressive or passive-aggressive communication has been your style up until now. If so, it's time to start working on a different approach that's more appropriate in the workplace. Put some effort into developing your assertive communication skills. Observe how other people deal with conflicts and the results they get. Then keep practicing your own skills. The more you practice, the easier it will become.

CONSIDER THIS

LEARNING TO COMMUNICATE THROUGH OBSERVATION

You can learn a lot by watching other people and noticing which communication techniques work for them, and which do not. Once you've observed an approach that appears to work, you can try it yourself to see if you get the same results.

Here's an example that occurs frequently. You notice a male customer and his companions seated at a table near yours in a restaurant. It's obvious that he isn't pleased with the food he was just served. You're wondering how he will react and what will happen. The following are four options.

Reaction #1: In a loud and angry tone of voice, he says to the waiter, "This isn't what I ordered! Either get it right or I'm not going to pay one dime for this food!" How well do you think this aggressive style of communication worked? Let's imagine a different approach.

(continued)

Reaction #2: The man says to his table companions, "I don't like this place. They get my order wrong every time I come here. Let's go someplace else." While the waiter isn't looking, he sneaks out of the restaurant, takes the other members of his party with him, and leaves nothing to pay for the food that's already been served. Is this *get-even* approach any better? Let's try again.

Reaction #3: In a pitiful, whining tone of voice, the man says to his companions, "This isn't what I ordered. But I don't want to make a scene, so I guess I'll just eat it anyway." Did this passive approach meet his needs? Let's try one more time.

Reaction #4: The man signals for the waiter to come over to the table. In a calm tone of voice he says, "I hate to complain, but I ordered french fries and got a baked potato instead. I was really looking forward to the fries. Could you take the baked potato back and switch it to fries for me? Thank you."

How well do you think this assertive approach worked? Consider each of the different approaches.

- How might the waiter have responded to the man's reactions?
- How might his table companions have responded to the man's reactions?
- Were the man's needs met? Why or why not?
- Which approach worked the best, and why?
- Which approach worked the least, and why?
- What could you learn by observing these interactions?
- Which approach would you use if you were in this situation?

By sharpening your observation skills, you can improve your assertive communication skills. Notice what works best for other people and try it yourself. The more you practice, the more skilled you will become.

Learn to "choose your battles wisely." Decide which conflicts are really worth tackling and which ones you should just "let go." Some battles aren't worth the effort. And be careful! Just because you're taking an assertive approach doesn't guarantee the other person will as well. Someone could turn aggressive on you. When communicating with a "difficult" person, make sure you can get out of the room quickly if you need to. If there's any concern about your physical safety, make sure there's someone else nearby who can come to your aid if necessary. Remember it's a crazy world out there. You never know when someone might be carrying a weapon or behaving in an aggressive or passive-aggressive manner. Here are some things to think about when confronting someone:

- Treat the other person with respect. Give him or her the benefit of the doubt until you've fully investigated the matter.
- Make sure you have complete, accurate information before confronting someone. Don't proceed on assumptions or unverified, third-hand information that might not be true.
- Stay calm and keep your anger and tone of voice in check.
- Arrange a suitable time and place to discuss differences. Never conduct this type of conversation in a public area.
- Don't go off "half-cocked" only to later regret something you've said or done.
- Listen carefully and make sure you understand the other person's point of view.
- Aim for a win-win solution.
- Take safety precautions. You may be able to control your own behavior but you cannot control the behavior of the other person.

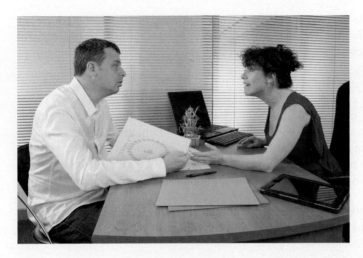

Figure 4-7 Discussing a disagreement to resolve a conflict (*Sylv1rob1/Shutterstock*)

Once you fully understand the other person's point of view and he or she understands yours, there should be a middle ground where both of you can compromise and feel like your needs have been met.

When you have a conflict with a coworker, resolve it quickly. Procrastination only makes things worse. But calm down first and make some rational decisions about how to handle the matter. Attack the issue, not the person. Remember that you cannot change other people; only they can change themselves. All you can do is make your best effort at communicating appropriately. If necessary, ask another person with good conflict resolution skills to serve as an intermediary.

If one of your superiors is the "difficult person," proceed cautiously! Remember to respect his or her position of authority. Weigh the pros and cons of addressing the situation head-on or just learning to live with it. If you decide to discuss the matter with your superior:

- Plan in advance what you're going to say, how you're going to say it, and what response you'll give to how he or she might react.
- Practice delivering the message in advance and consider role-playing the situation first with someone you trust.
- Listen carefully, watch for a win–win resolution, and be open to receiving some constructive feedback that might help you form a more positive relationship with your superior in the future.
- If the matter is still unresolved and you cannot move forward, speak with a human resources representative or another person in authority in your company.
- If the situation is serious and cannot be resolved, you may need to transfer into another position.

Effective communication and conflict resolution skills will serve you well in all aspects of your life. Avoid letting other people "press your buttons." When you hear yourself saying, "She makes me so angry!" stop and think about that statement. You have a choice as to whether to be angry or not. Allowing other people to "make you" angry means you are handing over control of your behavior to someone else. Is that really what you want to do? Find ways to maintain control of your own behavior and don't allow other people to push you into doing things or saying things that you would rather not do or say.

People who use an aggressive or a passive-aggressive style of communication at work may be viewed as **workplace bullies** (employees who intimidate and belittle coworkers). These rude and unprofessional workers use verbal and nonverbal language to demean and intimidate other people. They rarely show respect, good manners, or civil behavior. Bullies create a hostile work environment, and may be guilty of harassment and various forms of workplace violence. If you encounter a workplace bully, using conflict resolution skills probably won't help much. Document the aggressive behaviors in writing, and file a report with the appropriate person.

There's obviously a lot to think about when communicating with people in person. Let's examine the many pitfalls of communicating with people electronically.

Communication Technologies

In today's highly technological world, communicating by telephone, voicemail, fax, email, texting, and social media offers several efficiencies and convenience. But technological communication also creates the need for caution, especially when using email, voicemail, and texting, which have the possibility of being seen or heard by more people than the intended recipient.

Since a major part of communication in health care is by telephone, let's start there.

Telephone

The telephone is an important communication tool between you and those you serve. All health care settings require good telephone communication skills. You may be asked to answer the telephone, take a message, or respond to a request. Always follow good communication standards when answering an incoming or placing an outgoing call. Telephones at workstations are reserved for business use only. Personal calls must be done on your break or before or after your scheduled hours.

When communicating by telephone:

- Demonstrate open, honest, and respectful communication.
- Present ideas, information, and viewpoints clearly.
- Listen actively and seek to understand others.
- Use good telephone manners.
- If the doctor asks you to screen calls at an office or clinic, answer the phone and identify the caller, or use caller ID, and then politely notify the caller that the doctor is unable to speak at the moment. Then offer to take a message so the doctor can return the call.

Demonstrate the following behaviors when on the telephone:

- Answer the telephone cheerfully.
- Use a pleasant, caring, and sincere tone of voice.
- Answer the telephone on the first ring, if possible.
- Speak clearly and courteously.
- Remember to thank the caller when a call is returned.

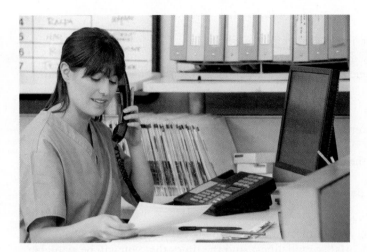

Figure 4-8 Communicating by telephone to convey test results (*Monkey Business Images/Shutterstock*)

- Identify yourself and give your title (such as, "This is Monica, nurse assistant.").
- Identify your department or doctor's office (such as, "Dr. Smith's office").
- Thank the caller for calling.
- Allow the caller to hang up first to ensure that the caller has said everything he or she wanted to say.

Use appropriate words and phrases such as:

- May I have your name, please?
- Would you repeat that, please?
- How may I assist you?
- I'm sorry; I didn't understand.

Avoid inappropriate words and phrases such as:

- What's your name?
- What did you say?
- What do you want?
- Huh?

Tips to be prepared:

- Have the necessary materials handy (pencil, message pad, and telephone numbers).
- Before placing a call, prepare questions, gather the information you'll need, and determine the appropriate action to take.

When placing a caller on hold:

- Ask the caller if he or she can hold, and wait for a response.
- Check every 30 seconds to see if the caller wants to continue to hold.
- Ask if you may take a message.
- Transfer the call as soon as possible.

When transferring a caller:
- Explain where you are transferring the caller and to whom.
- Give the caller the number you are transferring to.
- If possible, stay on the telephone and introduce the caller to the person receiving the call.

When writing a message:
- Record the time and date.
- Write the caller's name clearly (verify spelling) and the telephone number (read back the number).
- Summarize information with the caller by repeating the message.
- Sign or initial the message.
- Record the action you take to deliver the message.

When leaving a message:
- State whom you are calling for, your name and where you are calling from, your message (remembering to follow confidentiality guidelines), and the times that you will be available for a return call.
- Document the date, time, and message left.

For safety reasons, the health care facility where you work will probably have restrictions on use of your personal cell phone in the workplace. Cell phones can cause interference with medical equipment, including ventilators and pacemakers. Cell phones also may set off alarms on medical machines. You need to be aware of your employer's policy on how, where, and when employees, patients, and guests can use their phones. You may have to ask a patient or family member to turn off their phone. If so, politely explain the facility's policy and the need for it.

Despite the problems associated with using cell phones in health care environments, an increasing number of facilities are moving toward a text-based communication system for nurses and other caregivers. As with any other type of communication, when texting you must pay attention to what you are doing, use appropriate language, and be courteous and polite.

Voicemail

Voicemail is a convenient method of communication when you need to leave a message for someone. When delivering messages by voicemail, the receiver hears your words and your tone of voice, but your body language is still invisible. You need to speak slowly and clearly to be sure your message is understood. When you need to be absolutely certain that your message has been conveyed and received accurately, it's best to have a face-to-face conversation with the person. The second best option is a live telephone conversation. Anyone who receives a voicemail message from you can forward that message to someone else without your knowledge or permission. These types of situations can be highly embarrassing and may accidentally reveal sensitive, confidential information to people who should not have access to it.

Fax

If you need to send a patient's record to another provider, you may need to use a facsimile or fax machine. A fax transmission is a way to send or receive printed pages or images over telephone lines by converting them to and from electronic signals. You may work on a computer or have access to a printer that is connected to a phone line so that you can send and receive faxes directly from your computer or printer. In order to send a fax, you must have a telephone number used for faxes by the person to whom you want to send the documents.

There are a few things you should remember when sending a fax:

- Use a cover page. A cover page is the first page of a fax that gives the receiver important information about the fax. It should include your name, contact number, number of pages being sent, the name of the recipient, and any other important information.
- Confirm that the intended recipient received the fax. Since a fax often contains important patient information, call or email the recipient to ensure that he or she has received it.
- Remember that you may be dealing with confidential information. If you are sending confidential or potentially sensitive information, call ahead and let the recipient know to be ready. Using an online fax may help avoid security issues, as it lets users send and receive faxes from the privacy of their own computers.

Email

Email is an important method of communication in health care. When sending emails you should choose your words carefully. Sarcasm and humor should not be used in a business email because they may lead to miscommunication or misunderstandings. Although texting abbreviations are becoming a common form of language, texting abbreviations should not be used in your email or written communication at work unless approved by your employer. Many health care workers are not familiar with texting abbreviations. The use of unauthorized abbreviations in health care can cause serious problems related to patient care and medical records.

Remember that any message you send is permanent and may be forwarded to others. Do not use a business email address to send trivial or highly sensitive information. Before you hit *send*, follow these guidelines to write a professional email:

- Begin with a salutation.
- Include short, simple, and straightforward information. If a message is long, discuss the topic in a short email and use an **attachment** (a file linked to an email message) to provide details. You may also break up a longer email that has many topics into multiple, shorter emails that discuss each topic separately.
- Read your email aloud to check the tone of your message. Using *please* and *thank you* with requests ensures a polite tone.
- Proof the content for spelling and grammar mistakes. Use upper- and lowercase when writing. (Use of all caps implies yelling.)
- Include important contact information at the end of your email (your name, position, organization, telephone number, email address, and perhaps fax number).
- Include a subject on the subject line of the email.
- Use features such as *carbon copy* and *blind carbon copy* when appropriate. Carbon copy (cc) is used to send a copy of your email to another recipient. For example, you may send an email to a patient, but carbon copy a doctor on the email so that he or she knows what was sent to the patient. Blind carbon copy (bcc) is used when an email is sent to multiple people. Blind carbon copy allows a recipient to read the message; however, the recipient cannot see the other email addresses to which the message was sent. This is beneficial because it protects the recipients' email addresses and eliminates clutter in the email.
- When replying to an email message, be careful with *reply* and *reply all* functions. Don't select *reply all* unless it is really necessary for everyone who was included in the original message to receive your reply.

Respond to incoming emails within 24 hours. If you need more time to respond, call or email that you are looking into the matter and will get back to the person as soon as possible. Also be sure to answer all questions when responding to an email. When sending an email with questions, allow one or two days for a response. If you need an immediate response, you may want to call the person.

In health care, memorandums (memos) are used as reminders, to persuade an action, to issue a directive, or to provide a report. Memorandums can be delivered via email. When sending a memorandum via email, be sure to:

- Confirm the memorandum looks as intended in print and on the screen.
- Use fonts and graphics that are clear on all recipients' computers.
- Ensure that attachments are readable by all recipients.

Social Media

As mentioned previously, be especially careful posting personal information on social networking sites such as Facebook, Twitter, Instagram, and Snapchat. Once personal information or photos of you have been posted on social media, they can't be retrieved. Anyone who has access to your online information can manipulate the content and share your information with anyone they care to. So-called "privacy settings" aren't necessarily effective and way too many people are learning this lesson the hard way.

In general, there is little or no professional reason for you to communicate by social media and many reasons, as just stated, for not doing so. Health care companies are instituting new policies to govern their employees' use of social media and other online sites.

Texting

A text message has been described as a cross between a phone call (because it is sent from one cell phone to another) and a Twitter message (because there is a limit to the number of characters that can be used, normally 160 characters for a text message). It is also something like a voicemail message (short and transmitted by phone, but written rather than spoken).

So when you send a text message, keep in mind all the guidelines we have just discussed for communicating by telephone, voicemail, email, and social media.

Tips for Using Electronic and Other Communication Technologies

Here are some more basic factors to remember when communicating electronically at work:

- Slow down and think about what you are doing. Once a message has been sent electronically, it cannot be cancelled. Anyone who receives your message can send it on to someone else without your knowledge or permission.
- Keep your messages short and to the point. Omit information that could be embarrassing if it falls into the wrong hands, or result in a violation of confidentiality and privacy standards.
- Be especially careful when forwarding messages. Before you click on *send*, double-check the content of the *entire message* and confirm to whom it is being sent.
- Avoid using fancy fonts, smiley faces, and **emoticons** (combinations of keyboard characters used to convey the sender's emotions, such as :-) to represent a smile).
- Electronic communication isn't foolproof. You cannot be certain your message was received and read without following up. People receive scores of email messages at work every day. Sometimes a message is accidentally deleted before it has been read. People may become overwhelmed with too many messages and never open some of them. Some people who are assigned email accounts at work never use them.
- Every time you prepare to send a message, ask yourself how you would feel if your message appeared in the newspaper or showed up on your supervisor's computer screen. Never send an electronic message when you are angry or emotionally upset.

Keep in mind that electronic communication leaves a documented "trail" of messages. If you're angry with someone and send an emotionally charged message by email, text, or voicemail, the receiver has documented evidence of your communication and could use it against you. If you had had a live telephone conversation with the person or met with him or her in person, there would be no documentation unless someone recorded the conversation.

Computer security is major issue in today's world. Protect the security of your passwords, don't share passwords with anyone, and avoid using the same passwords at work that you use at home. Many companies require employees to change their passwords on a regular basis. Security can be compromised, so the potential exists that nonauthorized people could gain access to your email correspondence and your company's private and confidential information. Be sure to follow company policies that protect the security of computer systems and confidential information. Failure to do so could result in a breach of confidentiality, a violation of HIPAA and the HITECH Act laws, and embarrassment for you and your employer.

Written Communication

So far, we've focused on verbal, nonverbal, and electronic communication. Let's take a look at written communication skills.

Health care workers must be able to communicate effectively in writing. Some jobs rely more on written communication than others, but most everyone can benefit from improving their writing skills. Poor written communication skills can impede advancement in your career. Even if your job doesn't involve extensive writing, how you express yourself through written communication still has an impact on your work and your reputation.

In addition to jotting down telephone messages, communicating by email, and documenting patient information in charts and other records, health care workers need effective writing skills in order to compose:

- Memos, letters, and other correspondence
- Patient education materials
- Business reports
- Meeting agendas and notes
- Technical information
- Financial proposals
- Planning documents
- Research findings

There are several elements of effective written communication to keep in mind. These include:

- *Appearance.* Documents should be professional in appearance and easy to read.
- *Content.* Information should be accurate, up-to-date, and appropriate for intended readers.
- *Professionalism.* The appearance and content of the document should reflect the professionalism of the writer and his or her employer.
- *Relevance:* Documents should convey material that is interesting, meaningful, and of value to readers.
- *Sources.* Content should be factual and based on credible sources of information; when appropriate, sources should be referenced.
- *Organization.* Information should be concise, well organized, and include a brief introduction and summary.
- *Terminology.* Documents should use language and terminology that readers can easily understand and interpret.

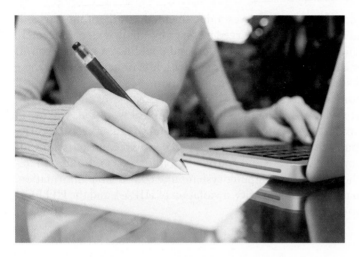

Figure 4-9 Practicing writing skills to make some improvements (*KieferPix/Shutterstock*)

- *Mechanics.* Writing should reflect proper spelling, grammar, and punctuation.
- *Illustrations.* Documents may include drawings, photographs, graphs, charts, tables, and so forth to help describe or explain the content.
- *Compliance.* Content must follow guidelines and meet legal requirements.
- *Distribution/access.* Access to documents that contain confidential and private information should be limited to authorized readers.

Here are some tips to improve your written communication:

- Keep your goals in mind. Know what you're trying to accomplish, and the reason why.
- Know your audience. Identify who you want to reach, the best way to reach them, and the reactions you are hoping to get.
- Create an outline. Organize your thoughts, identify the topics, and list your information in the proper sequence.
- Use complete sentences. Use words for numbers one through nine (such as *five*). Use numbers for quantities of 10 or more (such as *25*).
- For letters, include all of the components (date, subject line, salutation, body of the letter, closing, signature, and the sender's contact information).
- Use plain white paper and a standard black font.
- Print your document (such as a letter) on company or organization letterhead when appropriate.
- Follow company or organization policies when using a logo in a document.
- Proofread your work. Have another person review your document before sending or submitting it in case you missed something.
- Use the spell-check function on your computer but don't rely on it. Spell check won't catch words that are spelled correctly but used incorrectly. For example, the words *to*, *too*, and *two* will all pass as correctly spelled, but each word has a different meaning. Spell check may not work when it comes to medical terms.
- Make sure that medical terms are spelled correctly. Changing just one letter in a word can change the entire meaning. If you fill out forms to schedule tests or treatments for patients, order patient supplies, or process bills or other kinds of paperwork, make sure you can spell medical terms correctly.

- Use references such as a regular dictionary, a medical dictionary, a thesaurus, and a *Physician's Desk Reference (PDR)*.
- Use only standard medical abbreviations to avoid confusion.
- Do not use texting (text messaging) abbreviations.
- For long documents, include an executive summary and one or more separate attachments to reduce the length of the body.
- Include contact information and *next steps* to assist the reader in following up, if appropriate.

Depending on your job, your written documents may include charts, graphs, or tables. These illustrations help readers better understand the relationships between numbers and other data, and give meaning to information. Charts, graphs, and tables can be constructed on paper or via computer software. Health care workers should not only be familiar with how to create charts, graphs, and tables but also how to use and interpret them.

Public Speaking and Presentation Skills

No discussion about communication in health care would be complete without addressing the topic of public speaking. Few challenges in life are more anxiety-producing than having to get up in front of a group of people and make a presentation. But public speaking skills are important, especially if your job requires you to give updates at meetings, make announcements to the rest of the staff, or teach coworkers something new. You may be invited to speak at a workshop or conference as a representative of your company or your professional group, so developing your presentation skills is important.

Becoming comfortable with public speaking is like facing any other fear—the more you do it, the better you'll get, and the more comfortable you will become. Start out small with a group of supportive people and build from there. Make sure you're well prepared, organized, and familiar with the subject matter. Learn as much about your audience in advance as you can and tailor your presentation to meet their needs. Expect questions and comments; have your responses in mind. It's okay to admit that you're nervous. Most of the people in the audience will be glad it's you up in front of the group instead of them.

Here's some helpful information about the elements of effective public speaking:

- *Room setup.* Arrange the room so that audience members can easily see you, hear you, and view any visual aids that you might be using.
- *Goals.* Keep your goals in mind and make sure your audience knows what they are. If you want your audience to focus on something specific, make your intent clear.
- *Handouts.* If you're using an agenda and/or handouts, provide them in advance or at the beginning of your presentation. Allow space on the pages for people to take notes if they wish to do so. Depending on the setting, you might want to provide notepads and pens.
- *Introduction.* If audience members don't already know you, be sure to introduce yourself. Include personal and professional information that's relevant to your subject.
- *Content.* Keep the needs of your audience in mind. Your presentation should cover accurate, factual, up-to-date information that's interesting and relevant to your audience.
- *Organization.* Your content should be well thought out, with topics following a logical sequence. Your audience should be able to follow along from the beginning to the end of your presentation.
- *Notes.* Have an outline or some notes handy, along with a list of points that you want to make, but don't read your notes. Look at your audience and speak directly to them.

- *Eye contact.* Depending on the size of your audience, try to make eye contact with everyone. Don't direct all or most of your comments to just one person or one side of the room.
- *Language.* Use language and terms that your listeners can easily understand and interpret. Use proper grammar and avoid slang and unprofessional language.
- *Behavior.* Avoid irritating gestures and movements, such as waving your hands, crossing your arms, tapping your feet, pacing across the room, and sticking your hands in your pockets.
- *Visuals.* Use PowerPoint slides, handouts, or other visual aids that will help audience members understand your comments.
- *Participation.* Encourage audience participation whenever possible. Engaging people will help you hold their attention and they will be more likely to remember what happened during the session.
- *Group dynamics.* Manage questions and comments by audience members. Don't let a few people control the discussion or consume too much time.
- *Rules.* Stay within your allotted amount of time. If you end your presentation too early you'll look unprepared. If you run too long you'll inconvenience other speakers and your audience members. If your presentation is sponsored by a company or organization that has guidelines for its speakers, make sure you follow them.

Here are some tips to improve your presentation skills:

- Practice your presentation ahead of time. Ask family members or friends to serve as audience members and give you some helpful feedback.
- A few days before your presentation, stop by the room where you will be speaking. Familiarize yourself with the layout of the room and the location of light switches and other controls. If possible, practice using the microphone, projection equipment, and audio controls.
- Provide a comfortable environment for your audience. Make sure the room isn't too hot or too cold. If your presentation is scheduled during meal time, consider offering refreshments or encouraging people to bring their own.
- Arrange seating so that everyone may comfortably face the speaker. If people are seated at round tables, encourage them to turn their chairs around to face the front of the room.
- If you're using visual aids that appear on a screen at the front of the room, don't turn your back on your audience. Have a copy of your visuals in front of you so you may continue to face your listeners.
- Make sure that handouts and visual aids are professional in appearance and content.
- When considering what to wear, remember these two statements: "When you look good, you feel good" and "Professional image is in the eye of the beholder." Dress comfortably and select clothing that's appropriate for the setting and the audience. What might the audience expect in terms of a professional image? Don't overdress or underdress for the occasion.
- Avoid overused words and phrases such as "um," "uh," "like," and "you know."
- If you don't know the answer to an audience member's question, admit it. Offer to follow up with the person after the session.
- Take advantage of the expertise within the audience. Members may have some good ideas and experience to share.
- Show your sense of humor. If you make a mistake, admit it and laugh at yourself.
- Keep the session moving. If you lose your place or forget what you were going to say, just move on. Chances are your audience won't realize what happened.

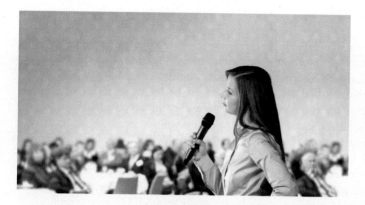

Figure 4-10 Using public speaking skills (*Halfpoint/Shutterstock*)

THE MORE YOU KNOW

DEVELOPING YOUR PUBLIC SPEAKING SKILLS

Based on surveys, people fear public speaking even more than getting cancer or dying. Learning to give effective oral presentations is just like developing any other skill—you need practice and more practice to become competent and confident.

There are lots of opportunities to develop your skills. The formal route would be to join an organization such as Toastmasters International. In operation since 1924, Toastmasters has 15,400 clubs in 135 countries. Clubs hold one- to two-hour meetings depending on the location. Instead of listening to lectures by an instructor, Toastmaster participants complete a series of "speaking assignments" to improve their public speaking skills. They give presentations and lead meetings in a "no-pressure atmosphere" and receive helpful feedback from other members.

Other options for developing your public speaking skills include volunteering to serve on committees at work, school, church, and in your community. Committee work often includes leading discussions, facilitating meetings, and giving informal reports. You could also join a health care professional group and gain valuable experience in both giving and listening to presentations.

If the thought of public speaking scares you, there's no time like the present to start building your skills. Who knows? One day *you* may become a highly paid, in-demand public speaker yourself.

Some people are *born speakers* while others are not. If you fall into the "not a born speaker" category, then expect sweaty palms, wobbly knees, shaky voice, and a stomach *tied in knots* until you become comfortable speaking in front of a group of people. A fear of public speaking can be detrimental to your career, so the sooner you start honing your public speaking skills, the better.

Your personality type, generational characteristics, background, and culture all impact how you form interpersonal relationships and communicate and work with other people. The next chapter explores cultural competence and how it applies in patient care settings.

REALITY CHECK

How well you interact with other people is where "the rubber meets the road" in health care. From the first day you walk in the door to begin your new job, your people skills will be front and center. You might be the highest-skilled person in your entire company when it comes to the hands-on, technical skills of your job. But if you fail to form and maintain effective working relationships with your coworkers, your high degree of competence will soon be overshadowed by your lack of interpersonal skills. If you get labeled as a loner, troublemaker, or complainer, other people won't want to work with you and your supervisor will regret hiring you. Once this happens, you'll need to either change your ways or change your job and start over again.

Complying with etiquette and netiquette standards and using good manners isn't difficult. In fact, treating other people in a polite, considerate manner should just be common sense. But too many people have forgotten the lessons they learned as children, and they've become adults totally focused on themselves. If you want to succeed in health care, you have to put the needs of other people ahead of your own. It's not about you. It's always about the patient—no matter what your job involves. Forming interpersonal relationships, serving as a good team player, and displaying manners and effective communication skills will go a long way in preventing conflicts and working well with other people.

For More Information

Etiquette and Manners
Emily Post
www.emilypost.com

Public Speaking Skills
Toastmasters International
www.toastmasters.org

Conflict Resolution
Association for Conflict Resolution
www.acrnet.org

Health Literacy
U.S. Department of Health and Human Services
**www.hrsa.gov/publichealth/healthliteracy/
healthlitabout.html**

Robert's Rules of Order
www.robertsrules.com

KEY POINTS

- Work hard to develop and maintain positive relationships with other people.
- Consider coworkers your internal customers and treat them with kindness and respect.
- Display a friendly attitude, cooperate with people, and create a positive work environment.
- Be inclusive and welcome people into your group.
- Treat other people as they want to be treated.

- Show loyalty to your coworkers and your employer.
- Practice good etiquette and manners and treat everyone with courtesy.
- Remember the standards for netiquette when communicating online.
- Develop effective team skills and use group norms when necessary.
- Strive to achieve consensus when making group decisions.
- Be aware of body language and the nonverbal messages you send.
- Listen carefully to make sure you hear and understand what's being said.
- Hone your assertive communication skills and use them to resolve conflicts.
- Use caution when communicating electronically.
- Sharpen your written communication and public speaking skills.

LEARNING ACTIVITIES

Using information from Chapter Four:
- Answer the Chapter Review Questions
- Respond to the What If? Scenarios

Chapter Review Questions

Using information presented in Chapter Four, answer each of the following questions.
1. Explain the concept of interdependence among health care workers.

2. List three ways to strengthen relationships at work.

3. List two ways to demonstrate loyalty to your coworkers.

4. Explain the role of courtesy, etiquette, and manners in the workplace.

5. List three examples of netiquette when using digital communication.

6. Give examples of two types of health care teams.

7. Describe how group norms can help facilitate meetings.

8. Explain why consensus is important but difficult to achieve.

9. List the four essential elements for communication to take place.

10. Describe how illiteracy impacts patient care.

11. Explain two of the factors that may influence your communication with other people.

12. Explain why labeling is a barrier to communication.

13. Describe the role that body language plays in communication.

14. Explain why conflict resolution is important in the workplace.

15. Name the four styles of communication.

16. Describe each of the four styles of communication including the likely outcome of each style.

17. Identify the importance of assertive communication.

18. List three types of communication technologies.

19. List three problems that may occur when communicating electronically.

20. Explain why it's important for health care professionals to develop their public speaking and presentation skills.

What If? Scenarios

Think about what you would do in the following situations and record your answers.

1. Your supervisor has given you a project to complete. There's no way you can possibly get it done by yourself in time to meet the deadline. Your coworkers have expressed willingness to help, but you're used to working alone.

2. Three coworkers approach you, angry about a new policy. They're rounding up support to complain to management and want you to get involved.

3. A new person joins your work group. She's much older than everyone else and no one seems to like her. It's time to go to lunch and your coworkers leave her behind.

4. At an employee recognition dinner, the head of your company calls you to the stage to praise you for creating a new inventory tracking system. Although three of your coworkers helped you a lot, their names aren't mentioned.

5. Your company offers a six-month, part-time equipment repair course free of charge to employees. Those who enroll get to attend the classes on paid time. The company also pays the fee for course graduates to become certified as equipment repair technicians. After completing the course and becoming certified, you spot an advertisement recruiting certified equipment repair technicians for a company that competes with your employer and pays more.

6. You've been on call the last two weekends and it's your turn to be off. At the last minute, a coworker asks if there's any way you could take call for her this weekend. Her brother was seriously injured in a car accident and needs her help taking care of his children for a couple of days. You don't have any plans yourself, but you've already taken call two weekends in a row.

7. One of your coworkers is really beginning to annoy you. He takes longer breaks than he's supposed to and seems to disappear when there's work to be done. This morning, he kept a patient waiting for 20 minutes while he made several personal phone calls. When you remind him he has a patient waiting, he says, "Mind your own business! I'll get to him when I'm ready!"

8. You hear through the grapevine that a coworker has been spreading gossip about you. You're so angry that, as soon as she walks in the room, you're anxious to tell her just what you think of her behavior.

9. One of your coworkers is on corrective action for misspelling several medical terms on patient records. Unless she passes a medical terminology test by the end of the month, her job could be in jeopardy. She's lost her confidence and isn't sure if she can do it.

10. Your teammate finds out that you expressed doubts about his competence on a recent 360-degree performance evaluation initiated by his supervisor and now he wants to speak with you. You value your relationship with him but you're leaving on vacation early tomorrow morning and you're in a hurry to get home. Your teammate has already left work for the day. Sending him a text message from home tonight would be the quickest way to explain your input on his performance evaluation.

11. A patient has returned to your practice three times in the past month. You keep reminding him of the importance of taking all of his medications at the proper time but he isn't following the instructions.

12. You wrote an email message expressing anger about your supervisor and sent it to a coworker. A few days later your coworker admits that she accidently forwarded your message to your supervisor and your supervisor's boss.

5

Cultural Competence and Patient Care

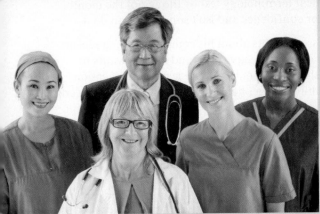

How far you go in life depends on your being tender with the young, compassionate with the aged, sympathetic with the striving and tolerant of the weak and strong. Because someday in life you will have been all of these.

—George Washington Carver (1861–1943), agricultural chemist

(Rawpixel.com/Shutterstock)

CHAPTER OBJECTIVES

Having completed this chapter, you will be able to:

- Give three examples of diversity in addition to age and gender.
- Explain how bias can result in health care disparities for members of minority cultural groups.
- List two things to do when cultural tension arises.
- Explain why health care workers need to be culturally competent.
- Describe the difference between stereotypes and generalizations.
- Explain what is meant by the cultural competence continuum.
- Describe two ways that online patient portals can improve health care.

- Explain how a person's personality type can affect his or her work.
- Give an example of how generational differences can cause problems at work.
- List four types of health care customers.
- Describe the purpose of the American Hospital Association's brochure, "Patient Care Partnership: Understanding Expectations, Rights and Responsibilities."
- Explain the purpose of the HCAHPS survey.
- List five ways to provide good customer service for hospitalized patients and their visitors.

KEY TERMS

advance directive

advocates

cultural competence

cultures

dictate

discrimination

emancipated

empathetic

expressed consent

extenders

extroverts

generalizations

HCAHPS

healing environments

health disparities

implied consent

incapacitated

introverts

noncompliant

norms

patient portals

political correctness

role models

stereotypes

surrogate

transparency

Diversity and Cultural Competence

Diversity and Culture

One of the challenges in forming effective working relationships is getting along with people who you might see as different from you. You're probably familiar with the term *diversity* as it relates to racial differences (Caucasian, Black, Asian, etc.). Diversity includes other kinds of differences as well, based on cultural influences such as gender, age or the era in which you grew up, ethnic background, sexual orientation, religious beliefs, socioeconomic status, physical or mental conditions, occupation, neighborhood, family size, language, and more.

Cultures are formed when groups of people share the same values and **norms** (expectations or guidelines for behavior). We all belong to multiple cultural groups at the same time. Depending on the situation, different cultures may take priority. For example, while you may belong to a large, rural, religiously focused family that holds well-established values about education and professionalism, your generational cultural norms might take priority over your religious culture when deciding how to dress appropriately for work.

Cultural groups share values and beliefs about what's most important to them. People in the nursing culture, for example, value disease prevention and keeping their patient safe. Cultural norms are the rules that members accept as normal: "the way we do things around here." These rules are learned (taught) and aren't usually written down, but they're well understood by members of the cultural group. Members of each cultural group instill their norms and values by way of customs, rituals, use of language, rewards and punishment, and modeling appropriate behaviors. Although they generally fall in line with the norms, behaviors by individuals of the cultural group may vary considerably. (Indeed, there is usually more diversity within a cultural group than between cultures.)

How do values, norms, and behaviors influence a particular cultural group? Let's take a look at the value of "respecting your body and health." Some of the norms or rules that apply to "respecting your body and health" might include focus on disease prevention, follow sound medical advice, eat nutritious food, exercise regularly, and avoid smoking. Although members of the cultural group share the same core value ("respecting your body and health") and understand the common norms, individuals will follow the norms with various behaviors. For example, using the *value* of respecting your body and the *norm* of eating nutritious food might mean *behaviors* of eating only organic for some, or vegetarian for other individuals, or a mixture of lean protein and veggies with treats of high-fat, sugary desserts for others.

Why is it important to understand the difference between values, norms, and behaviors? Because it's easy to make judgments about other people based on their behaviors when you filter

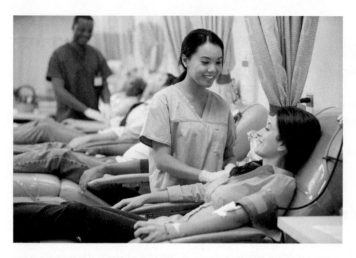

Figure 5-1 Diversity at work in health care (*Monkey Business Images/Shutterstock*)

those behaviors through your own cultural norms. You can't always identify another person's values or norms by their behaviors. This is where the cultural problem occurs. Once you start making judgments about other people, your decisions as well as your actions can become biased. Research shows that biased decision making by health care professionals can lead to **health disparities** (unfair misdiagnosis and treatment) among members of minority cultural groups.

Let's apply an example of how all of these concepts can play out at work. When you have a patient who doesn't take her prescription drugs as directed, you might label her as **noncompliant** (refusing or failing to follow instructions) and assume that she doesn't care about her body or her health or preventing disease. Perhaps you come from a medical culture where taking a prescription drug is readily accepted and you would expect the patient's behavior to be in line with that (your) norm. However, the patient who may not take the prescription drug as directed probably *does* value her body and her good health. She may have had a cultural upbringing with a norm of avoiding taking drugs of any kind. So when her behavior includes failing to take her prescription drugs as advised, her behavior is falling in line with her cultural norm, *but not yours*. You know that her condition would be greatly improved with the medication. Tension can creep into the interaction. (You're working hard and have given her reliable advice and direction that really would help. From your point of view, she is resistant, noncompliant, and unreasonable in her rationale for not taking the drug.) So, in response, you may have a tone of impatience, may disregard her preference for considering holistic solutions, may work with her a bit less, and may even blame her at some level for her condition. You may even disregard symptoms of something else because she has already demonstrated not complying with medical advice (even though the other symptoms may not need a prescription-related treatment). Actions are taken (or avoided) based on cultural differences, and a disparity has occurred. Yet the patient shares the same value as you of caring about her health, demonstrating that behaviors are unreliable in assessing a person's values.

When cultural tension arises, it is usually because of different expectations around the cultural norms, not the values. When there is cultural tension, what can you do?

- Examine the assumptions about the behaviors relating to values; look to discover how the norms differ. Learn to understand and accept the existence of different sets of cultural norms.

- Focus on discovering the values you and the other person share. Many core values are shared. Finding the shared value can lead to a deeper understanding of the cultural dynamics and the resulting behaviors, and lead to different solutions.
- Mutually work toward behavioral change, with more collaboration, because the values have not been challenged.

Think about it. Would you want someone else trying to change your values? No, of course not. But if you realize that you both have similar values and you both might need to change your behaviors or expand your cultural norms to get a good result, it might be easier to find ways to work together.

CASE STUDY

Carla told her manager about the social media etiquette discussion at the staff meeting and her interest in developing some new policies to help everyone understand the issues and behavioral standards involved. Not only did Carla's manager like the idea, she had been thinking the same thing herself. The manager had recently attended a workshop on the topic and everyone agreed that something needed to be done. The network's human resource director was forming a new committee to draft a set of new policies and Carla's manager asked if Carla would like to participate as a member. Of course, Carla said yes. Later on, thinking back on the conversation, Carla was reminded of something she had learned early in her career. People who perform well and come up

with good ideas to help the practice function even better are often rewarded with additional work assignments. That was okay with Carla. Helping the practice and its employees provide even better patient care was at the heart of everything she did.

When the network's human resource director convened the first meeting of the new Social Media Policies and Procedures Committee, Carla was struck by the size and makeup of the group. Looking around the room, she noticed a diverse cross-section of not only the network's staff but also its patient base. People representing various age groups as well as an array of racial and ethnic backgrounds and genders and sexual orientations had been added to the team. The HR director started the meeting by explaining that

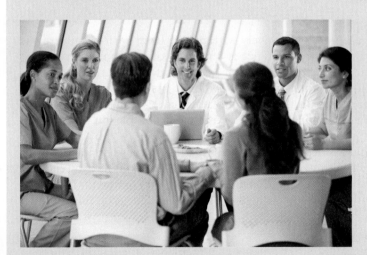

Figure 5-2 Meeting with a diverse group of staff members (*Monkey Business Images/Shutterstock*)

(continued)

the use of social media has broad implications for the network itself as well as for its staff members, doctors, and patients. Developing fair and effective policies and procedures requires input from everyone. Recognizing the diversity within the team, the director led a discussion about group norms and, once developed, the norms were posted on the wall to remind everyone of the guidelines under which they would operate.

As the meetings got underway and the group progressed with its work, personality differences emerged along with conflicting opinions and ideas. Variations among age groups became evident. Younger employees reported frequent use of social media while some of the older staff members mostly voiced their complaints. The sessions reminded Carla of how difficult updating the dress code policies had become from year to year. But over time the social media group came together with some common ground and the policies and procedures were drafted. After a lengthy review by various network departments and some employee focus groups, the documents were approved and circulated for everyone to read. Carla covered the material at her next in-service session and, for the most part, the information received a positive response from the staff.

Carla had learned a lot over the years by serving on different teams. Her first committee assignment was on the network's newly formed Patient Satisfaction Committee. Back then, collecting data from patients as a means of improving customer service had been voluntary. Once patient satisfaction data became a requirement and leaders understood that involving patients in the decision-making process was the key to motivating people to improve their health, the group changed its name to the Patient Engagement Team and broadened its efforts. The results had led to significant improvements but overall the network wasn't quite where it wanted to be with its patient engagement goals just yet.

Things were going well until one day when a transgender woman arrived at the practice for her doctor's appointment. After a brief encounter with a staff member at the check-in window, followed by the sound of laughter and an exceptionally long wait hoping to see a doctor, the patient asked to speak with someone in management. Carla got the call.

What should Carla do to make sure the patient's needs are met and she is treated with dignity and respect? What would you do if you were in Carla's place?

Cultural Competence

Cultural competence (the ability to interact effectively with people from various cultures) is crucial for health care workers. Cultural competence is a process of continual learning by being open to how their cultures influence people. Become confident in your ability to manage your responses to different cultures, including your own cultures. Cultural competence supports teamwork and helps ensure that decisions about patient care are made in an ethical and unbiased manner and without **discrimination** (unfair treatment of a person or group on the basis of prejudice).

Cultural competence is not about **political correctness** (eliminating language or practices that could offend social sensibilities about cultural groups such as race and gender). When you encounter conflict that is caused by cultural differences in behaviors and norms, try to find the core value behind the norm. Once you've identified the core value that people share, focus on this common ground to help resolve the conflict.

Here are some key strategies:

- Examine your own cultural norms first. Be aware that you experience other cultures through your own filters. Accept multiple approaches to "the way we do things around here."
- Be prepared to adjust your filters. If you don't understand another person's culture, ask him or her to share some information. Listen for understanding rather than defending your way.

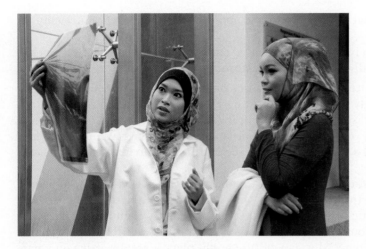

Figure 5-3 Diversity in the health care workforce (*EncikAn/Shutterstock*)

- Your goal isn't to avoid judgment or prejudice. Your goal is to acknowledge that judgment and prejudice exist and to learn to manage them. Remember that judgment and prejudice are thoughts that can be changed before taking action.
- Expose yourself to cultures that are different from yours. Stay, even if you feel uncomfortable. Discomfort is a sign that you're learning something.
- Learn to distinguish between **stereotypes** (beliefs that are mainly false about a group of people) and **generalizations** (facts, patterns, and trends about groups of people that are backed up by statistics and research findings).

Cultural competence occurs on a continuum. It begins with a lack of awareness and concludes with inclusion and integration. Here are the stages:

- *Unaware.* (You are truly unaware of a cultural situation.)
- *Denial.* (You say, "Oh, that doesn't really happen here." Or, "What? I thought that ended years ago.")
- *Defensiveness.* (You defend your own position as *the right one*. You say, "Oh, yeah? Well that's not as bad as what happened to me or my people." Or, "If your cultural group would work harder, you would be able to live like us.")
- *Repulsion.* (You say, "How could they live like that?" Or, "There's no way I could accept those people.")
- *Pity.* (You say, "If only they would . . . they could improve their lives. Or, "It's so sad those people live the way they do. It's too bad their lives aren't more like mine.")
- *Minimization.* (You say, "I don't care if someone is black or pink or green." This minimizes the impact that color or some other characteristic may have had on a group of people.)
- *Tolerance.* (You say, "Well, I guess I just have to put up with this person or group of people.")
- *Admiration.* (You say, "I admire people from [cultural group]. They've had to fight hard for justice.")

- *Acceptance.* (You recognize that diversity exists and appreciate the benefits that diversity brings.)
- *Inclusion and integration.* (You recognize the essential nature of diversity and actively seek ways to include and integrate diversity. You advocate for diversity.)

Think about where your cultural competence lies on this continuum and adjust your filters and behaviors accordingly. Be aware that in every new situation, you may be in a different stage of competence. Listen to your own thoughts to get a sense of your attitude and cultural perspectives. When you feel like someone is being hypersensitive, research historical events that may have had a lasting impact on the cultural group in which the person identifies.

Applying these concepts at work is really important because you need a variety of people with diverse perspectives to get the work done. If you're developing a new policy for your department, for example, you might look at the situation differently than a coworker who is much younger or older than yourself. A single woman might have a different perspective than a married man. Someone from a Mexican culture might place a greater value on a particular issue in the policy than someone from a Brazilian culture. An entry-level employee with life experience may offer different valuable insights than a seasoned, formally educated professional. All points of view must be taken into consideration to accommodate our diverse workforce. Let's start by examining differences in personality preferences.

PROFESSIONALISM ONLINE

DIVERSITY IN SOCIAL MEDIA AND ONLINE RESOURCES FOR PATIENTS

If you're looking for common ground among diverse groups of Americans, the widespread use of social media is a good place to start. According to an August 2015 report from the Pew Research Center by Maeve Duggan, the use of social media cuts across factors such as gender, race, age, and location. Of all U.S. adults who go online and use the Internet, 72% use Facebook, 23% use Twitter, 28% use Instagram, and 25% use LinkedIn.

About 70% of Facebook users log on daily, 21% weekly, and 9% less often. Among all online adults, who uses Facebook on a frequent basis? Here are some demographics:

- 77% of women
- 66% of men
- 70% of White, non-Hispanics
- 67% of Black, non-Hispanics
- 75% of Hispanics
- 82% of people ages 18-29
- 79% of people ages 30-49
- 64% of people ages 50-64
- 48% of people ages 65 and over
- 74% of people in urban settings
- 72% of people in suburban settings
- 67% of people in rural settings

To view the entire report, go to: www.pewinternet.org/2015/08/19/the-demographics-of-social-media-users/

Online Resources for Patients

In addition to communicating via social media, the Internet offers many resources for patients and opportunities to improve patient care. Online **patient portals**, for example, enhance patient involvement by giving people 24/7 access to their personal health information. Patients can communicate with their caregivers; check lab and test results; review medical records and clinical summaries; access information on diagnoses, medications, allergies, and immunizations; and view their medical bills and make payments all via secure websites. More than half of health care providers now offer patient portals and receive financial incentives for doing so via health care reform initiatives.

The Internet also offers vast amounts of information on all types of medical conditions, diseases, injuries, medications, and treatment options, leading to patients who are better informed and more engaged in their care than in the past. There's no doubt that digital technology can improve patient care and enhance patient–caregiver communication. But a whole host of problems can also arise. The challenge is how to use digital technology to its fullest potential without harming patients or health care providers.

Let's start with hacking. Although patient portals and electronic health records are set up on secure websites, they can still be hacked. Health care providers and health insurance companies have become primary targets for identity theft, releasing personal data such as the names, addresses, Social Security numbers, and birthdates of millions of Americans. Hackers can use and sell this information to get fake passports, take out loans, apply for credit cards, and file fraudulent tax returns. The problem appears to be getting worse. Over a recent five-year period, cases of identity theft via medical records have doubled. In just a three-year span, almost 30 million medical records were hacked. When such breaches of confidentiality are discovered, companies typically offer people free credit monitoring services for a period of time to help detect some types of criminal behavior.

Consumer Ratings and Online Information

Patients increasingly surf the Internet to find detailed information about their doctors and caregivers. Consumer ratings are now easily accessed online, providing feedback about doctors, malpractice claims, and performance reviews. Keep in mind that people can hide their identities and post anything they want

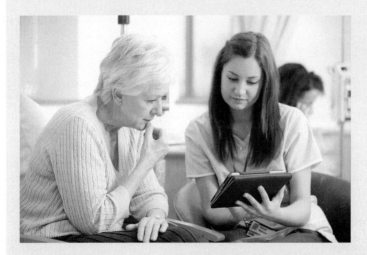

Figure 5-4 Explaining the benefits of a patient portal (*Monkey Business Images/Shutterstock*)

(*continued*)

to say about a particular doctor or health care provider whether the information is accurate and truthful or not. Once false or negative information is posted, it's very difficult to get it deleted. Efforts are underway to improve accountability and **transparency** (open, clear, and capable of being seen) when posting such information, and professional organizations and licensing boards are joining forces to establish fair standards.

Patients, doctors, and health care workers now have access to more detailed information about one another than ever before, and it's changing the way we interact and feel about each other. Online information includes where we live, where we travel and vacation, and details about our children, hobbies, sexual orientation, religious affiliations, and political preferences. Patients may Google you, so make sure that the information you post about yourself, as well as the information that other people share about you, supports your professional reputation. If patients find videos or photos of you smoking cigarettes, taking illegal drugs, or engaging in other unhealthy habits, they might be less likely to try to curb those habits themselves.

This bears stating again: Don't put any content, photos, or other information about patients on your Facebook page or other social media sites that could lead to embarrassment, anger, or HIPAA violations. Even if you haven't identified the patients, they could still identify themselves by what you've said about them. Remember, it's a small world out there. Some of your friends might be the friends of your patients, and they, too, could identify the patients you've described online.

Don't Google your patients! Discovering personal details about patients could lead to judgments, bias, and health disparities in how you relate to your patients at work. Differences in religion, politics, or sexual orientation, for example, should not affect the care you deliver unless it directly relates to the patient's health status. This is just one example of why you must avoid blurring the boundaries between personal and professional roles. Don't contact patients outside of business needs. Don't respond to Facebook "friend" requests from patients. Don't solicit patients to buy cookies or other fundraising products from your children. And don't socialize with patients after hours. Maintaining professional boundaries has become more difficult because social media are so intertwined in our lives. But it's absolutely critical in protecting your professional reputation and the trust that patients must have in their caregivers.

Personality Preferences

Just as you are a unique person with your own personality and individual preferences, so are the people with whom you come in contact. Personality types or preferences vary widely and they influence how people interact with one another and how they participate (or don't participate) in a group setting. Personality types also influence how people size up situations, make decisions, and approach their work.

Learn as much as you can about your own personality type and gain some insight into the personality types of the people that you work with. There are many personality assessments available through the Internet and career counseling centers. Here are a couple of examples.

The Myers-Briggs Type Indicator (MBTI)

The MBTI is based on Carl Jung's psychological theories about how people differ in perception and judgment. Perception is how people become aware of things and take in new information. Judgment is how people arrive at conclusions based on what they have perceived. The MBTI focuses on eight sets of preferences and identifies 16 different personality types based on those preferences. For example, some people are **introverts** (people who predominantly focus inwardly) while others are **extroverts** (people who predominantly focus outwardly). Some people want to make decisions and bring closure to their work while others prefer to remain open to more options and new approaches.

Keirsey Temperament Sorter–II (KTS-II)

The KTS-II is another widely used personality assessment. Based on Dr. David Keirsey's theory, behavior can be described in one of four "temperament groups," with each group subdivided into four "character types." The temperament groups and character types align with the 16 different MBTI personality types. According to Dr. Keirsey, temperament is based on a combination of personality traits, behavioral patterns, values, etc. Each temperament has its own characteristics. For example, some people talk about reality and everyday life—facts, figures, news, etc. Other people talk about the abstract world of ideas, dreams, and beliefs. Some people behave in a practical manner that is focused on getting results. Other people behave in a cooperative manner that is focused on social interactions more so than outcomes.

There is no "right" type or "wrong" type on either the MBTI or Keirsey assessments—just different types. By becoming aware of your own personality type and the types of other people around you, you'll be in a better position to understand differences and make the most of them.

Generational Differences

If you've had a job working with people from different age groups, you've probably already experienced some generational differences. Let's take a look at the characteristics of the four generations found in today's workforce.

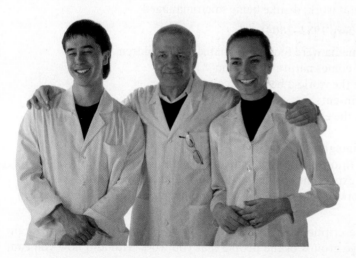

Figure 5-5 Different generations working together (*Tatiana Belova/Shutterstock*)

The Silent Generation (born 1923–1944)

- Arrived during the Great Depression and World War II
- Believe in working hard, paying your dues, and clean living
- Value stability and security; resist borrowing and debt
- Don't like surprises; prefer clear lines of authority (reporting to one boss)

The Baby Boomers (born 1945–1964)

- Largest generation; post–World War II baby boom
- Every life stage has been trendsetting; their impact can't be ignored
- "If you have it, flaunt it" attitude
- Competitive, stylish, bossy, and curious
- Like shopping, leading, creating a vision; dislike paying debts and growing older
- Economy was growing; plenty of job opportunities after college
- Tend to stay in their jobs; double Gen-Xers in number, so Gen-Xers may have trouble "moving up the ladder"

Generation X (born 1961–1981)

- Unlike Baby Boomers, they arrived almost unnoticed
- The economic boom was fading; saw their parents struggle with employment
- May have been "latchkey kids" who are independent, figure things out on their own
- The cynical generation; invented the term "whatever"
- Broken homes and divorce were common; may have been raised by two sets of parents
- Value friends, relationships, and loyalty
- Caught in the middle of economic change and companies in transition
- Naturally impatient; thrive on change
- Expect to be respected; but it may take time before they develop respect for other people
- Like surprises, fun, and humor at work; dislike being micromanaged

The Millennials/Generation Y (born 1982–2004)

- Arrived when society and the media were focused on babies and children
- Grew up with technology, so it comes naturally to them
- Want to get involved and make the world a better place
- Caring, honest, optimistic, clean-cut
- Like shopping, friends, family, the environment; dislike dishonesty and unbalanced lifestyles
- Respond to leaders who show integrity
- Like to be challenged, try new things, and learn in a hands-on manner
- Want to continually learn and expect the workplace to provide that opportunity
- Work isn't their life, they fit work into life; will leave an organization if work/life balance and growth aren't included

As you can tell by reading these descriptions, generational differences can have a big impact in the workplace. Think about the age groups of the people that you work with and how you can make the most of these generational characteristics. As you progress in your career and gain some leadership skills, familiarity with generational differences will become even more important as you figure out how to motivate, challenge, and reward each individual.

BY THE NUMBERS_____

THE GENERATIONAL DIVIDE BETWEEN MILLENNIALS AND BABY BOOMERS

There's more than just an age difference between Millennials and Baby Boomers. It starts with labels. Less than half of adults between the ages of 18 and 34 identify themselves as *Millennials*, while nearly 80% of those between 51 and 69 years of age see themselves as *Baby Boomers*.

Let's take a look at the Millennial generation:

- Millennials comprise the most educated generation in the United States, with 34% having a bachelor's degree or higher.
- By the year 2020, one in three adults will be millennials.
- About 70% of Millennials have never married. When they do marry, about 15% of them marry someone from another race or ethnicity as compared with just 3% of Baby Boomers in the 1960s. Half of Millennials think that interracial marriage is a positive step for society as compared with just 30% of Boomers.
- A larger percentage of Millennials is delaying starting a family and purchasing a home as compared with Baby Boomers at the same age years ago.
- Many Millennials are willing to forgo a promotion or take a pay cut to have more flexibility in where, when, and how they work. They would rather earn much less pay doing a job they really like than to earn much more pay doing a job they intensely dislike.
- Millennials prefer a team-oriented workplace as opposed to working as an individual.
- Almost 30% of Millennials do not affiliate with an organized religion, and half are political independents.
- Despite their college degrees, Millennials rank below their peers in other countries in the areas of math, literacy, and high-tech problem-solving skills.
- About 40% of Millennials have at least one tattoo.

When it comes to the Baby Boomer generation:

- Another Baby Boomer turns 50 years of age every seven seconds.
- In 1957 when the "boom" reached its peak, about eight Boomers were born every minute.

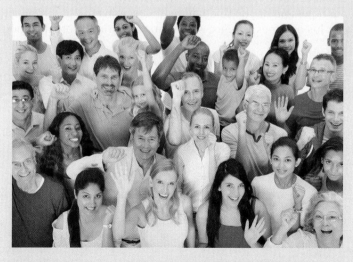

Figure 5-6 Millennials and Baby Boomers celebrating together (*Rawpixel.com/Shutterstock*)

(continued)

- Almost two-thirds of Baby Boomers ages 50–61 plan to delay retirement, mostly because they want to keep working.
- Baby Boomers will likely become the longest-living generation in U.S. history. Average retirees will have a pension income for about 24 years.
- Baby Boomers are more likely to have a home computer than Millennials, and almost as many Boomers own smartphones as do people younger than they.
- More than 80% of Boomers communicate via texting and are much more likely to own a digital tablet than members of other generations.
- Only 15% of Baby Boomers have a tattoo.

Respecting Differences

Diversity and respect go hand in hand. Regardless of whether you're working with people just like yourself or people who are different from you, respect is the basis for getting along well with everyone. Once you understand how people differ from one another and you realize there aren't "good people" or "bad people"—just "different people"—you can learn to respect everyone regardless of their differences.

Much has already been said about the need to show respect for people. But it's especially important to show your respect for employees who work in service and support roles such as housekeepers and food service workers. The health care culture places great value on its highly educated clinical caregivers such as registered nurses, doctors, and pharmacists. But lower-skilled workers often feel like they're at the bottom of the ladder, sometimes treated as if they're almost invisible. As a result, they may feel underappreciated and taken for granted. Take time to acknowledge their efforts and let them know that you value and respect the work they do.

The same is true for people above you on the occupational ladder. You may see highly educated people failing to give subordinates (including you) the credit they deserve. Try to give them the benefit of the doubt and don't take their lack of appreciation personally. When people function under stress, they don't always take time to thank other people for their efforts. Always respect authority. Even if you dislike your supervisor as a person, or you find fault with his or her job performance, it's still important to show respect for his or her experience and position within the organization.

CONSIDER THIS

OCCUPATIONAL CULTURES

In health care, another type of culture is the occupation in which you work. Registered nurses, for example, have a culture based on their educational background, where they work, what functions they perform, and the knowledge and abilities they possess. Physicians have a culture too, as do medical technologists, maintenance workers, and so forth.

In health care organizations, there's a hierarchy based on these cultures and it sometimes causes problems. One example is **extenders** (people whose job is to assist other workers who have more education or higher credentials). Patient care assistants, patient care technicians, and nursing assistants are examples of nurse extenders. Sometimes called "unlicensed assistive personnel," these employees lack the training and credentials that RNs have but they work alongside RNs. Housekeepers and phlebotomists may also be assigned to work on patient care units. Sometimes extenders and other employees may have trouble fitting in and feeling like they're part of the team.

As mentioned earlier, cross-training has become common in health care. Since multiskilled workers are trained to function in more than one discipline, they often work in more than one area. They may encounter multiple cultures and might not feel totally accepted or comfortable in any one of them.

Health care teams are often composed of workers from different occupational cultures. Surgical teams, for example, include surgical technologists, surgical nurses, surgeons, and anesthesiologists. These teams are supported by schedulers, surgical attendants, instrument technicians, and others. Each type of worker has a different education level and scope of responsibility but all of them play important roles in the operating room.

Anytime someone "different" enters a group, he or she may experience difficulty fitting in and being accepted by others. This is a common problem when dealing with diversity. Do differences have to create difficult challenges? Is it really a problem if your coworkers are younger or older than you, of a different gender, or from a different race or ethnic group? Does it really matter if some have more education than you or less?

Everyone needs to work a little bit harder to get to know one another and figure out how to use differences to the group's advantage. The point is you're all there for the same purpose—to provide high-quality health care. Focusing on the mission of patient care gives diverse groups of workers some common ground to build upon.

Diversity is an absolute necessity because the world would be a stagnant and boring place if everyone were alike. Health care professionals serve a diverse array of patients. Ideally, the health care workforce should be as diverse as the patient population so that workers could see things from the patient's point of view. This is why many health care companies try to recruit new employees who possess some of the same diverse characteristics as their patients.

Working with Patients

Most of what you need to know when working with patients is covered in other classes that are directly related to your discipline and the types of patients with whom you will work. The remainder of this chapter focuses on patients as customers, exploring some of the factors involved in ensuring a high level of patient satisfaction. We also take a look at how to apply customer service standards when working with visitors, guests, vendors, and doctors—all of whom are considered customers of the health care industry. Depending on your job, you may deal with some or all of these different kinds of customers.

Before taking a closer look at customer service and the role it plays in patient care, let's examine patients' rights and responsibilities.

Patient Rights and Responsibilities

Patients, doctors, and health care professionals must work as a team to ensure quality health care services. Hospitals and other health care facilities have policies and procedures in place to facilitate this type of collaboration. Effective communication, respect for personal and professional values, and sensitivity to diversity are important factors in providing optimum care while protecting the rights of patients.

The American Hospital Association (AHA) published "A Patient's Bill of Rights" in 1973 and later revised the document in 1992. Hospitals were encouraged to tailor this Bill of Rights to their own communities so that patients and their families would be aware of, and understand, their rights and responsibilities. In 2003, the AHA replaced its Bill of Rights with a new brochure titled "Patient Care Partnership: Understanding Expectations, Rights and Responsibilities" to make the information easier to understand and to emphasize the importance of collaborative effort between the patient and his or her health care providers.

In situations where the patient is legally incompetent, under the legal age of full responsibility, or lacks decision-making capacity, someone else such as a family member or close friend may be designated to act as the patient's **surrogate** (substitute) to exercise the patient's rights on behalf of the patient. To the extent permitted by law and by hospital policy, hospitals are expected to

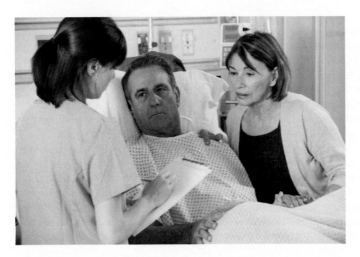

Figure 5-7 Discussing rights and responsibilities with a patient (*Monkey Business Images/Shutterstock*)

honor a patient's **advance directive** (a written instruction such as a living will recognized under state law relating to the provision of health care when the individual is permanently or temporarily impaired by a mental and/or physical condition) regarding his or her treatment and care.

The following information is from the AHA's brochure, "The Patient Care Partnership: Understanding Expectations, Rights and Responsibilities." This information is given to patients upon admission to the hospital to help explain their rights and how to exercise their rights.

What to expect during your hospital stay:

- High quality hospital care.
- A clean and safe environment.
- Involvement in your care.
- Protection of your privacy.
- Help when leaving the hospital.
- Help with your billing claims.

When you need hospital care, your doctor and the nurses and other professionals at our hospital are committed to working with you and your family to meet your health care needs. Our dedicated doctors and staff serve the community in all its ethnic, religious and economic diversity. Our goal is for you and your family to have the same care and attention we would want for our families and ourselves.

The sections explain some of the basics about how you can expect to be treated during your hospital stay. They also cover what we will need from you to care for you better. If you have questions at any time, please ask them. Unasked or unanswered questions can add to the stress of being in the hospital. Your comfort and confidence in your care are very important to us.

High quality hospital care. Our first priority is to provide you the care you need, when you need it, with skill, compassion and respect. Tell your caregivers if you have concerns about your care or if you have pain. You have the right to know the identity of doctors, nurses and others involved in your care, and you have the right to know when they are students, residents or other trainees.

A clean and safe environment. Our hospital works hard to keep you safe. We use special policies and procedures to avoid mistakes in your care and keep you free from abuse or neglect. If anything unexpected and significant happens during your hospital stay, you will be told what happened, and any resulting changes in your care will be discussed with you.

Involvement in your care. You and your doctor often make decisions about your care before you go to the hospital. Other times, especially in emergencies, those decisions are made during your hospital stay. When decision-making takes place, it should include:

- Discussing your medical condition and information about medically appropriate treatment choices.
- Discussing your treatment plan.
- Getting information from you.
- Understanding your health care goals and values.
- Understanding who should make decisions when you cannot.

Discussing your medical condition and information about medically appropriate treatment choices. To make informed decisions with your doctor, you need to understand:

- The benefits and risks of each treatment.
- Whether your treatment is experimental or part of a research study.
- What you can reasonably expect from your treatment and any long-term effects it might have on your quality of life.
- What you and your family will need to do after you leave the hospital.
- The financial consequences of using uncovered services or out-of-network providers.

Please tell your caregivers if you need more information about treatment choices.

Discussing your treatment plan. When you enter the hospital, you sign a general consent to treatment. In some cases, such as surgery or experimental treatment, you may be asked to confirm in writing that you understand what is planned and agree to it. This process protects your right to consent to or refuse a treatment. Your doctor will explain the medical consequences of refusing recommended treatment. It also protects your right to decide if you want to participate in a research study.

Getting information from you. Your caregivers need complete and correct information about your health and coverage so that they can make good decisions about your care. That includes:

- Past illnesses, surgeries or hospital stays.
- Past allergic reactions.
- Any medicines or dietary supplements (such as vitamins and herbs) that you are taking.
- Any network or admission requirements under your health plan.

Understanding your health care goals and values. You may have health care goals and values or spiritual beliefs that are important to your well-being. They will be taken into account as much as possible throughout your hospital stay. Make sure your doctor, your family and your care team know your wishes.

Understanding who should make decisions when you cannot. If you have signed a health care power of attorney stating who should speak for you if you become unable to make health care decisions for yourself, or a "living will" or "advance directive" that states your wishes about end-of-life care, give copies to your doctor, your family and your care team. If you or your family need help making difficult decisions, counselors, chaplains and others are available to help.

Protection of your privacy. We respect the confidentiality of your relationship with your doctor and other caregivers, and the sensitive information about your health and health care that are part of that relationship. State and federal laws and hospital operating policies protect the privacy of your medical information. You will receive a Notice of Privacy Practices that describes the ways that we use, disclose and safeguard patient information and that explains how you can obtain a copy of information from our records about your care.

Preparing you and your family for when you leave the hospital. Your doctor works with hospital staff and professionals in your community. You and your family also play an important role in your care. The success of your treatment often depends on your efforts to follow medication, diet and therapy plans. Your family may need to help care for you at home. You can expect us to help you identify sources of follow-up care and to let you know if our hospital has a financial interest in any referrals. As long as you agree that we can share information about your care with them, we will coordinate our activities with your caregivers outside the hospital. You can also expect to receive information and, where possible, training about the self-care you will need when you go home.

Help with your bill and filing insurance claims. Our staff will file claims for you with health care insurers or other programs such as Medicare and Medicaid. They also will help your doctor with needed documentation. Hospital bills and insurance coverage are often confusing. If you have questions about your bill, contact our business office. If you need help understanding your insurance coverage or health plan, start with your insurance company or health benefits manager. If you do not have health coverage, we will try to help you and your family find financial help or make other arrangements. We need your help with collecting needed information and other requirements to obtain coverage or assistance. (*From The Patient Care Partnership: Understanding Expectations, Rights and Responsibilities. Copyright © by American Hospital Association.*)

HOT TOPICS

RESIDENTS' RIGHTS IN NURSING HOMES

The Omnibus Budget Reconciliation Act (OBRA) was passed in 1987 to implement certain basic patient rights and guidelines for nursing home care facilities. Patients who live in nursing homes are called *residents*. This Nursing Home Reform Act states that:

1. Each resident must be fully evaluated upon admission and each year after in regard to health, memory, hobbies, habits, and so forth.
2. A plan must be created to maintain and possibly improve the resident's condition.
3. Patients have the right to be seen by a doctor. If they can't find one on their own, the medical director of the nursing home will help them find one.

4. Patients have a right to be informed about treatment, and to refuse if desired.
5. Patients have a right to privacy and a right to complain without fear of reprisal.

OBRA also contains the Resident's Bill of Rights, which is similar to the Patient's Bill of Rights. The Resident's Bill of Rights specifically addresses:

- Free choice of doctor, treatment, care, and participation in research
- Freedom from abuse and chemical or physical restraints
- Privacy and confidentiality of medical records
- Accommodation of needs and choice regarding activities, schedules, and health care
- The ability to voice grievances without fear
- Organization and participation in family/resident groups and in social, religious, and community activities
- Ability to manage their personal funds and use personal possessions
- Unlimited access to immediate family, and can share room with spouse if both are residents
- Access to information about medical benefits, medical records, deficiencies in the facility, and sources of **advocates** (people who speak or write in support of something or someone) for the residents
- The ability to stay in the facility and not be transferred or discharged except for medical reasons, failure to pay, or if the facility cannot meet the patient's needs

In addition to rights, patients have several responsibilities. Patients or their surrogates must be active participants in the care process. In order to fulfill their responsibilities, patients should do the following:

- Provide honest, complete, and accurate information about their past illnesses, hospitalizations, medications, and other matters related to their health.
- Ask questions and seek clarification when they don't fully understand the information or instructions they're given.
- Make sure they understand the risks and benefits of any procedure before giving their consent.
- Comply with treatment plans; alert their caregivers if they expect to have a problem doing so.
- Provide their caregivers with copies of advance directives if they have them.
- Provide necessary information for their hospital or doctor to file insurance claims.
- Fulfill their financial obligations; pay their medical bills on time or arrange payment plans when necessary.
- Show respect for their providers, for example by keeping appointments and showing up on time.
- Recognize that their lifestyle, behaviors, and personal choices have an impact on their health.

THE MORE YOU KNOW

PATIENT CONSENT

Before patients can be examined and treated they must give their consent. **Expressed consent** is when patients either sign a consent form or give verbal permission for the care. **Implied consent** is when patients give permission for care through an action, such as removing their clothing and putting on a patient gown. An invasive procedure, such as surgery, requires a signed consent. The signed consent form is evidence that the patient agreed to the care after having been informed of the risks involved.

(continued)

Consent forms must be written in a language that the patient understands. Based on the Doctrine of Informed Consent, the following information must be included:

- The procedure to be performed
- The doctor who will perform the procedure
- The person administering the anesthesia, when applicable
- Potential risks to the patient from having, or not having, the procedure
- Potential alternative treatments and their risks
- Verification that the patient has had his or her questions answered
- Exceptions or exclusions requested by the patient

Patients must be made aware of their diagnosis, if known, and the purpose, advantages, and risks of the procedure. Specialized consent forms are used for procedures such as blood transfusions, invasive procedures such as biopsies and lumbar punctures, chemotherapy, and cardiac or pulmonary stress testing.

Consent forms must be signed and dated by the patient or his or her representative. Patients must be mentally competent and at least 18 years of age to sign their consent form. If the patient is less than 18 years old, a parent or guardian will sign for the patient. If the patient is mentally incompetent or **incapacitated** (permanently or temporarily impaired by a mental and/or physical condition), the form will be signed by the patient's representative. Minors under the age of 18 who are **emancipated** (legally considered an adult) may sign their consent forms. Minors who are emancipated are married or otherwise responsible for paying their own bills, and have a court order stating they are emancipated. Minors who are in the armed services or undergoing care for a sexually transmitted disease or a pregnancy, or are being seen for birth control, abortion, or drug or alcohol abuse can sign their own consent forms.

Consent must be *informed*, meaning the patient must be told about the risks and benefits of the procedure plus any alternative treatments to be considered. Patients must be told about how much pain and discomfort to expect, and what their recovery or follow-up care will involve.

Patients should never be forced or threatened to sign a consent form, and they have the right to refuse the procedure. Patients near death due to cancer, for example, may refuse chemotherapy treatments because of the side effects, or patients may refuse blood products (transfusions) due to their religious beliefs. When patients refuse treatment, they must sign a refusal-of-consent form stating they were given information about the risks of having, or not having, the procedure. Patients who don't understand the procedure, or who can't read the form, should not sign a consent form.

Patients must give consent before their medical information can be released to other parties, such as physician specialists, insurance companies, and the patients' family members. Upon reaching 18 years of age, the patient's medical information cannot be shared with anyone, including his or her spouse, parents, or guardian without the consent of the patient.

Customer Service

Some people cringe at the thought of referring to patients as customers. But health care is a business and patients are the customers. It's important that health care customers be pleased and satisfied with the services they receive. So much of what is being done to improve patient care relies on technology. But it's important to remember that health care is a hands-on service industry where "high touch" is just as important as "high tech." Technology can never replace the human element when it comes to caring for patients.

Like coworkers, your customers are a highly diverse group of people. They represent all personality types and a wide variety of differences. Some will be easy to get along with, others will be more difficult, and some will be downright nasty. Some patients will appreciate your efforts while others will not. But they all deserve to be treated with respect and good manners.

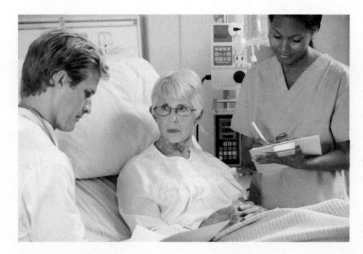

Figure 5-8 Ensuring a positive hospital experience (*Monkey Business Images/Shutterstock*)

Applying what you've learned so far in your interactions with patients is where "the rubber meets the road." Remember the difference between hard skills and soft skills? Everyone expects you to be competent (hard skills)—that's just a given. What will set you apart as a professional is how you behave (soft skills).

Working in direct patient care is a privilege. It's an honor to have another person entrust his or her health and safety to you. It's also an awesome responsibility. Today's patients have high expectations regarding how they will be treated by health care workers and they have choices as to where to obtain health care services. Patients won't hesitate to go someplace else for their care if they believe they haven't been treated well. Dissatisfied patients will complain to their doctors and before long, the doctors will start referring their patients elsewhere.

When patients have a decision to make about where to go for their health care, they assume that most, if not all, of the hospitals and doctors in town provide quality care. What differentiates one health care provider from another often comes down to customer service and the patient's experience. The patient's satisfaction with his or her experience has become a top priority and it's carefully measured and tracked over time. Health care companies provide customer service training for their employees and operate "service excellence" programs to raise their patient experience scores.

The Patient Experience

Hospitals have collected patient satisfaction data for their own internal use for many years. But until the **HCAHPS** survey (pronounced H-caps; Hospital Consumer Assessment of Healthcare Providers and Systems) was recently introduced, there was no standard approach for all hospitals to use in collecting this data and sharing it with the public. HCAHPS uses a 27-question survey to collect data about the patient's perception of the quality of his or her hospital experience. The survey is given to a random sampling of adult patients with a variety of medical conditions between two days and six weeks after they've been discharged from the hospital. The survey can be conducted by mail, telephone, or a combination of the two. Questions solicit feedback regarding communication with the nurses and doctors, pain management, cleanliness, noise levels, details about medications, etc. Patients are also asked to rate the hospital overall and whether or not they would recommend the hospital to other patients.

The HCAHPS system focuses on creating a culture of "always"—always delivering quality care to every patient during every encounter. Since data collection methods are standardized and hospitals post their results on a public website (*www.hospitalcompare.hhs.gov*), patients and other stakeholders have access to meaningful comparative data. Public reporting of survey results provides incentives for hospitals to improve the patient experience and become more transparent in sharing their outcomes. Patient satisfaction data plays a major role in health care reform since hospitals now have financial incentives to achieve and improve their scores. In addition to hospitals, doctor's offices, emergency departments, and other providers also use survey tools to collect data to measure their patients' satisfaction.

RECENT DEVELOPMENTS

HEALING ENVIRONMENTS

Green initiatives, which focus on protecting the environment, are leading to more **healing environments** (physical spaces designed to reduce stress, ensure safety, and uplift the spirits of patients, visitors, and staff) in hospitals and other health care settings, offering beneficial effects for both patients and workers.

Research has shown that the quality of the environment can improve the healing of patients and the morale and efficiency of staff. Calming spaces designed with carefully chosen colors, lighting, and building materials can lift the spirits of seriously ill patients and reduce the stress of busy health care workers. Green initiatives, which help save energy and reduce waste, are well timed since many health care organizations are gearing up to build new hospitals, clinics, and nursing homes to replace outdated facilities and respond to the increasing demands of the Baby Boomer population.

Developers are designing energy-efficient utility plants, improving waste management and recycling efforts, and incorporating recycled materials, natural sources of light, and live plants and trees.

Being There for Patients

When you work in direct patient care, the patient should be the focus of everything you do. It's not about you, your department, or your schedule for the day. It's *always* about the patient. When you arrive for work, remember this. Today is just another typical day for you. But for your patients, it could be a day that they will never forget.

Patients will tell scores of people about their experience and how they were treated. Patients don't miss much—they hear and notice everything going on around them. If there's tension among the staff, they pick up on it. If a piece of equipment doesn't work, the restroom hasn't been cleaned, or the lettuce on the cafeteria salad bar is rotting, they notice. Patients spend a lot of time (too much time) waiting. It's amazing how much information a patient can acquire just sitting in a waiting room or lying on a cart headed for surgery. If you think the patient can't overhear your phone conversation down the hall, think again.

When people become patients, they're vulnerable and at their worst. They're in pain and anxious, worried, confused, and overwhelmed with the medical experience. Many patients feel helpless, having to turn themselves over to strangers who will make decisions about their care. They're concerned about what might happen to them, how their lives will be affected, how their children and spouse will fare in their absence, and a whole host of other issues. Patients need reassurance and confidence that they're in good hands. As mentioned previously, how you look, communicate, and behave can have a tremendous impact on their feeling of security. Always introduce yourself and explain the rationale for whatever procedures the patient might be undergoing.

Every thing you say and do makes an impact on patients. A small act of kindness on your part may be huge to your patient. Patients tend to pick their favorite caregivers. Upon returning, they may ask to have the same person take care of them again. Some caregivers "go the extra mile" and those are the people that you want your patients to remember. Think back to the discussion about "being present in the moment." You must be able to filter out everything else going on around you and concentrate on "being there" at that precise moment for that patient. The connections that professionals make with their patients are not the result of just acting or performing a duty. The ability to connect with patients is a reflection of the caregiver's personal values and professional priorities—an indication that caring for others comes straight from the heart. Isn't this the kind of person that you would want taking care of you and your loved ones?

TRENDS AND ISSUES

HEALTH CARE PROFESSIONALS AS ROLE MODELS

Adopting healthy habits is not only good for you as a health care professional, it's also good for your patients. Take smoking, for example. Research shows that patients who smoke are less likely to stop smoking if their caregivers smoke. Although doctors, nurses, and respiratory therapists encourage their patients to refrain from smoking, their efforts are less successful when the caregivers don't practice what they preach. Patients view their caregivers as educators and trusted **role models** (people that others aspire to be like). When their caregivers continue to smoke despite the overwhelming evidence that smoking is hazardous to their health, then patients are less likely to follow the advice they're given. Therefore, one of the best strategies to reduce smoking among the general public is to reduce smoking among health care professionals.

According to the Centers for Disease Control and Prevention, smoking causes harm to almost every organ in the body. One out of every five deaths in the United States each year is related to smoking. You might know that smoking causes lung cancer, emphysema, and other respiratory diseases. You might not know that smoking can also cause many other cancers, including cancers of the mouth, larynx, pharynx, esophagus, bladder, kidney, pancreas, cervix, and stomach. Smoking also puts people at a higher risk for coronary heart disease and stroke. Women who smoke when they are pregnant can damage the health of their fetus. Older women who smoke are more at risk for osteoporosis.

If you don't smoke, don't start. Cigarettes are highly addictive, so it's difficult to quit smoking. If you smoke now, you really should quit. Many employers and health insurance companies have programs to help smokers overcome their addictions. Other resources are widely available online to help smokers kick the habit.

Remember what you've learned about valuing differences and diversity. These concepts apply to patients and your other customers, too.

- It's not your place to be judgmental. It doesn't matter if your patient is wealthy, poor, homeless, elderly, a transvestite, a celebrity, or a criminal. Each patient should receive the same level of respect, quality of care, and customer service.
- Protect your patients' dignity, self-respect, and personal possessions.

- Refer to patients as "Mr." or "Ms." instead of "honey," "sweetie," or "dear." You may think calling someone "honey" is a sign of caring, but keep in mind that many patients (and other customers) object to these kinds of terms.
- Be compassionate and **empathetic** (able to relate to another person's emotions and situation).

Anticipate your patients' needs and be prepared to meet them. No request or concern is too trivial. But if a patient asks you for a drink, food, medication, or help walking to the restroom, don't fulfill the request unless your job includes these duties. Always refer any matter that is outside of your scope of practice to the patient's nurse or another caregiver in the area and make sure the appropriate person follows through.

When communicating with patients, use terms they can understand. If they ask you a question you aren't capable of answering or aren't authorized to answer, refer the question to the appropriate person. Use your listening skills and watch for body language and nonverbal communication. When obtaining patient information, use feedback techniques to ensure accurate communication. Reflect on what the patient has said, restate the information in your own words, and clarify that what you *think* you heard is actually what the patient said.

Display sensitivity when scheduling appointments for patients, recognizing that people must balance many priorities in their lives. Be empathetic when discussing financial matters with patients, including their billing records and arrangements for making payments. Communicating with terminally ill patients and their family members requires a high degree of empathy and sensitivity. People go through several stages of grief starting with shock and denial, and ending with acceptance. As they move from stage to stage, they may voice their anger and suffer from depression. As a health care professional, you must be understanding and provide support whenever possible. Patients and family members have end-of-life decisions to make and this requires a close, respectful, and trusting relationship with caregivers.

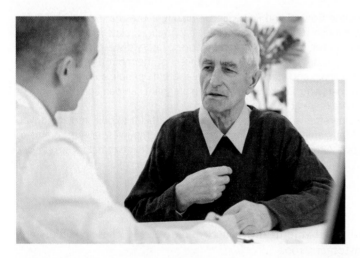

Figure 5-9 Communicating clearly to make sure the patient understands his treatment options (*Lucky Business/Shutterstock*)

When people are caught up in emergency situations, they are especially vulnerable due to the physical and emotional factors involved. It's important to calm people down, not just the injuried person but the other people around them. Depending on your job, you may find yourself in some very difficult and emotional situations where you must remain calm yourself while attending to the needs of those around you. This is especially true of emergency services personnel such as EMTs, paramedics, and firefighters. Being present at a fire or at the scene of a bad automobile accident can be a horrific experience for a health care worker. Keeping your own emotions under control while providing emergency care can be quite a challenge.

When working with patients, protecting their privacy is always a key issue. Here are some things to remember:

- Never read a patient's medical record unless it's part of your job.
- Never divulge information about a patient's medical status to the patient's family members, clergy, or other visitors without the patient's permission.
- Confine the exchange of confidential information to a "need to know" basis when discussing patients with other health care professionals.
- If you have patients who are celebrities, leaders in your organization, or coworkers, make sure you protect their privacy and give them every consideration you would give other patients.
- Never ask questions or make comments in a public area that might embarrass a patient or violate privacy. For example, a medical assistant should never raise his or her voice to ask Mr. Jones, who is sitting in the public waiting area, whether he remembered to bring his stool sample!
- Avoid the temptation to give your own personal opinion when a patient asks, "Which doctor in this group is the best?" or "Which doctor would you take your child to?"
- Don't discuss your own medical history, or the medical histories of your family members, with patients.
- Always stop and think—if *you* were the patient, how would you want to be treated?

Patient Visitors

No discussion of customer service would be complete without mentioning the patient's visitors—their family members and close friends. A patient's family is his or her "lifeline" to their normal life. When the patient invites other people to be a part of his or her medical experience, these other people become part of the patient's "team." Remember that "family" may mean something very different to the patient than to you. Accept who they identify as family and help them become a part of the patient's team.

Patients need families and friends to help them through difficult situations. Having clergy present may help. Sadly, not all patients have a support system. Some patients will complete their entire hospital stay with no family or visitors present. These patients need some special compassion and attention from their caregivers. Other patients have large families and lots of friends and sometimes this can cause problems. Policies regarding hospital visiting hours have always been controversial. Some hospitals strictly enforce limited visitation while others have abandoned visitation limitations altogether. The problem is that visitors don't always use common sense. If a person is sufficiently sick or injured to require hospitalization, then he or she needs rest and shouldn't be overtaxed with too many visitors. On the other hand, maintaining connections with family and friends is an important part of the healing process. Sometimes it's up to the caregiver to enforce limitations on visitors to carry out the wishes of the patient and what's best for his or her recovery.

THINK ABOUT IT

CAMPING OUT AT THE HOSPITAL

Families of seriously ill patients may literally "camp out" at the hospital. They want to be as close to their loved one as possible, and for as much time as possible. Spouses may spend the night in their loved one's room, even though it's very uncomfortable. Families bring things from home to comfort the patient, such as favorite foods, flowers, and personal items. They may bring clothes and toiletries because they are "living there" for the time being.

The patient's room could become cluttered with people and things. Try to avoid viewing this as an inconvenience to you and remember—this is the patient's and his or her family's "home away from home" for the time being. Providing family support is an important part of customer service and patient care.

When a patient is hospitalized for several days, the patient and his or her family spend hours and hours, and days and days, waiting. Their lives are on hold until their medical situation is resolved and they can resume their normal routine. With so much time on their hands, they notice when the free coffee down the hall isn't strong enough, the upholstery on the chairs is threadbare, and the elevator doors close too quickly. When it's finally time to eat, there's never an extra wheelchair available to push grandma down to the cafeteria. The patient's room is too hot or too cold. The meal tray was supposed to be delivered 20 minutes ago and when it finally arrived, the milk was white instead of chocolate. The TV remote control doesn't work the way it's supposed to.

Patients and families may become irritated when they don't get medical information about the patient's condition and treatment plans quickly enough. Doctors make rounds on the patient care units when it's most convenient for them. Families will stay in the room all day and refuse to leave even for meals for fear of "missing the doctor" when he or she makes rounds. They may pressure you for information that you don't have and ask for answers that you cannot give. It's enough to make a sane health care worker crazy!

Try to give your patients and their family members the benefit of the doubt and remember that their lives are in limbo. They're temporarily living in suspended animation, in some surreal world usually not by choice. They're uncertain about what's going to happen next and no one has all of the answers. Take a deep breath and remember why you went into health care. Give them some slack and rejoice that *you*, unlike your hospitalized patients, get to go home in a few hours.

Avoid the temptation to give personal advice or to express your own religious beliefs. When appropriate, generate some humor and laughter. Be positive whenever you can. Even tiny improvements in the patient's condition mean a great deal to the patient and his or her family members. Here's where your optimistic "the glass is half full" attitude can be helpful. Perhaps the patient's blood pressure and heart rate haven't settled down during the past hour. But they haven't worsened either. Maybe the patient isn't well enough to be transported to radiology for a chest x-ray. But he can sit up in bed and have a portable radiograph taken in his room. Maybe the patient's IV supply can't be completely disconnected, but the dosage has been reduced. Look for things to be happy about and express them. Optimism and a positive

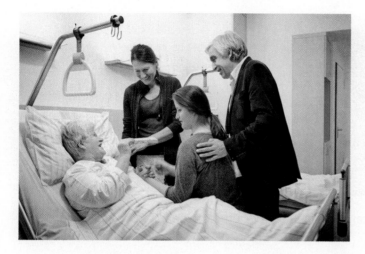

Figure 5-10 Family members are part of the patient's health care team (*Upixa/Shutterstock*)

outlook on the part of caregivers are important to patients. A positive frame of mind can lead to improvements in a patient's condition. When undergoing high-risk procedures, patients who are optimistic and more relaxed may have better outcomes. If a patient thinks his or her medical team has given up, he or she may give up, too. But don't give patients "false hope" or "get their hopes up" inappropriately. Some of your patients won't get better. Some won't leave the hospital alive.

You may be called upon to help prepare someone for death. The patient and his or her family will have difficult decisions to make. They will need privacy and time to talk, cry, and express their love and other emotions. They may have to "say goodbye" as the cart is wheeled out of the room on its way to surgery, facing the prospect of never seeing their loved one alive again. Those are the moments that your patients and family members will remember forever, and you are a part of it. Just as you may help usher in a new life in labor and delivery, you may also be present when someone passes. Both are humbling experiences that you cannot begin to imagine until you go through them yourself.

Working in an outpatient setting such as a doctor's office or clinic presents some unique challenges. Here are some things to keep in mind to provide good customer service and a positive experience for outpatients:

- When a patient approaches the check-in window or registration desk, he or she should be greeted by a friendly and welcoming face, not just a "robot" asking for an insurance card and any changes in the patient's information.
- Don't ask a patient why he or she is there in front of other patients. If possible, escort the patient to a private area to ask these questions. Provide a sign-in sheet for the patient to add his or her name.
- When checking in a patient, do not yell, "Mr. Smith, do you have insurance?" in front of the other patients. Mr. Smith could become embarrassed if his answer is no. This invasion of Mr. Smith's privacy could also be a HIPAA violation.

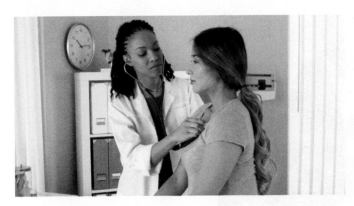

Figure 5-11 Undergoing a physical exam in a doctor's office (*Rocketclips, Inc./Shutterstock*)

- When patients arrive, they may be nervous and feeling ill. Engaging in some casual conversation ("It seems especially hot today" or "Has the traffic slowed down yet?") may help put them at ease. Patients need to be treated as individuals and not just "the man in exam room one."
- With regard to patient satisfaction, the main thing that people complain about is how long they have to wait. Most patients are willing to wait a reasonable length of time. But patients can become very upset when they're sitting in a waiting room listening to or watching employees socializing, eating and drinking, or otherwise playing around. Patients may think that such behavior is the reason why they must wait so long. If you need to have a personal conversation with a coworker, make sure that the patients in the waiting room can't hear you.
- If you know there's going to be a delay before someone is called into an examination room, inform the patient so that he or she doesn't think they've been ignored or forgotten. If you notice that a patient in the waiting room has become angry or unruly, escort the person to an exam room to avoid upsetting the other patients.
- Pay attention to patient names and arrival times. This can sometimes be a challenge in a very busy facility, but it's important to make sure that no one is forgotten. Patients may arrive with another person such as a friend, family member, or someone who provides the patient's transportation. Keep in mind that the patient may or may not want that person in the exam room with them. Always check with the patient before escorting another person into the exam room.
- Be familiar with your facility's policies and procedures regarding on-site visits by drug company representatives (drug reps). Don't take a drug rep in to meet with a doctor ahead of scheduled patients, especially if the patients have been waiting for awhile. Don't discuss drugs with the drug rep in front of patients, and don't discuss the patients with the drug rep.
- Dress codes in outpatient facilities have become a bit more relaxed in recent times but employees must still maintain a professional image. Many facilities don't allow "casual

days" where employees can wear denim jeans or casual clothing. Outpatient workers often deal with bodily fluids such as blood and urine, so wearing their personal clothes at work may not be acceptable. This is why outpatient facilities typically require staff, including front-office and other nonclinical workers, to wear scrubs.

- The use of inappropriate or "street language" is never acceptable around patients, coworkers, or other people in the facility. Patients will judge the quality of the facility and its staff by the behavior of those who work there.
- Remain in your work area and be readily accessible when needed. Don't make doctors or other staff members waste their time looking for you.
- Depending on your job, you may be "the eyes and ears" of the doctors with whom you work. Pay attention to details and be prepared to meet the doctors' needs. For example, if the patient is there to have his or her medications refilled, have details regarding the prescriptions ready when needed.
- Do your best to keep the workflow moving. If things fall behind schedule, patients may have to wait longer and could become upset.

Patients who receive health care in outpatient settings are on a quest for information. After seeing their doctor in his or her office and undergoing diagnostic tests, patients want to hear the results of those tests as quickly as possible. They also have questions about the results and next steps. All too often, patients receive a postcard in the mail or a brief phone call from the doctor's nurse or medical assistant directing the patient to pick up a prescription at the pharmacy. Patients may not have the opportunity to get all of their questions answered until returning for a follow-up doctor's visit several weeks later.

If part of your job is calling patients to inform them of test results, have sufficient information at hand to answer their questions. Today's health care consumers are often well informed. They don't just want to hear, "Your results were slightly elevated." They want details and actual numbers so they can go online and learn more about their conditions and potential treatment options. In situations where you can't provide all of the information requested, don't be surprised if the patient asks to speak with the doctor. Some doctors willingly take phone calls while others may do so begrudgingly or not at all. Depending on your job, you may be in an assistant role to the physician, a liaison between the patient and his or her doctor. Do your best to meet the patients' needs while still working within your scope of practice.

Working with Doctors, Guests, and Vendors

When working with doctors, you'll encounter people from various cultures, with different personality types and communication styles. You'll work with doctors that you really like and respect and others that you would avoid if you could. Some doctors will take an interest in you, answer your questions, and explain procedures as they are performed. They'll "go the extra mile" for their patients and they'll express appreciation for their staff. Other doctors may appear smug, dispassionate, indifferent, or downright rude. To save time, they may **dictate** (to read aloud and record patient information for medical records) in front of a patient during an office visit rather than converse directly with the patient. (Yes, unfortunately this really happens.) As a worker, they may treat you as if you're invisible or unimportant. One day a doctor will be friendly, and the next day he or she will be grumpy. A doctor may appear angry when speaking with you, yet his or her anger may actually have nothing to do with you at all.

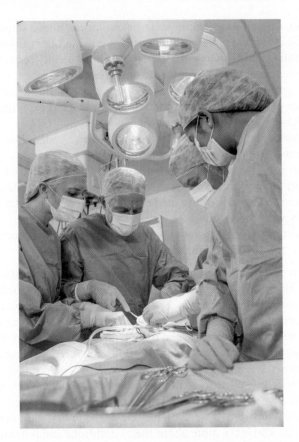

Figure 5-12 Displaying competence and confidence in working with doctors
(*Spotmatik Ltd/Shutterstock*)

Even though some doctors will be demanding and intimidating, try to keep in mind that doctors are just people, too. They have hopes and dreams, feelings and fears, frailties and flaws just like everyone else. Much of the time they're in a hurry and under a great deal of stress. Some of them literally hold life and death in their hands on a daily basis. Practicing medicine is an enormous responsibility and it takes its toll. Until you have walked in a doctor's shoes, you have no idea what their jobs are like.

Occasionally a doctor may ask you to do something that's outside of your scope of practice. He or she may mistake you for a different type of worker or may not be familiar with your training and job duties. If this happens, speak up! Don't just go ahead and do something you aren't qualified to do because a doctor asked you or told you to. Say politely, "That's not within my scope of practice but I'll go get someone who can help you." If you are competent and apply your best communication and customer service skills, you'll likely get along just fine with the doctors.

Guests in your facility are also customers and they, too, are a diverse group of people. Some may be lost or stressed out, running late for an important meeting or a job interview. Others may be in the building to attend a conference or keep an appointment with someone in management. The most frequent request that you'll get from guests is help with directions.

- If you work in a large building, make sure you know your way around so you can give good directions to other people.
- If you have the time or are headed in that direction anyway, offer to walk with the person to make sure he or she gets to their destination.
- If someone is waiting to see your supervisor or someone else in your area and you have access to coffee or a soft drink, offer the person a beverage.
- If you know someone is going to have to wait for awhile, let the person know and explain why.

Do whatever you can to make guests comfortable. Your customers will appreciate even a small gesture of kindness.

The last group of customers is vendors. Vendors are people who work for companies that your company does business with. Vendors might be salespeople from a patient supply company, insurance agents, drug company representatives, or people who work for advertising agencies or temporary services. Just like other customers, they too should be treated with respect, manners, and good customer service.

REALITY CHECK

This chapter includes several terms and concepts that may be somewhat confusing—cultural competence, values, norms, behaviors, culture, discrimination, prejudice, disparities, political correctness, and so forth. Here's the bottom line. Learning to work with diverse groups of people will probably require a significant amount of time and experience before you begin to feel confident and competent. This is especially true if you've lived in a "sheltered environment" most of your life without experiencing people from many different cultures. If you expect to excel in your role as a health care professional, you must learn to not only get along with people who are different from you, you must learn to embrace differences and make them work to everyone's advantage.

Each time you encounter someone who is different from you, stop and think before you act. Are you judging this person based on your own cultural values and norms? If so, you're normal. It's human nature for people to judge other people based on their own values and prejudices. But don't allow these judgments to guide your behavior because the assumptions you've made about the other person might not be accurate. Remain open-minded and try to see things from the other person's point of view. If you find that difficult, ask the person for help. Most people enjoy talking about their backgrounds and the cultures in which they grew up and live. Don't hesitate to help other people learn more about you. Everyone has insights to share. You might be surprised what you'll learn.

Working effectively with patients, families, doctors, guests, and vendors requires respect for diversity and cultural competence along with many of the other skills you're learning by reading this text. Whether you work in a hospital or outpatient setting, understanding what your patients are going through and supporting good customer service will go a long way in providing a positive experience and meeting the needs of those you serve.

For More Information

Research on Cultural Competence in Health Care
Agency for Healthcare Research and Quality
U.S. Department of Health and Human Services
www.ahrq.gov/research.cultural/htm

Personality Assessments
MBTI Assessment
www.myersbriggs.org
Keirsey Temperament Sorter Assessment
www.Keirsey.com

Patient Rights
The Patient Care Partnership: Understanding
Expectations, Rights, and Responsibilities
American Hospital Association
www.aha.org

Patient Satisfaction
HCAHPS
CMS/Centers for Medicare and Medicaid Services
**https://www.cms.gov/Medicare/Quality-
Initiatives-Patient-Assessment-instruments
www.hcahpsonline.org**

Hospital Compare Website
www.hospitalcompare.hhs.gov

Social Media Usage Rates
Pew Research Center
**www.pewinternet.org/2015/08/19/
the-demographics-of-social-media-users**

KEY POINTS

- Develop an appreciation for diversity and differences among people.
- Examine your own cultural norms and avoid letting bias and prejudice govern your behavior.
- Expose yourself to cultures that are different from yours and share information about your culture with other people.
- Avoid Googling your patients and if patients Google you, make sure the content they find supports your professional reputation.
- Identify your personality type and the personality types of the people that you work with and consider how your similarities and differences can be assets at work.
- Find ways to take advantage of occupational and generational differences in the workplace.
- Treat all customers with respect; show special respect and appreciation for service and support workers.
- Focus on customer service strategies that result in high levels of patient satisfaction.
- Track patient satisfaction scores where you work and submit suggestions for improvement.
- Filter out the distractions around you in order to "be there" for your patients when they need you.
- Be especially empathetic with people who are terminally ill or involved in emergency situations.
- Extend good customer service to the patients' family members, friends, and other visitors.
- Apply customer service standards when interacting with doctors, guests, and vendors.

LEARNING ACTIVITIES

Using information from Chapter Five:
- Answer the Chapter Review Questions
- Respond to the What If? Scenarios

Chapter Review Questions

Using information presented in Chapter Five, answer each of the following questions.

1. Give three examples of diversity in addition to age and gender.

2. Explain how bias can result in health care disparities for members of minority cultural groups.

3. List two things to do when cultural tension arises.

4. Explain why health care workers need to be culturally competent.

5. Describe the difference between stereotypes and generalizations.

6. Explain what is meant by the cultural competence continuum.

7. Describe two ways that online patient portals can improve health care.

8. Explain how a person's personality type can affect his or her work.

9. Give an example of how generational differences can cause problems at work.

10. List four types of health care customers.

11. Describe the purpose of the American Hospital Association's brochure, "Patient Care Partnership: Understanding Expectations, Rights and Responsibilities."

12. Explain the purpose of the HCAHPS survey.

13. List five ways to provide good customer service for hospitalized patients and their visitors.

What If? Scenarios

Think about what you would do in the following situations and record your answers.

1. A hospitalized patient has a medical condition that you suffered yourself six months ago but the patient isn't aware of this. He asks if you have any idea what he can expect from his treatment plan.

2. You just moved from Maine to Southern California to start a new job. The majority of your clinic patients are immigrants from across the border. You've never been to Mexico yourself, but you remember that your parents didn't like the Mexican family who lived next door when you were growing up in Maine.

3. Your supervisor is 30 years older than you. He constantly looks over your shoulder to make sure you're doing things correctly. If he would just give you the chance, you could download some new software to improve your office's financial records and make things quicker and easier to report.

4. Several people from your unit, including you, have been cross-trained to work in three different areas. Since all of you rotate on a weekly basis, none of you feel as if you really "belong" anywhere.

5. One of your patients scheduled for a procedure this morning has just informed you that she refuses to have the treatment.

6. You've heard a rumor that people who were hospitalized where you work were not as satisfied with their care as the people who were treated in the other two hospitals in town.

7. One of your patients seems depressed. She can't go home yet but her vital signs have improved considerably and she has regained her appetite.

8. A representative from a drug company has arrived to meet with one of the doctors in your office. But the doctor just got called away to deal with an emergency and you have no idea when she will return.

9. Late this afternoon you took a phone call from a doctor in the sports medicine clinic who is upset about the delay in getting an x-ray report for a patient scheduled for surgery early tomorrow morning. The doctor got angry and called you unreliable even though you are just the receptionist who answers the phone.

10. One of your patients said he saw a video of you on Instagram and was surprised to see you drinking at a gay bar. You didn't know the video had been taken or shared.

Professionalism and Your Personal Life

6

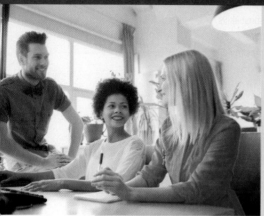

We make a living by what we get,
but we make a life by what we give.

—Winston Churchill (1874–1965),
British prime minister

(Syda Productions/Shutterstock)

CHAPTER OBJECTIVES

Having completed this chapter, you will be able to:

- Explain how personal skills affect your success as a health care worker.
- Describe how your personal image affects patient care.
- List five appearance and grooming factors that result in a professional image.
- Explain how stereotypes impact first impressions.
- List three examples of annoying and troublesome personal habits.
- Describe how grammar and vocabulary impact your professional image.
- Explain the importance of maintaining professionalism after hours.

- List three health and safety concerns with social media.
- Describe the importance of self-care for health care workers.
- Give two examples of how employers are encouraging employees to become healthier.
- Describe three time management techniques.
- Describe three financial management techniques.
- Describe three stress management techniques.
- Explain why the ability to manage change is so important in health care today.

KEY TERMS

adaptive skills

adversity

body mass index (BMI)

body mechanics

dress code

grammar

health risk assessments

health screenings

immunizations

infectious diseases

invincible

malnutrition

personal financial
 management

personal image

personal management
 skills

personal skills

posture

procrastinate

resilience

self-care

stress management

taboo

time management

well groomed

Personal Image

In previous chapters we discussed how professionalism brings together who you are as a person and how you contribute those characteristics in the workplace. We examined work ethic, character, morals, relationships, communication skills, diversity, and many other related topics. Now it's time to explore the connection between your personal life and your professional life.

You're just one person. It stands to reason that if your personal life is out of control your professional life will suffer. Good **personal skills** (the ability to manage aspects of one's life outside of work) free you up to concentrate on your job and your career. Of course, many of your personal skills transfer to the workplace and influence your reputation as a professional. This includes your **personal image** (the total impression created by a person), personal health and wellness, and the ability to manage your time, finances, and stress and adapt to change.

What does it take to have a well-orchestrated personal life that puts you on the right path to success in your career? Let's examine some personal skills and the impact they have on professionalism and success in the health care workplace.

One of the first things people notice about you is your personal image. Personal image includes your appearance, grooming, and **posture** (the position of the body or parts of the body); personal habits; and the **grammar** (the system or structure of a language; the generally accepted rules of speech and writing) and the acceptability of the language you use. What kind of an impression do *you* make on people?

- Are you **well groomed** (personally clean and neat)?
- When you come to work, are you dressed properly to perform the duties of your job?
- Do your appearance and posture convey pride, competence, and professionalism?
- Do any personal habits detract from your image?
- How does your grammar or the language you use impact your personal image?

Appearance and Grooming

Your personal image is especially important in patient care. Patients need to have confidence in their caregivers. They want assurance that the people caring for them are competent and professional. How would *you* feel if *your* caregiver had a ripped uniform, dirty shoes, oily hair, grimy fingernails, body odor, or bad breath? Would you wonder if that person's unprofessional appearance might also indicate a lack of pride or competence in his or her work?

Other people besides patients are affected by your personal appearance. Family members and friends who visit patients also need reassurance that their loved ones are being cared for by

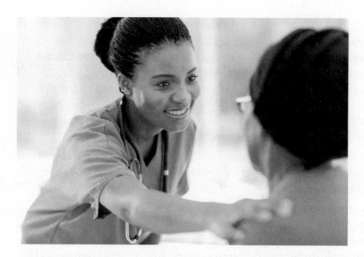

Figure 6-1 Displaying a positive personal image (*Michaeljung/Shutterstock*)

professionals. Vendors, guests, and other people who come into your workplace expect to see employees supporting a professional environment. Your coworkers and supervisor expect you to uphold the company's professional standards, too.

Then there's you. When you *look* good, you *feel* good. Setting high standards for your personal appearance not only conveys an image of professionalism to others, it reinforces your pride and self-esteem. How can you expect others to view you as a professional if you don't look like or feel like a professional yourself?

Dress Code Standards

Most employers have a written **dress code** (standards for attire and appearance). Dress code requirements vary among different settings depending on the duties involved. For example, dietary workers have a different dress code than administrative assistants. Be sure you're familiar with the dress code for your job and do your best to comply with it.

Consider the following as a general "rule of thumb." If you don't wear a uniform, select clothing that's appropriate for the duties of your job.

- Your clothes should be clean, pressed, and fit properly. Avoid clothing that is wrinkled, frayed, too short, too tight, too baggy, or too revealing. Avoid clothes with wild colors and prints. Don't wear shirts or tops with messages printed on them unless approved by your employer.
- Avoid visible skin on your torso below the neckline of your shirt or top. This means no visible tummies, breasts, or back skin. No short shirts, no short skirts, no low-rise pants, and no undergarments that are visible through your clothing.
- Your shoes should be clean, polished, and closed-toe. You must wear socks (not no-show footies) or stockings. No bare feet, slippers, flip-flops, sandals, or open-toe shoes.
- Keep makeup, jewelry, and other accessories to a minimum and in good taste. In some health care professions such as dental assisting, no jewelry is allowed. Avoid brightly polished fingernails and acrylic artificial nails.

- Long hair should be pulled back and secured to avoid sanitary or safety problems. Facial hair should be groomed and neatly styled.
- Never wear perfume, aftershave, or scented lotions. Aromas may not be welcome among patients and coworkers and might aggravate breathing difficulties.
- Poor posture can undermine a professional image. Sit up straight, stand erect, and don't slouch.
- Wear your employee identification badge as prescribed in your company's dress code.
- Avoid nontraditional hairstyles and colors and facial piercings; cover up tattoos.

Remember, you don't come to work to set new fashion trends or win a beauty contest. Your clothing and accessories should support getting your work done efficiently and safely while instilling a feeling of confidence among those you serve.

- Save your evening wear, party attire, sportswear, and the latest fashions for after hours.
- Shorts, capris, leggings, cropped pants, tight pants, tank tops, bare-back tops, miniskirts, midriff tops, athletic attire, sweatshirts, sweatpants, T-shirts, painter pants, bib overalls, spaghetti-strap dresses, reflective clothing, see-through fabrics, low or revealing necklines, spandex tops and pants, untucked shirttails, and visible undergarments are not acceptable.
- On "casual days," remember that you're still in the workplace. If your job involves contact with patients and other customers, avoid wearing blue jeans, T-shirts, or other questionable attire even on casual days.
- Health care employers may ban any type of clothing made of denim including scrubs, skirts, shirts, pants, dresses, and jeans regardless of the color.
- Sunglasses should not be worn unless for medical reasons. The use of head coverings is limited to those that conform to religious customs or job-specific regulations.

Keep in mind that what constitutes a professional image to one person might be quite different from that which constitutes a professional image to another person. In other words, professional image "is in the eye of the beholder." Such differences often relate to the age and generation of the beholder. Appearance factors that may seem appropriate for your age group may be disturbing to other people, especially those older than you. This includes such things as nose jewelry, nontraditional hairstyles and colors, and tattoos.

THINK ABOUT IT

CONTENDING WITH CONSERVATIVE DRESS CODES

The health care industry is going through a period of rapid and unprecedented change in how care is delivered, who delivers it, and how businesses are run. But health care is still an industry that changes slowly when it comes to some social aspects such as dress codes and standards for attire and appearance.

What's considered *normal* in the rest of the business world may be considered *extremely liberal* among health care employers. For example, in most health care settings women must still wear socks or stockings that cover their ankles and shoes that cover their feet. This means that *no-show footies* are not considered socks, and *flip-flops* and *sandals* are not considered shoes. Although tattoos are becoming more accepted in some health care settings, many employers still require that tattoos be covered at all times. Nose jewelry and other body piercings may be fashionable in public, but still remain **taboo** (banned from social custom) in many health care companies.

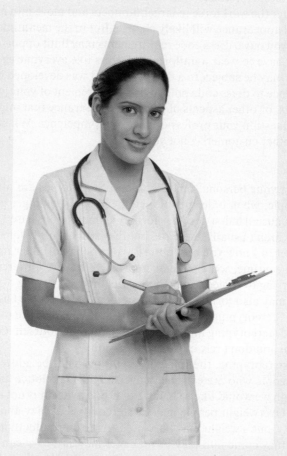

Figure 6-2 Starched white nurse's uniform with cap (*Imagedb.com/Shutterstock*)

In some cases, dress code requirements relate to the need for infection control. If you work with patients, for example, you may be instructed to not wear nail polish, false nails, or gels because bacteria and germs can hide between the nail and the polish and spread **infectious diseases** (conditions caused by viruses, bacteria, fungi, or parasites that can be passed from person to person).

If you think the health care dress codes of today are old-fashioned, keep in mind that not too long ago female nurses had to wear white, starched, uniform dresses with caps on their heads. Facial hair on men was highly discouraged. Women had to wear skirts at work because slacks were considered unladylike and unprofessional. Only surgery employees could wear scrubs.

In today's health care settings, the white starched uniforms and caps of years past are pretty much gone. Facial hair on men is rarely an issue as long as it's well groomed. Women wearing pants to work is the norm, and the majority of caregivers wear scrubs. Standardizing scrub colors and styles helps patients and other people identify RNs, LPNs, nurse aides, support staff, technologists, and other types of health care workers.

So when it comes to health care dress codes, the times are changing but changing slowly. Maintaining a professional image today means complying with your employer's unique set of standards for attire and appearance.

Based on history, the dress codes of tomorrow may be less rigid than those of today. As younger generations enter the workforce in larger numbers and move into management positions, standards for attire and appearance will likely change. But in the meantime, depending on where you work and what job you have, dress code requirements may limit opportunities to express your individuality. You may have to wear a uniform and dress like everyone else in your department, practice, or office. You may be subject to a dress code that was developed by people significantly older than you. Adherence to dress code policies is a requirement of your job. Always think twice about attire, accessories, or other aspects of personal appearance that might make someone else feel uncomfortable or question your professionalism or competence. When you're at work, it's all about the patient and other customers—not you.

Stereotypes

Stereotyping can affect your personal image at work. Stereotypes are often based on personal appearance. For example, when older people see members of younger generations with facial piercings, tattoos, and unusual hairstyles, they form first impressions based on the stereotypes they hold. First impressions aren't usually accurate, but they still occur. If someone negatively stereotypes you, once they get to know you and observe your behavior, their impression will improve over time. But in the meantime, some patients may ask to have a "different" health care worker take care of them, referring to someone who better fits their stereotype of a professional-looking person. Young people may also form first impressions of older people based on stereotypes and inaccurate judgments. Stereotyping is a fact of life. But if you're aware of it, you can counteract its impact. Try to avoid stereotyping and judging other people yourself. Give everyone you meet the benefit of the doubt and don't rely on first impressions.

When discussing stereotyping, the topic of weight needs to be addressed briefly. Although it's a sensitive issue, people who are extremely overweight may notice an adverse affect on job opportunities. Although we would like to believe that body weight is not a factor in employment decisions, it happens. Overweight people may be stereotyped as lazy and unable to muster self-discipline. Yet in reality, one's weight may have no bearing on productivity and self-control. The issue of limited space may come into play. A manager may say, "We can't consider him for this job because the space he would have to work in is too cramped and confining for him to function properly." In surgery, there may be concerns about an obese nurse or surgical technologist contaminating a sterile field when working in a cramped environment. In radiology, equipment controls may be housed in cubicles too confining for a large person. In jobs requiring heavy lifting or frequent physical activity, employers may feel that such activities could jeopardize the health and safety of an overweight worker.

Although it's unfortunate that a person's body weight could have a negative impact on his or her career, it is a fact of life. If you are seriously overweight and wish to do something about it, work closely with your family physician to plan a safe and healthy course of action. If you're content with your weight, or for medical reasons are unable to reduce your weight, be on the lookout for employment opportunities where weight is not a factor.

Personal Habits

Your habits are also part of your personal image and they can sometimes be annoying or troublesome to those around you. Here are some suggestions:

- Don't wear noisy shoes or jewelry that jangles.
- Don't chew gum, pop your knuckles, or bite your fingernails.

- Don't play jokes and childish pranks on coworkers.
- Avoid making a mess when eating or drinking in your work area.
- If you have a hearing loss, get fitted for hearing aids; asking people to repeat things can become annoying.
- Don't play music loudly enough for other people around you to hear it.
- Don't forward chain email messages to coworkers.
- Don't use business computers for personal purposes.
- Don't use personal cell phones or other personal mobile devices during work hours.
- Don't congregate with coworkers in patient or visitor areas before or after your shift.

In terms of other dos and don'ts, remember to practice good etiquette and manners.

Health care companies are smoke-free. If employees must smoke, they're directed to designated "smoking huts" or they stand outside the building, huddled together on public sidewalks. As you might imagine, this doesn't present a very professional image to the public. Some health care employers have a total campuswide ban on smoking and won't allow employees on-site if their clothing smells like smoke. If you must smoke:

- Make sure you're familiar with your company's smoking policies.
- Confine smoking to designated areas to protect others from secondhand smoke.
- Avoid taking too many smoke breaks or breaks that last too long.
- Don't appear for work smelling of cigarette, cigar, or pipe smoke. Many people are allergic to smoke. Patients are ill and the smell of smoke can be detrimental to their comfort.

Some employers require job applicants to undergo drug/nicotine screens and they won't hire people who smoke. Some employers charge higher premiums on health insurance benefits for employees who smoke. Just as obesity may have an adverse affect on job opportunities, so may smoking. It's hard to maintain your professional image when engulfed in a cloud of smoke or wearing clothing that reeks of cigarettes, cigars, or pipes. Many employers offer free smoking cessation classes for their employees. If you smoke and wish to quit, join a support group and get your doctor's advice.

Language and Grammar

In some cases, the language you use may annoy people at work. Don't refer to people has "honey," "sweetie," or "dear." Adult males are "men," not "boys" or "guys." Adult females are "women," not "girls" or "gals." Don't assume that an older female is a "Mrs." It's best to refer to females as "Ms."

Some language is totally unacceptable in the workplace, including obscene, vulgar language or cursing; sexually explicit or risqué comments; and terms that demean members of any racial, cultural, or ethnic group. "Street language" that might be acceptable after hours with your family or friends may be viewed as inappropriate by coworkers, patients, or visitors. Words such as "fart," "suck," "pissed off," and "ass" have become common in public but are still considered inappropriate in the workplace. Using the "f-word" or "n-word" at work can get you fired.

Telling jokes in poor taste and making "off-color" remarks is not a good idea, even during breaks. Remember the prior discussion about sexual harassment and creating an uncomfortable work environment for others? Even if you mean no harm, someone else's perception might be different than yours. Always be respectful of other people's points of view and avoid using language and remarks they might find offensive.

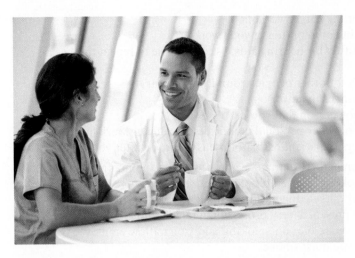

Figure 6-3 Using appropriate language at work (*Monkey Business Images/Shutterstock*)

Grammar also plays a role in your personal and professional image. Poor grammar is a warning signal, indicating a lack of education and refinement. It's not uncommon for people to mismatch the subject and verb in a sentence. Here are some examples:

- "We was there" should be "We *were* there."
- "I seen you do that" should be "I *saw* you do that."
- "Me and him" should be "He and I" if they are the subject of the sentence, but "him and me" are correct as objects. (It is correct to say, "He and I are working on those records so please give that information to him and me.")
- "Her and I" should be "she and I" if they are the subject, "her and me" if they are the object. (Correct: "She and I work at the hospital." "Those notebooks belong to her and me.")
- "She don't know" should be "She *doesn't* know."

Poor grammar is learned and reinforced by the people with whom you associate. Poor grammar starts with your family when you are a child and is influenced by your friends and coworkers. Contemporary music, advertisements, and the media can also reinforce poor grammar (as with the lyric, "It don't matter to me"). If the people who are close to you use incorrect grammar, you may too, without even realizing it. Just being aware of the need for good grammar can help. If your grammar is weak, work toward improving it. You might be surprised how much your grammar, good or bad, can affect your personal and professional image.

Remember the old saying, "You only get one chance to make a good first impression"? In health care, *every* impression you make is important. To patients and other customers, *you* are the company you work for. If you appear less than professional, so might your company. Put together a total personal package that portrays a professional image. It's a big part of your job and it can make or break your reputation as a professional.

Maintaining Professionalism After Hours

At first you might not realize it, but even when you're away from work your behavior can affect your professional image. For example, how do you answer your telephone? What kind of impression does your recorded telephone message make on people who call you? Don't assume that every caller is a friend, family member, or stranger trying to sell you something. What if your supervisor or a potential employer calls? Your telephone is an extension of your personal image so think about who might be calling you and the impression you want to make on them.

What impression does your ring tone make on people who hear it?

CASE STUDY

Carla invited a transgender patient who had asked to speak with someone in management into her office. She introduced herself, offered the patient a beverage, and then asked how she could be of assistance. The patient said she was there to see her new doctor for the first time and felt she had been disrespected by some of the employees in the front office. She said the worker at the check-in window had looked at her closely and responded with a grin and quizzical facial expression. After she had taken a seat in the waiting room, she said she heard employees behind the window laughing and assumed they were laughing at her. After waiting for more than 20 minutes to be called in to see her doctor, she said she became frustrated and felt she was being treated rudely and unfairly.

Carla asked a few follow-up questions to make sure she understood the patient's point of view and took notes during the conversation. She assured the woman that she would investigate the matter and take whatever steps necessary to address the situation. She apologized to the patient for the staff's failure to provide a respectful, positive experience in the practice and then personally escorted the woman to an examination room where she introduced the patient to her new doctor. As Carla was leaving the exam room, the patient thanked her for her assistance and for her professional response to the woman's concerns.

When things slowed down a bit, Carla called everyone who was working in the front office that morning into her office. She informed the three employees of her discussion with the patient and, using her notes, she described in detail why the woman felt she had been disrespected and treated rudely and unfairly by the front office staff. As the employees responded from their points of view, Carla listened carefully and documented their comments. No one admitted to having treated the patient with

disrespect. They said their laughter had nothing to do with the patient and that the delay in placing her in an exam room was due to unrelated circumstances. Carla wasn't sure who or what to believe, but she did know one thing—perception is reality to patients. The patient felt she had had a negative experience and that's what really mattered. Carla told the employees that a note would be placed in each of their personnel files documenting the incident. While no formal corrective action would be taken at this time, each employee needed to recognize the severity of the situation and take steps to make sure that all patients feel they have been treated with dignity and respect.

After the meeting, Carla contacted the network's patient advocate office and explained what had happened. Mandatory in-service training sessions regarding protocols for treating members of the LGBT (lesbian, gay, bisexual, transgender) community were scheduled for all doctors and staff members in the practice. During the sessions, the group learned that the correct use of pronouns (*he, his, she, her*) is very important when communicating with transgender patients, and that the number of doctors who specialize and are willing to care for transgender patients is highly limited. In fact, some states have no such doctors at all. Carla was pleased to hear that the doctor in her practice who cared for the woman she met last week had recently completed coursework to support transgender patients undergoing transition. She knew that, before long, the practice would be seeing more members of the LGBT community and was glad that the staff's in-service sessions were well timed. The speaker also mentioned that same-sex marriages are on the rise due to recent Supreme Court rulings. Staff members need to become competent and confident in relating to patients who might differ from themselves in terms of sexual orientation and gender identity.

(continued)

Following the formal presentation, ample time was allowed for questions and open discussion. Employee feedback indicated that the sessions had been informative and helpful. Staff members reported a higher degree of knowledge in interacting with members of the LGBT community and appreciated the insights they had gained.

A few weeks later on a Monday morning, things took a turn for the worse. When Carla arrived for work she could tell something was wrong and her manager was waiting for her in her office. The network's new social media policies had only been in place for a few weeks when a serious violation had evidently occurred. Carla's manager showed her several videos that appeared to have been taken in a bar or club and shared via several social media sites over the weekend. Two of the practice's physician assistants, a man and a woman, were featured engaging in what looked to be a sexually explicit "performance" in front of a sizeable crowd of onlookers. The two were scantily clothed; the woman was topless. There was no question as to their identities.

Carla was stunned by what she saw and knew instantly there would be repercussions. By now, everyone in the office had heard what had happened and had seen the videos. A quick investigation unraveled the facts. The PAs had been out of town attending a conference over the weekend and decided to go bar-hopping with some of their colleagues. They said they had too much to drink and couldn't remember much of anything that had happened that night. Several people in the crowd had taken videos of them without their knowledge or permission and shared them via social media with countless other people. Unfortunately, some of the people who saw the videos were coworkers, doctors, and patients of the practice.

What should Carla do about this unfortunate situation? What would you do if you were in Carla's place?

Your relationships, both at work and outside of work, can also have a positive or negative effect on your personal and professional image. The types of people with whom you associate are a reflection of your personal values and who you are as a person. What impact do the people with whom *you* associate have on your reputation?

It's a small world. You never know when you might run into your supervisor, a coworker, or someone who knows someone you know after hours. "So what?" you might ask. "If I'm not at work, what difference does it make? What I do on my own time is no one's business." While it's true that you are "off the clock," what you do after hours can make a huge difference. Your reputation goes with you *every place* you go. You never know who might be sitting across the room from you in a restaurant, bar, or some other public place. If you've had a few drinks and your voice gets loud, and if you spread gossip, reveal confidential information, or criticize your employer in public, these kinds of after-hours behaviors can cause serious problems at work. If you call in sick when you really aren't and then go out in public, you never know who you might run into. If someone sees you and word gets back to your supervisor, you wouldn't be the first person to get fired from a job under circumstances such as these. If you're arrested and spend the night in jail, don't be surprised if your employer finds out.

If your work group, department, or company has a special event after hours, the standards that govern acceptable behavior at work apply during those events, too. Always conduct yourself in a professional manner. Don't drink too much, engage in wild behavior, and then regret it the next day. It's hard to reestablish trust, respect, and your professional reputation after making some poor decisions the night before. Be very careful about what you post on Facebook, Twitter, and other social media sites and blogs. Sharing personal photographs and private information, posting complaints and gossip about coworkers and your employer, and making even casual

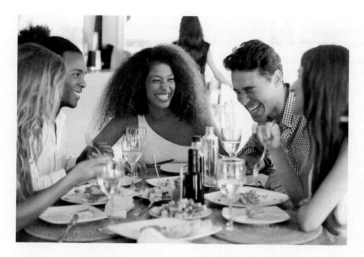

Figure 6-4 Socializing after hours (*Monkey Business Images/Shutterstock*)

comments about patients are easy ways to ruin your reputation and lead to corrective action or dismissal from your job.

Give serious thought to the pros and cons of dating someone you work with before you decide to do it. How might having a personal relationship outside of work impact both of you at work? What might happen when the relationship ends? Could the other person end up being your supervisor someday, or your subordinate? What issues related to sexual harassment might arise? If you're dating your supervisor and things go wrong, you may have to change jobs. If you "mix business with pleasure" with people who report to you, you may have difficulty supervising them later on. It's best to avoid these kinds of social relationships as they often lead to trouble.

The point of this discussion is to remember that you are just one person. You aren't one person at work and a different person outside of work, so do your best to maintain a positive image after hours, too. It is okay to "let your hair down" and have a good time, but don't let your guard down as well. Always think before you act.

PROFESSIONALISM ONLINE

HEALTH AND SAFETY CONCERNS WITH SOCIAL MEDIA

The use of digital devices and social media raise some issues related to your personal health, wellness, and safety. Let's start with health and wellness concerns.

It's not unusual to hear about people who have difficulty getting a good night's sleep because they won't (or can't) disconnect from their devices. They work on their device or computer for several hours before turning off the lights and then have trouble going to sleep. They wake up during the night, check their messages, and then struggle returning to sleep. They take a day off from work or leave home on vacation but continue to be tethered to their phones. These habits not only have a negative effect on personal health and wellness, they also take a toll on personal relationships with family and friends.

(Continued)

Some companies are instituting new policies that encourage or even require employees to disconnect when off-duty. It's not healthy to monitor and transmit work-related emails and text messages 24 hours a day, 365 days a year. There's a reason why employers don't want their staff members obsessed with emailing and texting at all hours of the day and night. They understand that people need breaks from their work to reduce stress, anxiety, and fatigue. Just a few years ago, staff members who emailed on days off and late into the night were thought to be hard workers and dedicated to their jobs. But today, many employers realize that such practices are unhealthy.

The light created by computer screens resembles daylight. Viewing a computer screen two hours before bedtime can interrupt sleep patterns. Spending too much time with your head lowered looking down at a device without taking frequent breaks is causing back and neck pain and vision problems. Everywhere you look, people are stumbling along sidewalks, bumping into other people, crossing streets, and moving through stores looking down at their devices instead of watching where they're going. And worse yet, they're texting and checking social media sites while driving. Cell phone distractions are involved in at least 25% of all car crashes. Almost 50% of car crashes involve excessive speed. It's hard to be a competent, cautious driver when you aren't watching the road or paying attention to how fast you're driving.

When it comes to personal safety issues, the Internet and social media are full of predators. You never know who is really at the other end of a digital communication. People can be imposters. Participants in chatrooms are anonymous.

Online romance scams accounted for at least 10% of the $800 million attributed to Internet crimes in 2014, and those are just the scams that were reported. Many victims are too ashamed and embarrassed to admit they've been duped.

People on online dating sites can lie about themselves and hide their criminal histories. They find women on online dating sites and then quickly change to email or texting to continue communication. They come up with reasons why they can't meet in person and often won't talk by phone because of bad connections when secretly calling from other countries. They provide fake photos of themselves, often hacked from social media sites or online stock photo providers. They express love quickly and endear themselves to their victims. Once they've become the love of your life, they make up exciting stories about business ventures and exotic travel. Before long, they're asking for money for things like family problems, business investments, or tax issues—all of which are temporary and solved via a quick loan from you. These predators scam their naive victims for thousands of dollars. Reporting this type of fraud is important but it's almost impossible to track down the perpetrators and prosecute them, especially in other countries.

Dating scams is just one example of dishonesty and criminal activity online. When you consider other types of scams along with hacking, identity theft, stalking, invasion of privacy, and embarrassment it's obvious that people must be very careful with whom they connect.

It's a dangerous world out there and predators are just a click away. To file a complaint with the Internet Crime Complaint Center, go to *www.ic3.gov.*

Personal Health and Wellness

Health care is one of most physically demanding, emotionally draining, and stressful industries in which to work. Meeting the needs of patients, operating high-tech equipment, dealing with lean staffing, adhering to tight schedules, and handling life-and-death situations on a daily basis can result in high levels of stress. Lifting patients and heavy objects can cause back injuries and employees can catch infectious diseases from patients, visitors, and guests. So it's important to pay attention to your own health and wellness while caring for other people.

THE MORE YOU KNOW_____

SELF-CARE FOR HEALTH CARE WORKERS

Self-care (the actions that people take to establish and maintain their own physical, mental, and emotional health) is an important aspect of working in health care, yet it's often overlooked when people have so many other priorities to balance at work and in their personal lives. Taking care of your own health is the first step in readiness to care for other people. Make self-care an intentional habit by reminding yourself, "I need to take care of myself."

If your job involves direct patient care, or working in areas where patients are present, you may be exposed to a variety of infectious diseases. It's important to follow handwashing procedures and other precautions to guard against getting sick yourself. Use personal protective equipment such as gloves, masks, and gowns when called for and follow up quickly if you've been stuck with a dirty needle or exposed to an infectious disease.

Keep a journal or diary to track your physical, mental, and emotional health. When you notice negative or harmful patterns, take action. Be proactive. Don't wait to discuss any health issues with your doctor. Here are some more self-care tips to think about:

- Get plenty of physical exercise to strengthen your muscles and your cardiovascular and immune systems and help prevent obesity, diabetes, and heart disease.
- Schedule a routine physical examination at least once a year.
- Undergo routine **health screenings** (tests or examinations to find a disease or condition before symptoms may have appeared) and follow up on the results.
- Get an annual flu shot and keep your **immunizations** (vaccinations to protect against getting a disease) up to date.
- Avoid substance abuse including alcohol, tobacco, prescription drugs, and illegal substances.
- Practice effective **body mechanics** (proper body movements such as safe lifting techniques to prevent or reduce injuries).
- Get a sufficient amount of sleep.
- Practice good dental health and protect your eyesight and hearing.
- Eat a healthy diet and control your weight.
- Maintain adequate personal health insurance.

Health care costs are continuing to rise in the United States, causing financial difficulties for employers who provide health insurance benefits for their employees. As the cost of health care increases, employers must absorb the extra expense, charge employees more for their insurance, or reduce the level of benefits their employees receive. When you stop and think about it, health care companies are employers, too. As they increase their prices for the services they provide, they too must figure out how to handle the rising cost of health insurance for their employees.

These financial pressures have resulted in a variety of programs to encourage employees to become healthier. Employees in some companies get a discount on their health insurance when they meet certain health indicators. In other companies, employees are charged higher rates for their health insurance when they fail to meet certain health indicators. Either way you look at it, these financial incentives are generating visible improvements in the way health care workers manage their own health.

TRENDS AND ISSUES

NUTRITION AND A HEALTHY DIET

Eating a nutritious diet is one of the best ways to protect your health and avoid getting sick. But with today's busy lifestyles, it can be hard to find the time to prepare and eat healthy food. A proper diet includes the appropriate intake and absorption of vitamins, minerals, carbohydrates, proteins, fats, and water. An improper diet can lead to **malnutrition** (poor nutrition caused by an insufficient or poorly balanced diet or by a medical condition) and conditions such as anemia, obesity, diabetes, rickets, constipation, diarrhea, dehydration, anorexia nervosa, bulimia, osteoporosis, and dental problems. Think about your food choices and how they affect your body and health. Let's take a quick look at eating disorders.

The three main types of eating disorders are anorexia nervosa, bulimia, and binge eating. All three can affect a person's health including causing serious heart conditions, kidney failure, and electrolyte imbalance. The cause of eating disorders is not entirely clear. They seem to have a basis in biology but they are also affected by emotions, genes, and culture.

Eating is controlled by many factors including a person's appetite; the availability of food; family, peer, and cultural practices; and attempts at voluntary control. An eating disorder involves a serious disturbance in eating behavior, such as extreme reduction of food intake, severe overeating, or intentional vomiting.

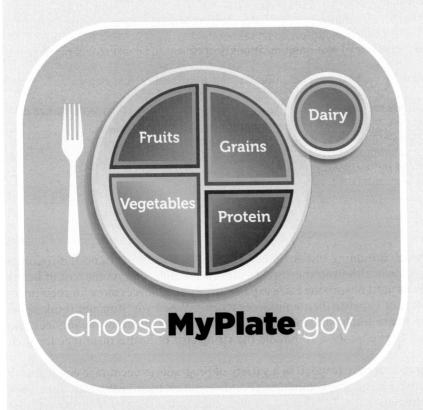

Figure 6-5 U.S. Department of Agriculture Choose MyPlate.Gov poster
(*From ChooseMyPlate.gov. Published by U.S. Department of Agriculture, © 2011.*)

Eating disorders frequently develop during adolescence or early adulthood and can often be found with other problems such as depression, substance abuse, and anxiety disorders. Women are much more likely than men to develop an eating disorder. Women's magazines, fashion trends, and some activities and professions promote dieting to achieve the *perfect* lean body. This can lead to pressure on women to be thin. Eating disorders are sometimes triggered by the stress of being unable to reach an unattainable goal. Males make up only about 10% of people with anorexia or bulimia.

People with eating disorders often don't recognize or admit they're ill. They may strongly resist getting and staying in treatment. Family members or friends can be helpful in making sure that a person with an eating disorder receives the necessary care. Eating disorders can be treated and a healthy weight restored. The sooner a doctor diagnoses and treats these disorders, the better the outcomes are likely to be. Eating disorders often have multiple causes and require a complex treatment plan. This may include medical care, psychological treatment, nutritional counseling, and medication. Ongoing research by scientists continues to advance the understanding and treatment of eating disorders. These are just a few examples how eating habits and diets can affect your health.

USDA Guidelines

In 2011, the U.S. Department of Agriculture (USDA) released MyPlate as a guideline to promote a healthy diet and to reduce obesity and the risk of chronic diseases. Using a *place setting* example, MyPlate illustrates the five food groups that your plate should contain. These dietary guidelines encourage people to eat more fruits and vegetables, whole grains, fat-free and low-fat dairy products, and seafood while reducing sodium, saturated and trans fats, refined grains, and added sugars. Reducing calories and increasing physical activity are also important aspects of the guidelines.

According to the USDA:

- Fruits and vegetables should cover half of your "plate" with grains and protein covering the other half. Half of the grains you consume should be whole grains.
- Eating seafood twice a week should provide your protein, along with beans, which are also a good source of fiber.
- Poultry and meat portions should be lean and small.
- Dairy products such as milk should be fat-free or low-fat (1%).
- Fatty foods such as ice cream, pizza, hot dogs, and cookies should be *treats* and not part of your daily diet.
- When eating packaged or frozen meals, choose low- or reduced-sodium options.
- Water is the beverage of choice as opposed to sugary drinks.

Employee Wellness Programs

Health care companies want their employees to set a good example for patients and the community when it comes to health and wellness. Many offer voluntary wellness programs that include:

- **Health risk assessments** (questionnaires that identify which health issues a person needs to focus on based on medical history and lifestyle)
- Health screenings that measure **body mass index (BMI)** (measure of body fat based on height and weight for adult men and women), blood pressure, blood glucose, and cholesterol
- Exercise, nutrition, weight loss, smoking cessation, and **stress management** (means of dealing with stress and stressful situations) classes
- Coaching and support provided by wellness counselors

Employers are offering healthier food choices in their cafeterias and vending machines, setting aside bicycle and walking paths on their campuses, planting gardens to provide fresh produce, and offering employee discounts on memberships at local fitness clubs. All of this is good news for health care workers who recognize the connection between a healthy personal life and a healthy professional live.

Personal Risk Factors

Another important element of your personal health and wellness is avoiding unnecessary risks that could lead to accidents, injuries, or death. Stop and think before doing something foolish that could cause harm to yourself or those around you. Pay attention to where you are, what you're doing, and what's going on around you. You're probably familiar with the statement, "If you see something, say something." Watch for situations where you may be in danger and take steps to protect yourself.

BY THE NUMBERS

LEADING CAUSES OF DEATH

Taking risks is a fact of life. You can't get ahead without taking a few risks along the way. Think of the thrill of a roller coaster ride: you want to hang on tightly yet let go and have fun! But when it comes to your personal life, you should avoid risks that might have serious consequences. The risks you take should be well thought out, calculated, and intentional.

A study published by *Time* magazine (July 6–13, 2015) reveals the risk factors that caused the deaths of the 2.6 million people who died in the United States in 2013. Here are some of the findings:

- Birth defects were the leading cause of death (20%) for infants under the age of 1, followed by premature birth (18%), and maternal pregnancy complications (7%).
- For people who died between the ages of 1 and 4, 32% died from accidents, 12% from birth defects, and 8% from homicide.
- For ages 5 to 9, the leading cause of death was accidents (31%), followed by 18% cancer and 7% birth defects.
- For ages 10 to 14, 27% died from accidents, 15% from cancer, and 13% from suicide.
- For ages 15 to 24, 41% died from accidents, 17% from suicide, and 15% from homicide.
- For ages 25 to 34, 36% died from accidents, 14% from suicide, and 9% from homicide.
- For ages 35 to 44, 22% died from accidents, 16% from cancer, and 15% from heart disease.
- For ages 45 to 54, 26% died from cancer, 20% from heart disease, and 12% from accidents.
- For ages 55 to 64, 34% died from cancer, 22% from heart disease, and 5% from accidents.
- For ages 65 and over, 26% died from heart disease, 21% from cancer, and 7% from chronic respiratory disease.

It's not surprising that birth-related problems were the leading cause of death for infants, and disease-related conditions were the leading cause of death for adults 45 and older. What is striking about these findings is that accidents were the leading cause of death for people between the ages of 1 and 44. Consider that many, if not most, accidents are preventable. For children ages 1–4, drowning is the top cause of accidental death. For ages 5–24, motor-vehicle accidents kill the most people. Think about these statistics the next time you are tempted to text, talk on the phone, or operate a device while driving.

Personal Management Skills

Personal management skills (the ability to manage one's time, personal finances, stress, and change) help keep your personal life in order and support your success at work. Attendance and punctuality are good examples of how your personal life can affect your job. After all, does it really matter how professional you look or how competent you are if you can't get to work on time and be there when you're supposed to be? Your ability to show up for work on a daily basis and keep your appointments is one important aspect of your job. If you have trouble managing your time, handling your finances, dealing with stress, or adapting to change, your personal life could have a negative impact on your job and on your career. Let's take a closer look.

Time Management

When it seems like there are never enough hours in the day to get everything done that needs to get done, **time management** (the ability to organize and allocate one's time) skills can be a big help in increasing your productivity and well-being. Here are some suggestions to help you balance work, family, and the many other priorities in your life:

- Use an electronic or pocket-sized calendar to record your work schedule, classes, appointments, and so on. Refer to your calendar every day and think about what's coming up tomorrow so you can be prepared. Don't schedule things too closely together, allow extra time for travel, and have backup plans for unexpected complications.
- Make lists of things that need to get done. If you become overwhelmed, decide which are the most important and which you can let go. Eliminate activities that waste time and learn to say "no" when you're overbooked.
- Don't **procrastinate** (to postpone or delay taking action). Letting things build up is a sure way to become overwhelmed and disorganized.

Identify your priorities and allocate your time accordingly. You can't create more hours in the day, but you can seize control and make better use of the time you have. After all, time is one of your most precious and limited commodities. Learning how to manage it appropriately can have a huge impact on your personal and professional lives.

Personal Financial Management

How well you manage another precious and limited commodity—your personal finances—can have a big impact on your personal and professional lives. Effective **personal financial management** (the ability to make sound decisions about personal finances) skills can help you pay your bills on time and avoid financial problems that could cause embarrassment at work. Current and potential employers may have access to your personal credit history and financial details, so it's important to make sure your affairs are in order.

Here are some suggestions to help you live within your means and avoid wasting money:

- Develop a budget, monitor your expenses, and know where your money is going. Keep your checking and savings accounts balanced. Match up paydays with the dates you pay your bills to avoid getting charged late fees.
- Read the fine print on loan and credit card applications. Avoid the high cost of doing business with companies that offer check-cashing services, payday loans, rent-to-own furniture, and income tax refund anticipation loans.

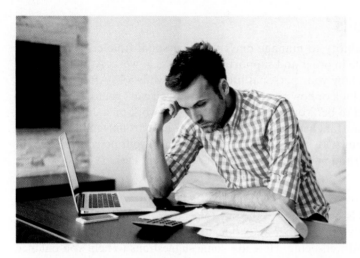

Figure 6-6 Reviewing the budget and paying bills on time (*Baranq/Shutterstock*)

- Limit credit card use to emergency situations or to make purchases that you already have the cash to cover. Pay the balance as soon as possible to avoid interest fees.
- Have a savings plan and stick with it. Put some money away for emergencies and other unexpected expenses. Start saving now for retirement. You'll be surprised how quickly small investments can grow over many years.
- Think twice before loaning someone money or cosigning their loan. If you must loan someone money, use a written agreement detailing their plans for repayment. Only loan money that you can afford to lose.
- If you find yourself deep in debt, get some help from a credentialed, qualified financial counselor. Follow through with the plan and don't give in to the temptation to spend money that you don't have.
- Ask if liability insurance is recommended for people in your profession. This is especially important for some types of licensed professionals.

Managing personal finances can be quite a challenge in today's world. Establish priorities for how you want to allocate your resources and make your financial decisions accordingly.

Stress Management

Health care jobs are among the most stress-producing occupations. Stress can affect your physical health as well as your mental and emotional health. Many physicians and researchers are convinced that stress is a contributing factor to several different diseases and abnormalities. Stress can make you sick and cause symptoms such as headaches, fatigue, sleep problems, diarrhea, indigestion, ulcers, hypertension, dizziness, hives, grinding teeth, skin disorders, and stuttering. Stress has been linked with heart attacks, high blood pressure, alcoholism, depression, and drug abuse.

People with "Type A" personalities are among the most susceptible to stress-related disorders. They are highly competitive, impatient high achievers with strong perfectionist tendencies. They often rush from place to place, work long hours, have an intense drive to get things done, become frustrated easily, and have trouble relaxing. When Type A personalities have a lifestyle that includes smoking, drinking, a poor diet, a lack of exercise, and obesity, they become targets for stress-related illness. If you're a Type A personality yourself, or if the stress you experience tends to affect your health in any way, don't wait until it's too late. Watch for the warning signs and seek help in dealing with it.

CONSIDER THIS

MAKING THE MOST OF YOUR TIME OFF

Depending on your job and where you work, you may be caring for more people, and sicker people, than in the past. This can translate into working more hours and longer hours, both of which can cause stress, anxiety, and fatigue. Working too many hours can harm your health, your relationships with other people, and your ability to concentrate and make good decisions. Taking breaks during your shift and scheduling time off from work to rest and to replenish your energy and emotional well-being are important self-care strategies for health care workers.

Employers often combine the time they allow for vacations, holidays, and sickness into one lump sum called *paid time off*, or PTO. As time passes, workers accumulate PTO hours and may request time off based on their work schedules and company needs. Time off for vacations and holidays can be anticipated in advance, but illnesses and injuries occur without notice. So it's important to save some of your PTO for unexpected situations when you need time off but haven't planned for it. It's also important to use some of your PTO for vacation time. Don't be a workaholic! Get away from work, leave work-related stress behind, and enjoy spending quality time by yourself or with family and friends.

Effective stress management skills can be quite valuable in both your personal life and at work. Managing stress is a key factor in your image as a professional. If you "blow up," "melt down," or run for the door at the first sign of stress, you may be letting down your coworkers and patients. Your ability to perform the duties of your job may be affected and your personal health and wellness may suffer. Good stress management techniques can help you keep everything in balance and add more enjoyment to your life. Here are some suggestions:

- Become aware of when, how, and why stress is affecting you; identify where the stress is coming from and seek ways to reduce or eliminate it.
- Identify someone you can talk with—a person who can relate to what you're experiencing and help you think through it.
- Try to keep work-related stress from affecting your personal life, and try to keep stress in your personal life from affecting your job and your work. This is easier said than done because, as mentioned previously, you are just one person.
- Maintain a healthy balance between work, recreation, and rest. Use your vacation time wisely. Learn to relax and schedule time for hobbies, sports, and other personal interests. Get plenty of sleep and exercise and eat properly.
- Use your conflict-resolution skills when necessary and avoid keeping negative feelings bottled up inside you.

An important part of managing stress is being well adjusted and finding happiness in life. Professionals have a positive self-image. They have high levels of self-esteem and self-respect and they know they are worthy individuals. Let's face it—it's difficult for others to have confidence in you if you don't have confidence in yourself.

- Look for the good in yourself, know your limits, and work within them.
- Be patient with yourself and with others. Avoid being a perfectionist—no one is perfect. Setting unrealistic goals is counterproductive and leads to disappointment, low self-esteem, and unnecessary stress.
- Set high but realistic standards for yourself and feel good about your accomplishments.

   Learn to manage your stress and find ways to achieve happiness at work and at home.

HOT TOPICS

FINDING HAPPINESS

Working with patients in a stressful environment can take a toll on your mental and emotional health. It's hard to feel happy when you encounter pain and suffering at work and hear about the horrific tragedies and events that impact people's lives around the world. According to research, about half of our potential for happiness is genetic, while the other half can be under our control. Human nature has a bias toward negativity, so people have to actively seek out happiness and contentment in their lives. Once again, thinking and acting with intention is the key.

It seems that happiness has little to do with wealth or power and more to do with how you interpret and respond to the events in your life. Often when people think back to their childhoods, they remember a simpler time—the happiness that comes from learning to bounce a ball or tie their own shoes. Children experience the joy of learning to read and write, conquering a fear, or mastering a new skill. But as people grow up, human nature kicks in. It's easy for adults to lose the joy of childhood when they become overwhelmed and distracted by the complexities of everyday life. People who become health care workers experience burnout from stress and exhaustion from working so many hours. People start wondering why they aren't as happy as they used to be and how they can regain a sense of joy and contentment in their lives.

The good news is you have the power to be happier by framing what's going on in your life in more positive terms. Cancer survivors often say that getting cancer was one of the best things that ever happened to them because facing death helped them discover what's really important in life. People with terminal illnesses who know they are about to die typically use their remaining time to enjoy family, friends, and the "small things" in life. Think about that. What's really most important in *your* life? What do *you* have to be happy about?

Here are tips to help you enhance the happiness in your life:

- Find a few minutes each day to relax and be quiet; free up your mind to think and ponder.
- Focus on the positives; find reasons to be happy and content with your life.
- Be mindful of what really matters the most in your life.
- If you have to adjust or learn something new, find reasons to embrace the change.
- Be forgiving and don't hold grudges; move on with a positive attitude.
- Count your blessings; remember for what you are grateful.
- Cry when you need to; laugh and smile as much as you can.
- Stay connected with other people; enjoy social time with family and friends.
- Take time to appreciate the small things in life; *stop and smell the flowers*.
- Set aside time for hobbies, sports, and other activities that bring you joy.
- Spend time outdoors; take a walk, ride a bike, watch the clouds and the sunset.

- Connect with nature; listen to the rain, enjoy a waterfall, and breathe in some fresh air.
- Take a hot shower or a warm bath; sip a cup of hot soup or tea.
- Volunteer your time and energy to help other people who could benefit.
- Challenge your brain to try something new; be creative and imaginative.
- Break your routine; go someplace you've never been and meet some new people.

So what's the secret to finding happiness? It's already within you.

Managing Change

In today's health care workplace, one of the most important personal management skills is the ability to adjust to change. Just when you think everything is arranged as it should be, something changes. You might acquire extra job duties, undergo cross-training, or be assigned to work in a different location. Your work schedule might get altered, your company might merge with another company, or your supervisor might change.

At the same time you're affected by changes at work, you're probably facing changes in your personal life as well. Family responsibilities, relationships with friends, and pressures involving finances, housing, and personal health can all cause many changes over the course of our lives. It's almost impossible to avoid change. If you're the type of person who resists change, you're going to face some difficult struggles working in health care. On the other hand, if you have effective **adaptive skills** (the ability to adjust to change), you'll be well prepared for the many changes that life will send your way. Years ago, health care workers were encouraged to *cope* with change. When the pace of change increased, people were encouraged to *manage* change. Now that change is occurring so rapidly, health care workers must *embrace* change and even *lead* change from time to time.

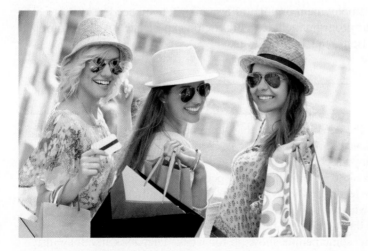

Figure 6-7 Enjoying time with friends (*Kamil Macniak/Shutterstock*)

RECENT DEVELOPMENTS

BUILDING RESILIENCE TO DEAL WITH CHANGE AND ADVERSITY

Just about the only thing you can count on with certainty these days is that things will change and, oftentimes, not for the better. That's why **resilience** (the ability to adapt and recover from stress and difficulty) is such an important factor in maintaining personal health and wellness for health care workers. Life is full of challenges and **adversity** (hardships; misfortune). If you're resilient, flexible, and adaptive to change, you can deal with your problems and avoid feeling overwhelmed or depressed.

Resilience is a skill that can be learned and strengthened over time. By training yourself to be intentional in your thoughts, you can focus on what's meaningful and positive in your life instead of viewing yourself as a victim. People who are resilient:

- Find healthy ways to deal with stress.
- Avoid coping mechanisms such as alcohol or drug abuse.
- Work through their emotions and feel a sense of control.
- Find confidence in their strengths and abilities.
- Use effective communication and problem-solving skills.
- Dwell on what's right with their lives rather than what's wrong.

Resilient people ask for help when they need it, and they help other people when they can. They maintain good relationships with their families and friends and they learn to overcome grief, sadness, and loss.

Change can be a positive influence in your life if you learn to accept it and let it open new doors for you. Having your job redesigned, for example, can be pretty scary. You might have to learn some new skills and take on additional responsibilities. But the more new challenges you face, the more you will grow. The more you grow, the better your chances for advancement. View change as positive and learn to make it work *for* you instead of *against* you. After all, do you really want your personal life and your career to be exactly the same five years from now as they are today?

Chapter Eight takes a look at employment opportunities and what you need to know to plan for career advancement. But if your program includes a practicum experience, let's take a look at what to expect in your practicum first—in Chapter Seven.

REALITY CHECK

It's time to take a close look at the personal image that you portray. Do your appearance, habits, language, and grammar lead people to view you as a professional? Or would patients, coworkers, and doctors question your competence because of your attire or the condition of the clothes you wear? Do you take into account how older people might react to your appearance? Or is your unsettling image leading patients to ask for "someone different" to take care of them? Are you careful about what you say at work and how you say it? Or is using "street language" offending people and damaging your reputation?

You might be amazed at how some people show up for work. They look like they just rolled out of bed, or never went to bed. It's obvious they either don't care what they look like or they don't have a clue how people are expected to dress in a business environment. Once you've made an impression such as this, it will be difficult to overcome people's opinions of you. Bare skin, visible undergarments, and spandex clothes are enough to shock your supervisor into putting you on corrective action and sending you home without pay. If any of this describes you, it's time to clean up your act and your appearance.

Your health care education and training will provide the knowledge and skills you need to support the health and wellness of your patients. But it's up to you to protect, maintain, and improve your own health. How healthy are you? What lifestyle factors are affecting your health and wellness? Are you physically, mentally, and emotionally fit? Do you eat a healthy diet and avoid the dangers of smoking, alcohol, and drugs? Do you get a physical exam every year and undergo health screenings? Are you aware of your family's medical history and taking proactive steps to watch for similar signs and symptoms yourself? Or are you taking unnecessary risks such as binge drinking, driving drunk, having unprotected sex, or texting while driving? Many young people tend to think they are **invincible** (incapable of being overcome), and that health problems and diseases are for *old people*. Nothing could be further from the truth. If you're serious about a career in health care, it's never too early to start focusing on your own health and wellness.

For More Information

Vaccines and Immunizations
Centers for Disease Control and Prevention
www.cdc.gov/vaccines/vac-gen/imz-basics.htm

Body Mass Index
National Heart, Lung, and Blood Institute
U.S. Department of Health and Human Services
**https://www.nhlbi.nih.gov/health/educational/
lose_wt/BMI/bmicalc.htm**

Time Management Strategies and Techniques
www.timemanagement.com

Stress Management
MedLine Plus
U.S. National Library of Medicine and
National Institutes of Health
https://www.nlm.nih.gov/medlineplus/stress.html

Personal Financial Management
Kiplinger
www.kiplinger.com

Health Risk Assessments
Heart Attack Risk Assessment
American Heart Association
**www.heart.org/HEARTORG/Conditions/
HeartAttack/HeartAttackToolsResources/
Heart-Attack-Risk-Assessment_UCM_303944_
Article.jsp**

USDA Guidelines for a Healthy Diet
MyPlate
www.choosemyplate.gov

Personal Risk Factors
"What Are My Risk Factors"
Time magazine, July 6–13, 2015
**http://backissues.time.com/storefront/2015/
the-answers-issue/prodTD20150706.html**

Internet Crime Complaint Center
Federal Bureau of Investigation and the National
White Collar Crime Center
www.ic3.gov

FBI Warnings of Online Dating Scams
**https://www.fbi.gov/sandiego/press-releases/2015/
fbi-warns-of-online-dating-scams**

KEY POINTS

- Do your best to keep your personal life in balance so that personal problems don't have a negative impact on your professional reputation.
- Adhere to dress code policies to portray a positive personal image.
- Avoid stereotyping other people and forming inaccurate first impressions.
- Avoid personal habits that annoy other people.
- Use proper language and grammar and avoid "street language" at work.
- Don't let your guard down after hours.
- Think twice before dating a coworker or your supervisor.
- Take advantage of health risk assessments and address any medical conditions uncovered.
- Use good time management skills and don't procrastinate.
- Keep your personal finances in order and live within your means.
- Identify the sources of your stress and take steps to reduce or eliminate them.
- Sharpen your adaptive skills and be open to opportunities that come with change.
- Consider the health and safety concerns of using digital communication and social media and protect yourself from online predators.

LEARNING ACTIVITIES

Using information from Chapter Six:
- Answer the Chapter Review Questions
- Respond to the What If? Scenarios

Chapter Review Questions

Using information from Chapter Six, answer each of the following:

1. Explain how personal skills affect your success as a health care worker.

2. Describe how your personal image affects patient care.

3. List five appearance and grooming factors that result in a professional image.

4. Explain how stereotypes impact first impressions.

5. List three examples of annoying and troublesome personal habits.

6. Describe how grammar and vocabulary impact your professional image.

7. Explain the importance of maintaining professionalism after hours.

8. List three health and safety concerns with social media.

9. Describe the importance of self-care for health care workers.

10. Give two examples of how health care companies are encouraging employees to become healthier.

11. Describe three time management techniques.

12. Describe three financial management techniques.

13. Describe three stress management techniques.

14. Explain why the ability to manage change is so important in health care today.

What If? Scenarios

Think about what you would do in the following situations and record your answers.

1. Your company's dress code allows denim jeans and T-shirts on Fridays for "casual day." Because you've been cross-trained to fill in for the customer service department when it is shorthanded, it's possible you could be asked to work at the information desk in the main lobby with little or no notice.

2. You've spent six months working out at a fitness center and look really good in tight blouses and short skirts. Hopefully, the cute guy who started working in medical records last week will notice you and ask you out.

3. Some of the employees with whom you eat lunch use street language and at times it can be overheard by other people in your company's cafeteria.

4. The only free time you have to jog on a regular basis is during your lunch break. Your break is long enough to get some good exercise, but you don't have time to take a shower before resuming work.

5. You and a group of coworkers decide to start meeting at a popular bar on Saturday nights to "let your hair down" and have a good time. On the very first night, one person in your group drinks too much and ends up in a fistfight with a stranger seated at the next table. You overhear the bartender calling the police.

6. It seems there are never enough hours in the day for you to get everything done that you want to do. You work full time, participate in two softball leagues, transport your children to sporting events, volunteer at a local charity, play basketball with your friends on Saturday afternoons, and take two courses each semester toward the degree you've been working on. Last week, you were late for work twice, called in sick the day your son's school was closed because of the weather, and had to cancel a dentist appointment at the last minute. You know your job is important, but so are your family, friends, and other activities.

7. You just received a raise, giving you an extra $25 in each paycheck. Then the telephone rang and you found out you qualified for a new credit card that you hadn't even applied for. With your pay raise and a $5,000 credit limit, you've got the money you need to buy that new smart television your children have been begging you for.

8. For the past month, you've been having headaches and difficulty sleeping at night. You're less patient with your children and have yelled at them several times. Even though you've been eating more than usual, you seem to have very little energy and can't keep up with physical activities. Yesterday, when your supervisor asked if you could work overtime, you blew up and yelled, "Are you kidding me? Why can't somebody else do it? Why does it always have to be me?"

9. You just found out that your health insurance premium at work is going up $50 a month. If you fill out a health risk assessment, undergo a physical exam, and fall within the healthy range for indicators such as blood pressure and body mass index, you can reduce your cost by $25 a month.

10. You met someone via an online dating site. After communicating by email for several months and becoming close friends, he tells you his mother is sick and asks you to loan him $5,000 for her surgery.

The Practicum Experience

7

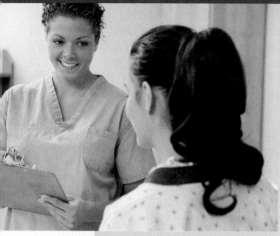

My interest is in the future because I am going to spend the rest of my life there.

—Charles F. Kettering (1876–1958),
inventor and engineer

(Tyler Olson/Shutterstock)

CHAPTER OBJECTIVES

Having completed this chapter, you will be able to:

- Identify the purpose of a practicum.
- List three benefits of a practicum experience.
- Identify three requirements to gain clearance for a practicum.
- Describe two ways to prepare for a practicum.
- Explain the connection between your performance on a practicum and securing an employment reference at graduation.
- Explain the value of keeping a journal during your practicum.
- Give three examples of protocol involving cell phones and social media during your practicum.
- Explain the importance of maintaining patient confidentiality during your practicum.
- List three safety factors to keep in mind when working in a health care facility.
- Identify three of the criteria considered when evaluating your performance and assigning a grade for your practicum.

KEY TERMS

drug screen	mentors	office politics	samples room
journal	observations	profane	

The Purpose of a Practicum

A practicum is a real-life learning experience obtained through working on-site in a health care facility while enrolled as a student. Schools and educational programs use different terms for the practicum experience such as clinicals, externship, internship, hands-on experience, professional practice experience, and so forth. But these terms all mean basically the same thing. Whether you're in medical assisting, surgical technology, radiography, medical technology, or another type of health care educational program, there's a good chance you'll be doing a practicum experience before you graduate. Some programs begin the practicum experience early in the curriculum, integrating classroom instruction with hands-on experience. Other programs complete classroom instruction first and schedule the practicum at the end of the program just prior to graduation.

The Benefits of a Practicum Experience

You may be thinking, "Why should I worry about my practicum? It's just another assignment to complete before I can graduate." In reality, your practicum is much more than just another assignment. In fact, it's probably *the* most important part of your education. Your practicum is an opportunity to apply the knowledge and skills you've acquired during the classroom portion of your training in an actual health care setting while still a student. If you perform well, your practicum could also result in an employment recommendation or a job offer when you graduate.

Students Compared to Employees

Practicum experiences vary in length, depending on the discipline you're studying and the program in which you are enrolled. Some practicums will be relatively short, lasting just a few weeks or months. Other practicums will extend over several months or a year or more. Since educational accreditation requirements don't permit students to be paid during their practicum, at times you may feel like "free labor." But keep one very important fact in mind: You are there as a *student* to learn and to hone your knowledge and skills. Even though the site supervisor will assign your work hours, break times, duties, and responsibilities, you are *not* there as an employee. There's a big difference between being at the site as a student and working there as an employee. You need to keep these differences in mind as you progress through the experience. Although you are a student in the facility, you must still comply with certain policies, procedures, and OSHA (Occupational Safety and Health Administration) standards to ensure a safe work environment.

Participating in a practicum is a privilege. Whether your practicum is in a hospital, outpatient clinic, physician practice, surgery or imaging center, or clinical lab, you are a guest in the facility. The site supervisor has the right to terminate your practicum at any point in time if he or she believes that your appearance, attitude, or performance negatively impacts the site's patients, visitors, doctors, or employees. So you must "prove yourself" in the early stages of your practicum to convince the site supervisor that you are prepared and personally committed to performing well. This is the time to apply everything you've learned so far to begin establishing your own reputation as a health care professional.

Identifying Preferences

Another benefit of a practicum experience is having the opportunity to explore what types of patients you'd like to work with after you graduate. It's not unusual to hear students say they want

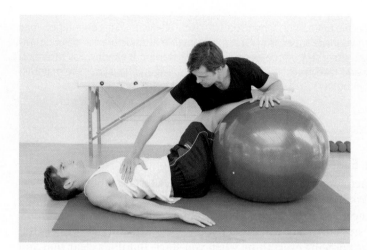

Figure 7-1 Practicing physical therapy skills (*Lightwavemedia/Shutterstock*)

to work in pediatrics (peds). Working with pediatric patients can be highly rewarding, but it takes a certain type of person to do this. Sometimes students have an unrealistic image of working with children. They imagine themselves holding and cuddling newborns and small children. They may not think about the children being sick or unruly, and their parents being anxious and upset. Experience shows that about half of the students who say they want to work in peds change their minds after a pediatric practicum. Radiography students who think they want to specialize in neurology procedures, or surgical technology students who think they want to scrub in on cardiovascular cases, may change their minds after working with these types of patients during their practicum.

The same may be true for different employment locations. Pharmacy technician students may think that working in a hospital pharmacy would be their first choice after graduation, and physical therapy assistants may set their sights on outpatient rehabilitation centers. But after their practicums, the pharmacy tech students might decide on retail pharmacies and the physical therapy assistant students might seek jobs in acute-care hospitals. There's nothing like "being there" to know for sure where you'd like to work and the types of patients and procedures with which you'd like to be involved. Your practicum can help you make those decisions before you apply for jobs and accept an offer.

CONSIDER THIS

SITE ORIENTATION

Health care employers are highly focused on customer service and patient satisfaction. Protecting their reputations to remain competitive is a high priority. Although you'll be a student in your practicum site, you might be issued a site ID badge to wear while you're there. The site's patients, visitors, and guests may assume that you work for the company. Your appearance, attitude, and behavior will impact the site's reputation, so it's important to be familiar with the site's mission, vision, and values and support them accordingly.

(continued)

Expect to participate in a site-specific orientation when you start your practicum. This orientation may be short, such as a conversation with your site supervisor. Or it might involve attending a full-day orientation session, possibly with some of the site's new employees who are just starting their jobs. Pay attention to what is covered in the orientation and take notes. It's time to apply yourself and help your site maintain and enhance its reputation in the community.

How Your Performance Will Be Evaluated

Your performance during your practicum will be evaluated based on criteria established by your school and educational program. You'll likely receive a grade based on your attendance, attitude, appearance, and overall performance, so it's important to do your best. The employees who work at the site will know that you're a student. They will expect you to be a little bit nervous at first and won't hold you accountable for knowing everything when you start. But if it's clear that you haven't been well educated prior to starting your practicum, your deficiencies will soon become apparent. Feel free to ask questions and show an interest in what goes on at the site. But don't ask the same question repeatedly. Remember the answer and jot it down on a small notepad to keep in your pocket.

Picture a practicum site with two students present. One student arrives early, is always visible, asks questions, and steps in to help. He takes notes and pays attention. The other student arrives late and is usually off in another area socializing with people, taking a smoke break, or checking her phone. She rarely asks questions, doesn't show much initiative, and always wants to leave early. It should be obvious which student will earn the highest grade. But what neither student knows is there's going to be a position opening up about the same time the practicum ends and the students graduate. Which student will get the job offer? In situations such as this, the practicum wasn't just "another assignment," it was actually a multiweek job interview.

HOT TOPICS

GAINING CLEARANCE

As a result of growing concerns about workplace theft and violence, sexual harassment, breach of patient confidentiality, and unauthorized sharing of private business information, health care employers are becoming very selective about who they accept for practicum experience. As a result, the requirements that students must meet to gain clearance are becoming increasingly restrictive.

To be cleared for a practicum, expect to undergo a criminal history background check, a **drug screen** (lab test to detect illegal substances), and a physical examination. If you have a criminal history, discuss the situation as soon as possible with your instructor. Certain types of minor offenses may be permissible depending on the details. Other, more serious offenses may prevent you from gaining clearance for a practicum and securing employment after graduation.

If you have questions about passing a drug screen, speak with your instructor as soon as possible. Employers won't tolerate having impaired students or employees in their facilities. Even if you pass a drug screen prior to starting your practicum, you can still be retested without notice at any time if your site supervisor or instructor thinks there might be a problem. If you attend school in a state that has legalized marijuana for medicinal and/or recreational use, you must still pass a drug screen to work in a health care facility. After all, alcohol consumption is legal in all 50 states, but you can't show up for work impaired. The same goes for marijuana. Also keep in mind that using prescription drugs and some over-the-counter medications can cause impairment on the job. Just stop and think—would *you* want *your* caregiver working under the influence of drugs or alcohol?

Certain vaccinations will be required to gain clearance for your practicum. You'll either have to submit documentation from your personal doctor that you've had the vaccinations, or you'll need to receive the vaccinations prior to starting your practicum. Requirements may vary from site to site but typically include vaccinations for mumps, rubella, varicella, measles, tetanus, diphtheria, and pertussis. You will probably be expected to get an annual flu shot. Depending on the types of patients with which you'll be working, you may also need the hepatitis B vaccination (or be required to sign a waiver form) and be fit tested for an N95 respirator. If your practicum is lengthy, expect to undergo an annual TB test. You might also be expected to provide proof of personal health insurance coverage during your practicum experience.

These clearance requirements aren't just for students starting a practicum. They're also a common part of the employment process prior to starting a new job.

Preparing for Your Practicum

Depending on your school and educational program, you may be assigned to a practicum site or you may have some choices. If you have choices, there are some important things to consider before making your decision.

Don't choose a practicum site where you or your family members are patients. It's best to choose a location where you can be viewed solely as a student. It's also preferable to choose a site where you don't know the patients. Having personal relationships with patients at your practicum site can create some issues with privacy and confidentiality.

Pre-Practicum Observations and Research

Some educational programs offer voluntary on-site **observations** (opportunities to view a "real-life" setting to take note of what happens there) for students to visit potential sites before selecting, or being assigned to, a practicum location. Other programs may require an observation and even a pre-practicum interview by the site before being assigned to a location. If your program offers voluntary observations, take advantage of the opportunity. Whether an observation is voluntary or required, you'll gain valuable information about the people who work there and the pace at which they work. Is it a friendly, service-oriented facility? How do the employees interact with their coworkers, patients, doctors, and visitors? Is the environment fast-paced or slow-paced? Which type of environment would be most comfortable for you? Some students prefer a fast-paced environment and get restless if things move too slowly. Other students prefer a slower pace and feel rushed if things move too quickly.

Regardless of whether you're assigned to a site or have some choices, it's a good idea to do some research before you get there.

- Review the company's website and printed materials. The more that you know about the site, the better prepared you will be and the more at ease you will feel on your first day.
- Ask for permission to contact the site ahead of time. Speak with the site supervisor and introduce yourself. Confirm your practicum start date, the hours that you'll be there, and the site's dress code. If there are days when you'll need to leave early for class or a prior commitment, discuss this with your site supervisor before your start date.
- Travel to the site a few days before your practicum starts. Note the travel time. What time do you need to leave home in order to arrive at your site on time? How much traffic should

you anticipate? What if the parking lot is full? What if your bus connection is running late? Imagine the "worst-case scenario" and have contingency plans.

- On your first assigned day, allow sufficient travel time to arrive at the site at least 15 minutes early so you'll feel more comfortable and less rushed. You don't want to arrive late or appear unprepared.

Remember, you *never* get a second chance to make a good first impression.

THINK ABOUT IT

OBSERVATIONS, PRACTICUMS, AND JOB OFFERS

Some practicum sites won't accept students unless they've done an observation there first. This pre-practicum observation gives students a chance to check out the site before starting their practicums. But more importantly, it gives the site a chance to check out the students before accepting them into the facility. If students make a poor impression during the observation, there's a good chance they won't be invited back for a practicum experience.

Many employers hire primarily from the pool of graduates who did their practicum at the site. In some cases, new employees who did their practicum at the site will start their jobs with higher pay. Think about it. If you did your practicum at the site that hired you, they've saved time and money because you're already oriented and ready to work. You're familiar with the staff, doctors, and patients. You know how the practice, department, or work unit functions and you can operate the equipment, perform the procedures, and process the paperwork. You can "hit the ground running" when compared with someone else who might need weeks or months of work experience to ramp up to the level from which you have started. This is just one more reason to impress the staff at your practicum site and aim for a job there at graduation.

During Your Practicum

As mentioned earlier, keep a small notepad with you and take notes. Write down questions that you may want to ask later on. When you think of a question, it may not be the appropriate time to ask it. For example, if you have a question about the way a doctor performed a certain procedure, it would be inappropriate to ask in front of the patient. Asking in front of the patient could make him or her feel uncomfortable, as well as the doctor. You may have questions that you want to hold until you meet with your program instructor again. During the course of a week, many things will occur and your notepad will really come in handy.

Keeping a Journal

Consider keeping a **journal** (a written record of personal thoughts and experiences) during your practicum. Some educational programs require keeping a journal and documenting certain types of information. Your program may be required to keep a copy of your journal in your student file. In such cases, it is best to record your personal thoughts and emotions in a separate document or notepad. (Refer to Appendix G for a Sample Practicum Journal.)

To protect patient confidentiality, do not mention patient names in your journal. Take a few minutes at the end of each day to record what happened, how you reacted, how you felt about it,

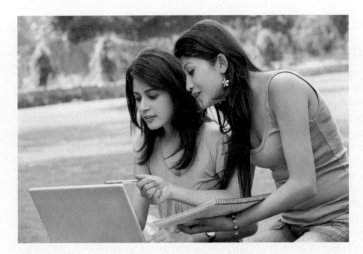

Figure 7-2 Updating journals at the end of the week (*India Picture/Shutterstock*)

and whether you could have handled it differently or better. Journaling can help you "regroup" your feelings, process your experiences, and reflect upon what you've learned. Write about both the good and not-so-good things that you see and experience. Record both the things you *do* and *do not* want to do again in the future. Sometimes you may hear an employee being impolite to a patient. Write down what you heard to remind yourself how others may perceive the things that you say.

You'll likely see some things being done in a different way than how you were taught. By recording this, you'll remember to bring it up when you meet with your instructor and class-mates later on. Expect to be nervous and busy at the same time. If you don't write things down, you may forget something important. If it's written in your journal, you'll have it as a reference whenever you need it. There are also some good pocket-sized reference books for different professions. Check with your instructor to find out if such a book might be helpful during your practicum.

Protocol

Your site will have policies and procedures outlining what you may, and may not, do as a student. This protocol will vary from site to site. Familiarize yourself with protocol at the beginning of your practicum and comply with all policies and procedures while in the facility.

Some patients are comfortable with having a student present during their procedure while other patients are not. Patients have rights that must be protected. So some sites will ask each patient in advance for permission to have a student observe or assist with their procedure. As a student on practicum, you also have rights including the right to observe and participate in proce-dures related to your educational experience. But the patient's rights *always* come first. If a female patient, for example, isn't comfortable having a male student present during her procedure, the male student must comply with the patient's wishes. In most sites, there are a sufficient number of other patients who are comfortable with having students present to ensure that the students' educational goals can be met. Make sure you know how your practicum site protects the rights of its patients and comply with protocol.

PROFESSIONALISM ONLINE

COMPLYING WITH YOUR PRACTICUM SITE'S PROTOCOL

When you get to the portion of your educational program that includes on-site experience, you don't want to jeopardize earning a good grade or securing a positive employment reference due to the inappropriate use of cell phones, digital devices, and computers during your practicum.

Find out how the site handles cell phones, digital devices, and computer use and comply with protocol. Sites typically don't allow students or staff to use personal phones or devices during work hours. In some situations, cell phones may interfere with technical equipment. If you use your phone as a watch when taking vital signs, for example, patients may question what you are doing and wonder if you are video- or audio-recording them. If you text in front of patients, they may assume that your personal messages are more important to you than doing your job and taking care of patients.

The cameras in cell phones can easily lead to HIPAA violations. Companies may prohibit employees, doctors, students, and vendors from taking photographs and videos of *anything* or *anyone* inside the facility or even outdoors on the property.

Most likely you'll be expected to either leave your phone and devices at home or stow them in your car, purse, backpack, locker, or a private area at the site. If your site supervisor gives you permission to have a cell phone on you for a good reason (for example, your child is sick and you're expecting a call from his doctor's office), place your phone on silent so you don't disturb other people. Avoid having your phone ring in areas where patients, visitors, or staff members can hear it, especially if your ring tone is loud or broadcasts music or annoying, unprofessional sounds.

Don't make or take personal phone calls or engage in texting during practicum hours. You're at the site to work and learn, not to interact with family and friends. Keep in mind that computers in health care facilities have strict security requirements. Unauthorized use can lead to disciplinary action. Never log on to a computer at your site without getting permission first.

Social media really has no place during your practicum. If you name the facility where you're doing your practicum, or mention factors that could reveal the location, you are inviting trouble. If the photographs, videos, or content on your social media sites are unprofessional and don't support the mission, vision, and values of your site, your practicum could be quickly terminated. If you mention the site's patients or otherwise violate confidentiality or privacy, you are setting yourself up for disciplinary action and potential prosecution.

This is no time to take risks just to share information with your family and friends. Employers take these matters *very* seriously. Be aware of your site's protocol regarding the use of cell phones, digital devices, computers, and social media and make sure you comply with it.

Privacy and Confidentiality

Protecting patient privacy is extremely important. If a patient must remove all or part of his or her clothing during a procedure, do everything you can to help the patient feel safe and comfortable. Make sure they understand how to properly wear and tie a patient gown. Use sheets and blankets to cover patients and keep them warm. Close doors to examination rooms and pull curtains to provide privacy. Protect patients from situations where they might be needlessly exposed.

Maintaining confidentiality according to HIPAA and HITECH Act rules is a top priority. While on practicum you may have access to patient medical records and other private information. You may even know some of the patients. What you see, hear, or read at the site

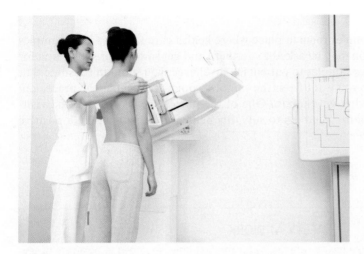

Figure 7-3 Practicing mammography skills while protecting the patient's privacy (*KPG_Payless/Shutterstock*)

must stay at the site. Never read a patient's medical record unless instructed to do so. You will undoubtedly see and do things that you'll want to tell your family and friends about later on. It's natural to be excited and want to share your experiences. But you must remember to never use the patient's name or provide any other descriptive information that could reveal the patient's identity.

Here's an example of an acceptable comment: "You won't believe what I did today. We removed a mole from a patient's arm. I got to prepare the patient for minor surgery and assist the doctor with the procedure." You described what you did without breaking confidentiality. Usually while on practicum, there will be times when you, your classmates, and the instructor meet to discuss what you've seen and done during the week. Again, this is a time to protect the confidentiality of the site's patients.

In addition to medical records, you may also have access to other information such as patient financial records or the site's patient charges or financial transactions. This information must also remain within the site and you should not discuss it with people outside the site. Private information is shared only on a "need-to-know" basis. This means the information is made available only to those people who need to know it to care for patients and conduct the site's business.

You may be rotating to different sites during your practicum and working in companies that compete with one another. Maintain the privacy of business-related information and use discretion when making comparisons among the different places you work. Remember what was said earlier—you are a guest at the site and the supervisor has the right to terminate your practicum at any point should your performance pose a problem. Violation of confidentiality or the unauthorized sharing of sensitive information is a legitimate reason for immediate termination. If you are terminated from your practicum site, you might find it difficult to gain access to another site and your quest for recognition as a health care professional will suffer a major setback.

Samples

Some sites have what's called a **samples room** (a place where health care facilities keep samples of drugs and medical supplies). You may be asked to go there and get samples of something for a patient. Just because the site gives samples to patients at no charge, you shouldn't assume that you can help yourself to whatever you want from the samples room. Remember the practicum student mentioned earlier who didn't get the job? One of the places she was discovered visiting frequently was the samples room. Needless to say, this behavior didn't support a positive reputation.

THE MORE YOU KNOW

SAFETY AT WORK

If your practicum involves working in a health care facility for the first time, you need to be aware of several safety factors. A portion of your site orientation will likely include information designed to ensure a safe work environment. This includes topics such as on-site hazards and how to respond to accidents and emergencies such as fires, chemical spills, workplace violence, weather-related incidents, disasters, and possibly even terrorism. As a student, your role in emergency response will be limited, but you need to be knowledgeable and ready to assist if called upon. Make sure you're familiar with your site's safety-related policies and procedures and comply with them.

Never take risks at work that could harm you or the site's patients, employees, or visitors. Do not under any circumstances bring weapons to your practicum site. Depending on your site, you might be working in areas that involve various types of risk factors. Health care facilities have injury and illness prevention programs and hazard communication programs to identify:

- Which hazards are present and how to prevent injuries from them
- How to use the hazard communication system
- Which chemicals are present and where they're stored and used
- How to respond to chemical and biohazard spills
- How to access and use personal protection equipment
- How to report and respond to a fire
- How to report an injury or illness during work hours and complete the necessary paperwork

Here are some basic safety tips to keep in mind to help prevent accidents at the site:

- Never run in the hallways; walk on the right-hand side of the hall.
- Use handrails when climbing or descending the stairs.
- Watch out for swinging doors.
- Don't play around; rowdy and childish behavior will not be tolerated.
- Always check labels; don't use anything from a container that's not labeled.
- Place litter in containers.
- Dispose of needles in designated sharps containers.
- Wipe up spills using gloves and other precautions when called for.
- Prevent situations that could lead to slips, trips, and falls.
- Avoid using malfunctioning equipment and report the situation to your supervisor.
- Don't use electrical cords that are damaged.
- Report any injury to yourself or others immediately.

Office Politics

No discussion about proper behavior while on a practicum would be complete without talking about **office politics** (clique-like relationships among groups of coworkers that involve scheming and plotting) and how to avoid them. If you've had more than one job, you've probably already discovered that all workplaces have office politics. Whether you're doing your practicum in a doctor's practice, long-term care facility, or hospital critical care unit, there will usually be coworkers who don't get along well with one another.

One employee may tell you something negative about another employee or complain about something that someone else has done. This happens frequently with students and it's easy to get caught in the middle. Stay neutral and don't get involved. Remember, you are not employed by the site and you probably don't have all of the facts. If you allow yourself to become involved in office politics, you could be labeled a troublemaker. The site supervisor may reconsider allowing you to remain there. You could be terminated from the site or lose your opportunity for a good employment reference or job offer at graduation. There's more to a practicum than just practicing your hands-on skills. Practicing your "people skills" and your "professionalism skills" are equally important in ensuring success.

One of the reasons why sites provide practicum experience is that having students present in the facility helps keep the staff "on their toes." Students tend to be inquisitive and ask lots of questions. They watch how coworkers interact with one another and with patients, visitors, and physicians. The employees at the site are all aware of this. They must be able to explain things, answer questions, and set a good example. This helps keep the employees focused on the correct ways to do things and cautious about their behavior.

More Than One Right Way

There is often more than one right way to do things, and your way might not be the only right way. For example, when you clean a room, do you dust or vacuum first? It doesn't matter because both ways

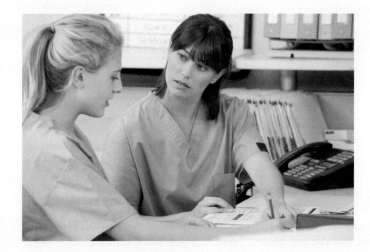

Figure 7-4 Reviewing notes and asking questions (*Monkey Business Images/Shutterstock*)

lead to the same result. If you observe a site employee doing something in a way that's different from the way you were taught, don't say, "That's wrong" or "You aren't doing that right" or "That's not the way we were taught." Instead, turn it into a learning opportunity. Ask the person to explain why and how he or she did it that way. You might learn a new technique that's easier and more efficient.

You will likely see different equipment in your practicum site as compared with your classroom or lab at school. This is one of the benefits of doing a practicum. You get to experience different technology before starting your job. You should approach this situation by saying, "This equipment is different from the one I was taught on. Would you please show me how this one works?" This sounds much better than saying, "I don't know how to operate this equipment. We didn't learn this in school." With the first example, you're indicating that you know the correct procedure but aren't familiar with the specific equipment. Medical equipment can be complicated to operate, mistakes can be expensive, and failure to use equipment properly can jeopardize patient care and patient safety. So make sure you know the correct way to use each piece of equipment.

You may also notice some things being done incorrectly during your practicum, such as not using gloves or other personal protective equipment when called for. Make a note of these situations and discuss them with your instructor and classmates when you meet again as a group. It's just as important to learn *what not to do* on your practicum as it is to learn the correct way to do things.

TRENDS AND ISSUES

THE VALUE OF MENTORS AND ROLE MODELS

Role models and **mentors** (wise, loyal advisers) can be helpful as advisers and/or references as you complete your education and apply for employment. Role models have the education, work experience, and professional reputation that you aspire to achieve yourself. You can learn a lot from a role model because that person has already traveled down the road on which you are starting. Mentors haven't necessarily achieved the same goals to which you aspire, but they can provide the insight, advice, and encouragement you need each step of the way.

Consider who might make a good role model or mentor for you and ask if he or she would be willing to serve. You might be surprised how quickly someone will say yes. Consider volunteering to serve as a role model or mentor for someone else. After all, everyone is on this road together.

Initiative

Once you've learned what is expected of you and you feel comfortable with the equipment and procedures, it's important to begin functioning with less direct supervision. If you are uncertain about something, by all means ask! But if you've been given a responsibility and it's "your job" to do it, then do it. If a patient has checked in and it's your job to escort the patient to the exam room and take their vital signs, then that's what you should do without waiting to be told. Don't make the patient wait. If you hear the phone ring and you've been instructed how to answer it, you should answer it. The more you can do, the better. The more you learn to do and the more cross-training you undergo, the more marketable you will become.

Keep one thing in mind. You are there to learn and to help, not to stand around and get in the way. Show initiative. One of the quickest ways to get labeled as unprofessional is to stand around doing nothing. Everyone from the receptionist to doctors will be watching your every move. Avoid spending too much time chatting with the staff. Be productive and help keep the workflow moving smoothly.

Language

Here's a story that actually happened in a large medical office. A medical assisting student reported to the office on the first day of her practicum. When she arrived, she couldn't remember the name of her contact person. As she was talking to the person seated at the receptionist desk, she became discouraged and used some **profane** (improper and contemptible) language. As it turned out, the "receptionist" was actually the office manager who was in charge of hiring for the practice. Needless to say, the student's practicum experience didn't get off to a good start, and there was no job offer from the site at graduation.

Unprofessional language should never be used in your practicum site. That is not to say you won't hear it yourself, because you will. But just because you hear the employees using profane language is no excuse to use it yourself. Put yourself in the patients' position. If you were sitting in the waiting room and heard the staff using profanity, how would *you* feel? What impact would it have on *your* opinion of the company? At each step of the way, put yourself in the patients' shoes. Even though you are there as a student, the patients will consider you part of the staff. Your behavior not only affects your own reputation but that of the site. Using profanity or any other type of unprofessional language will undermine both reputations.

BY THE NUMBERS

OPENING THE DOOR FOR FUTURE STUDENTS

Depending on the size of the town and the geographic area where you attend school, there may be a limited number of places where students can gain practicum experience. Some health care employers don't offer practicums. They strictly focus on patient care and don't have sufficient staff, time, space, or other resources to accommodate students. Facilities that do offer practicum experiences may only accept a limited number of students each semester or year and restrict their involvement to schools with which they have contracts. Schools that contract with employers for practicum experiences line up their sites in advance. Other schools expect students to find their own practicum site. A limited number of sites may result in competition among schools and students to gain access to the "best" sites for practicum experience. The "best" sites are those that not only welcome students but also provide a supportive learning environment, active supervision, and a sufficient number and variety of procedures to meet the students' educational needs.

It's not unusual for employers to hire graduates who have completed practicum in their facilities. They've had the opportunity to see those students in action, and they know which people would be a good match for the facility and which would not.

One way you can serve your school and your educational program is to perform exceptionally well in your practicum. If you prove to be a mature, serious, competent student who clearly appreciates being there and is willing to go above and beyond meeting the minimum requirements, you may actually *open the door* for other students to follow. On the other hand, if you *slack off* and give the impression that you're just putting in your time and don't really care about being there, the site may decide that working with students isn't worth the effort and may stop offering practicum experiences altogether.

This is an example of the ripple effect. Your attitude, appearance, and behavior during your practicum could have a far-reaching impact well beyond your ability to know it—for better, or worse.

Teamwork

While on practicum, avoid becoming part of a clique. Depending on how long you're there, you may start to feel comfortable with the staff and feel as if you "belong." Belonging is a good feeling, but there's a difference between "fitting in" and being part of a clique. "Fitting in" simply means that you work well with the staff and you are viewed as cooperative. Your personality may blend well with the personalities of the employees. But being part of a clique can work against you. Cliques stick together and don't associate with the rest of the staff. They're exclusionary and they impede teamwork. Employees in cliques are typically less productive because they spend too much time socializing and gossiping.

Supporting teamwork should be one of your goals. When everyone works well together, the site can function smoothly. During your practicum, pay attention to which employees are good team players. Note the difference between team players and nonteam players. You'll notice that nonteam players have to work harder to get the work done while team players pitch in and help each other out. Strive to be a team player and avoid cliques. This could become a major factor in getting a positive employment reference or a job offer at the end of your practicum.

There are several other things to consider during your practicum. Protect yourself and others from infectious diseases by applying everything you've learned about infection control and Universal Precautions. Know where to find personal protective devices and how to use them correctly. If you become ill during your practicum, stay home, call in to report your absence, and don't report for duty. Avoid spreading your germs to the patients and staff.

Patient Preferences

While on practicum, you may come in contact with patients who are familiar with the staff and uncomfortable with anyone who is "new," including students. Don't take this personally as it's very common. Some patients will refuse to tell the student (or a new employee) anything. If a student tries to obtain the patient's history, for example, the patient may resist and ask for someone with whom he or she is more familiar. Patients can bond with members of their health care team and reject the involvement of people they don't know. If this happens to you, don't argue with the

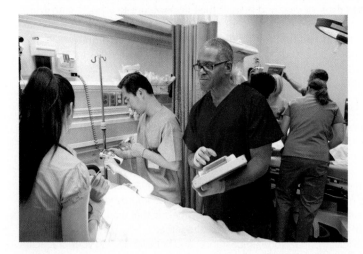

Figure 7-5 Developing teamwork skills in the emergency department (*Monkey Business Images/Shutterstock*)

patient. Explain who you are and why you're there. If the patient still insists on interacting with someone they know, simply excuse yourself and go get one of the staff.

Personal Issues

When you walk through the door to your practicum site, leave your personal problems outside. If you had a disagreement with your spouse or your child that morning, don't discuss it with the people working at your site. If you're upset, distracted, and not thinking clearly, you're more likely to make a mistake. Mistakes must be avoided whenever possible.

Never discuss your personal life or your own medical history with patients. You're there to focus on the patient's situation, not your own. The medical profession is a relatively "small world." People who work for one company often know their counterparts at other companies. They participate in the same professional associations and attend the same continuing education conferences. When they get together, it's not uncommon for them to discuss personnel issues. If you're doing your practicum at a site where you don't want to work after graduation, just keep in mind that the people who work at your site may know their counterparts at the site where you do want to work after graduation. Your performance and reputation as a student can easily spread from one place to the next without you ever knowing about it.

CASE STUDY

Carla and her manager knew there was nothing they could do to save the jobs of their two physician assistants. The PAs had become inebriated in a bar and were videotaped engaging in a sexually explicit act in front of a crowd of onlookers. The videos were posted on social media and shared with other people. Several coworkers, doctors, and even some patients had seen the videos and when the network's leaders became aware of what had happened, they called Carla's manager to voice their outrage. The embarrassing videos not only made the PAs look bad, they harmed the reputations of the practice and the network as well. Even though the employees in question didn't know they were being videotaped, and didn't share the videos themselves or give other people permission to do so, it didn't make any difference. In this case, the employees' behavior outside of work hours really did matter.

The policy was clear and the PAs had to be fired. Carla thought about how this unfortunate situation would affect the future careers of her two colleagues and she knew how difficult it would be to replace them. Highly skilled PAs are in high demand and the practice had just lost two of their best because of poor judgment. It was truly a sad day for everyone involved.

One of Carla's many duties as a supervisor was overseeing medical assisting students doing their internships in the practice. Even before her promotion, she had performed this role and always enjoyed it. Carla's practice was known to be the "best" practicum site for MA students in the area and she was proud of that reputation. Each group brought its own challenges, but for the most part the students were well prepared and eager to make a positive first impression. Not only did they need to complete their clinical education, they also hoped for a positive employment reference and, better yet, a job offer from the practice at graduation.

Some of the students did better than others and it all started at their orientation to the site. Carla went over all of the rules and regulations as set forth by their school, and also covered the protocol for students as mandated by the facility. She made it clear that failure to comply with these requirements could result in terminating the student's practicum at the site. "It's a privilege to be here," she said, "and you must remember that what's best for our patients always comes first."

There were usually at least a few minor infractions along the way. Carla had to inform students

(continued)

that flip-flops are not shoes according to network policy. Cell phones and devices cannot be used during practicum hours. Showing up for work on time does not mean arriving 15 minutes late. And no, you can't take whatever you want from the samples room or the office supply cabinet.

Carla always gave each student a copy of the book *Professionalism in Health Care: A Primer for Career Success* and covered the chapters during her weekly sessions with the group. She'd been given a copy of the book herself when she was an MA student and found the information to be really helpful. Now here she was, semester after semester, covering the same common-sense information with her own students.

One afternoon shortly after the current group had started their practicum, Carla was doing clinical work to maintain her MA skills. She saw one of the male students looking at an elderly female patient who was walking in the hallway to the restroom clothed only in a patient gown with the back portion flapping open. As Carla watched, the student pulled his cell phone out of his pocket and quickly snapped a photo of the patient.

What should Carla do about what she just witnessed? What would you do if you were in Carla's place?

Ensuring Success on Your Practicum

Achieving success, especially during a lengthy practicum, isn't easy. Working without pay can become frustrating and tiresome, especially when you're a student with bills to pay and family obligations to meet. If your practicum occurs at the end of your educational program, you are probably counting the days until graduation and your first paycheck. When you look at employment ads, you'll notice that employers prefer to hire applicants who have work experience. Once you've finished your practicum, you'll have that experience. You'll know how the real world operates. You'll have firsthand knowledge and insights to share during your job interviews. You'll be more polished in your communication skills and you'll present yourself in a professional manner. You didn't get paid for the hours you worked during your practicum, but the experience you gained is priceless.

Be sure to list your practicum experience on your résumé. Ask your site supervisor if you may use him or her as a reference. If you've had a positive experience, most supervisors will be happy to assist you in finding a good job. If you arrived on time, avoided unnecessary absences, and did your best to fulfill the goals of your practicum—all without pay—then your site supervisor will assume that you will work just as hard, or even harder, when you are getting paid.

If you secure a job prior to graduation, and especially if you're hired by your practicum site, don't make the mistake of slacking off just because you've already landed a job. Too many students have made this mistake. Once they have a job, they start arriving a few minutes late, take longer breaks than they should, or fail to show as much initiative. This behavior indicates that they were making a good impression just to get a job. Keep this in mind: The job that you already have becomes your reference for the next job you seek.

As mentioned earlier, you'll probably receive a grade for your practicum. When you use your practicum site supervisor as a reference, he or she will be contacted by employers and asked a series of questions about you and your performance. The following criteria are the types of things that will be considered when assigning your grade and providing an employment reference:

1. *Were you dependable?* Did you show up on time, ready to work? How many times were you absent? When absent, did you follow procedures for calling in? No matter how competent you are, if you aren't there, you aren't doing your job. Employers would rather have a less experienced employee with a good attendance record than an experienced employee with a poor attendance record.

2. *Was your appearance professional?* Were you dressed appropriately and well groomed? Did your appearance reflect a positive image to your patients and the site's staff? Avoid trendy clothing and appearance. Facial piercings, visible tattoos, and blue hair may be considered fashionable in some settings, but not on practicum. If you wear jewelry, make sure it's conducive to the work you're doing. Safety comes first when working with body fluids, equipment, and patients. Remember that some professions don't allow any jewelry to be worn for this reason.

3. *Did you display a friendly personality and good customer service?* Did you get along well with patients, doctors, and the site's staff? Were you cooperative with the staff and a team player?

4. *How well did you work under stress?* Did you maintain a calm demeanor and balance the priorities of your work appropriately? How well did you adapt to change and unexpected circumstances?

5. *How well did you perform your duties with limited supervision?* Did you demonstrate initiative or wait to be told what to do? Did you accept responsibility and perform your duties competently?

6. *Did you display a positive attitude and a desire to learn?* Were you motivated? Did you ask good questions? Were you eager to learn new procedures and practice what you learned?

7. *Did you display a professional image?* Did you apply everything that's been discussed in this book to make the very best impression you could possibly make?

If you can answer "yes" to all of these questions, you are well on your way to achieving a good grade, a positive employment reference, and recognition as a health care professional.

RECENT DEVELOPMENTS

SECURING A POSITIVE REFERENCE

When you apply for employment after graduation, you'll be asked to provide one or more references. References are people who know you and can provide information of interest about you. References can verify your education and training and your work experience. They can offer insight into your work ethic, attendance record, communication skills, customer service skills, and your capacity to acquire new skills quickly.

Your practicum site supervisor could serve as a valuable reference if he or she is impressed with you and your performance. Your supervisor's feedback would be valuable in helping employers determine if you're a good match for a job opening or not. Your supervisor will have *seen you in action* over a period of time working in a health care setting and can describe your level of interest, commitment, and motivation.

It's quite possible that your supervisor knows the people in other health care companies who do the hiring for those facilities. So it's very important to make a good impression during your practicum, not just to earn a high grade and an outstanding performance evaluation, but to also secure a positive reference for employment. Once you've begun working in health care, your reputation will travel with you from place to place.

At the End of Your Practicum

On the last day of your practicum, personally thank everyone at your site with whom you worked. Let them know how much you appreciate the opportunity to be there and the encouragement and support they provided. Within a few days (no longer than a week) of leaving, send them a typewritten thank-you letter, not a text or an email or voicemail message. Sending a thank-you letter is a courteous, professional way to convey appreciation, and a typewritten letter also demonstrates your written communication skills. Make sure you spell the person's name correctly and use good grammar. Believe it or not, a thank-you letter can be the deciding factor in who gets a job offer and who doesn't. (Refer to Appendix H for a Sample Practicum Thank-You Letter.)

If you apply everything you've learned so far in this book, you should have an exceptional practicum experience. You'll be well on your way to developing a professional reputation and landing a good job.

REALITY CHECK

Up to this point, if you haven't spent enough time gaining the knowledge and skills you need to be successful in your new occupation, your practicum experience will probably be disappointing. Your site supervisor is expecting you to be well prepared for your practicum. If you show up not knowing what you're supposed to know, your opportunity may be cut short. You may be sent back to your school to try to line up a different practicum site. If your skills are really weak, it's possible that no site may be willing to take you. Do you really want to get to this stage in your education only to be excluded from your practicum because you didn't take your studies seriously enough?

Employers that offer practicum experience aren't in business to serve students, they exist to serve patients. Having students on-site provides some benefits, but many employers won't take students for a variety of reasons. Supervising students, answering their questions, and showing them how to operate equipment takes time and results in an expense to the company. Students who perform poorly may damage equipment, waste supplies, and have a negative impact on the company's reputation and its patient satisfaction scores. So when an employer offers you a practicum experience, don't just take it for granted. The people who work at the site are taking a chance on you. If you perform poorly, you may be closing the door for future students who would like to do their practicum there. On the other hand, if you perform well, you may actually open the door for future students.

KEY POINTS

- Research the site in advance and visit there before your first day.
- Keep a journal and use a notepad to jot down things you want to remember.
- Arrive on time and avoid unnecessary absences.
- Show initiative; ask questions and remember the answers.
- Dress appropriately and display a positive attitude.
- Show respect and put the site and its patients first.
- Remember that you're a student at the site, not an employee.
- Follow HIPAA and HITECH Act rules to protect confidentiality.
- Follow protocol regarding the use of personal cell phones and devices, business computers, and social media.

- Don't use profane language.
- Avoid discussing your personal life with the site's patients and staff.
- Don't participate in office politics or become part of a clique.
- Send a thank-you note shortly after your practicum ends.

LEARNING ACTIVITIES

Using information from Chapter Seven:
- Answer the Chapter Review Questions
- Respond to the What If? Scenarios

Chapter Review Questions

Using information from Chapter Seven, answer each of the following.

1. Identify the purpose of a practicum.

2. List three benefits of a practicum experience.

3. Identify three requirements to gain clearance for a practicum.

4. Describe two ways to prepare for a practicum.

5. Explain the connection between your performance on practicum and securing an employment reference at graduation.

6. Explain the value of keeping a journal during your practicum.

7. Give three examples of protocol involving cell phones and social media during your practicum.

8. Explain the importance of maintaining patient confidentiality during your practicum.

9. List three safety factors to keep in mind when working in a health care facility.

10. Identify three of the criteria considered when evaluating your performance and assigning a grade for your practicum.

What If? Scenarios

Think about what you would do in the following situations and record your answers.

1. While escorting a patient to the exam room, she asks if her husband's tests results are back yet. You know that the results are back, but you don't have permission to give the results to anyone except the patient himself.

2. The telephones in the office ring continually. You notice the receptionist talking on the phone but most of the time she's involved with personal calls. In the meantime, the ringing telephones are ignored.

3. One of your patients is a friend of your mother. She's at the doctor's office to find out if she's pregnant. After she leaves, her pregnancy test comes back as negative. You've been unable to reach her by telephone to give her the results. The next day you see her at the shopping mall with her family.

4. You realize that your neighbor is a patient at your practicum site. You see her medical record and are wondering why she always looks so tired all of the time. Her records are right there and no one is watching.

5. During your practicum, a patient mentions that he would prefer that no one other than his doctor be present in the room during his medical procedure. It's a procedure you've never seen before and you would like to observe. The patient will be under the influence of medication and probably won't remember what happened during the procedure.

6. You're short on money and could use some drugs from the samples room. You notice there's an ample supply and they are given to patients free of charge.

7. While on your practicum, you notice that an employee has left work 15 minutes early every day for the past week. Two other employees who suspect this behavior but have not witnessed it themselves ask you to report it to the site supervisor.

8. You learned how to operate a new piece of equipment and would like to show your classmates what it looks like when you meet again as a group next week. Your cell phone is in your backpack and no one would notice if you took a quick photo during your lunch break.

Employment and Professional Development

8

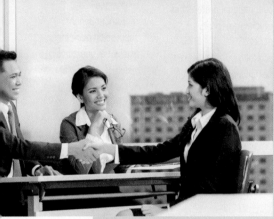

My mother said to me, "If you become a soldier, you'll be a general; if you become a monk, you'll end up as the Pope." Instead, I became a painter and wound up as Picasso.

—Pablo Picasso (1881–1973), artist

(Kzenon/Shutterstock)

CHAPTER OBJECTIVES

Having completed this chapter, you will be able to:

- List four questions to answer when identifying your occupational preferences.
- Explain the value of researching labor trends and projections.
- Identify three places on the Internet to find job openings.
- Describe four characteristics of a professional résumé.
- Name five things you should do when filling out a job application form.
- Explain why employers use preemployment assessments.

- Describe five ways to present a professional image during a job interview.
- Explain the importance of having a professional presence online.
- List two reasons why health care workers must engage in professional development.
- Describe four characteristics of effective leaders.
- Identify two ways to develop leadership skills.
- Describe the benefits of participating in a health care professional association.
- Explain the importance of having a career advancement plan.

KEY TERMS

behavioral questions	employment status	misdemeanor	preemployment assessments
career plan	exempt positions	networking	professional development
clock in and out	head hunter	nonexempt positions	references
cover letter	hire-on bonus	occupational preferences	retirement benefits
credit report	job application	official transcript	succession planning
dynamic	job boards	perks	traditional questions
employers of choice	labor projections	portfolio	vision
employment agency	labor trends	postsecondary	
employment benefits	legislative issues		

Job-Seeking Skills

Finding a job is the next step in applying what you've learned in school. Developing job-seeking skills will help you identify the best employment opportunities in the geographical area of the country where you want to live and work.

Identifying Occupational Preferences

Looking for and finding the right job for you requires planning and preparation. Start by identifying your **occupational preferences** (the types of work and work settings that an individual prefers). Your options will be somewhat governed by the occupation you've chosen. Consider hospitals, outpatient facilities, physician practices, home care agencies, community health clinics, rehabilitation facilities, mental health centers, public health organizations, school systems, long-term care facilities, imaging centers, laboratories, and surgery centers. You might be surprised at the variety of places where people with your education and skills can find employment.

There are several questions to be answered when identifying your occupational preferences:

- Do you want to work close to where you live now or move to another location?
- Do you want to work in the same place throughout the year, work seasonal jobs in different parts of the country, or rotate among different companies as a temporary worker?
- Do you want a full-time job (about 40 hours/week), a part-time job (about 20 hours/week), or a supplemental job with no guaranteed hours/week but with flexibility in work schedules?
- Are **employment benefits** (employer-paid insurance and retirement savings) important to you?
- Do you want a job where you can stay and grow with the company over time, or just a place to launch your career?
- Do you want a small organization where you can become multiskilled and work in more than one area, or a large organization where you can become a specialist?
- Do you want a job that pays well but may require compromising on some of your other preferences such as location, work schedule, or employment benefits?

Begin making some decisions about the kind of job you want:

- Geographical location (city, state, region, country)
- Type of employment setting (inpatient, outpatient, community-based, academic medical center, etc.)

- Size of the organization (small, large, statewide network, global company)
- **Employment status** (full-time, part-time, or supplemental employment)
- Work schedule/shift (days, evenings, nights, weekends, holidays, 10- or 12-hour shifts)
- Employment benefits (health, life, vision, and dental insurance; retirement and pension)
- Amount of compensation (pay) and paid time off for vacations and holidays
- Opportunities for advanced training, tuition assistance, and job promotions
- Required length of employment to be eligible for **retirement benefits** (employer-funded pension contributions)

Finding Employment Information

Once you've narrowed down your occupational preferences and know what kind of job you want, it's time to track down some labor and employment information.

BY THE NUMBERS

LABOR TRENDS AND PROJECTIONS

As you begin your job search, it's important to learn about the labor trends and projections for your occupation.

Labor trends (the general direction or development over time of workforce supply and demand) are forces that impact employers, workers, and job seekers. Using nursing as an example, the trend among hospital employers is to hire nurses with bachelor's degrees over nurses with associate's degrees. If you're planning a career in nursing, you need to know this. If you stop your nursing education at the associate's-degree level, you may be limited in where you can work. Labor trends are affected by workforce supply and demand. When there's a shortage of registered nurses, employers may be more open to hiring nurses with associate's degrees because there aren't enough nurses with bachelor's degrees to fill their positions. But when there's a surplus of registered nurses, or fewer nursing jobs to be filled, employers will likely hire candidates with bachelor's degrees.

Nursing is just one example. Labor trends vary from discipline to discipline, so it's important to research the trends for your specific occupation.

Labor projections (estimates of the number of positions that will need to be filled in the future) are important to consider when searching for your first job and later on when exploring options for career advancement. If you've chosen an occupation that may be shrinking in the future, your employment options could be more limited. Occupations referred to as *hot jobs* are typically those with the best employment opportunities.

Labor projections are presented as percentages and as actual numbers. It's best to look at labor projections presented as actual numbers because projections presented as *the percentage of growth* can be misleading. If the number of workers in an occupation is relatively small (13,000 audiologists in the United States, for example), then even a high percent of growth (e.g., 37%) will create a relatively small number of new jobs (4,810 additional jobs for audiologists). But if the number of workers in an occupation is higher (108,800 respiratory therapists, for example) then even a modest percent of growth (e.g.,19%) will create many more new jobs (20,672 additional jobs for respiratory therapists).

Labor projections vary from state to state, so it's important to find projections for the state in which you want to work. Understanding how to use labor projections is a key element in career planning. If your interests point you to a career with just a modest projected growth rate, that's okay. You might still decide to pursue that career with the knowledge that securing a good job could be more of a challenge.

Labor trends provide insight to the supply and demand for certain types of workers. Supply and demand changes over time and varies in different parts of the country. When there is a shortage of nurses, for example:

- The demand for nurses increases.
- There are more nursing jobs to fill than there are nurses to fill them.
- Nurses have an easier time finding a job and may have several job offers from which to choose.
- Salaries and benefits increase to help recruit nurses.
- Employers offer a **hire-on bonus** (extra compensation for accepting a job offer) to recruit more nurses.

Conversely, when there is an oversupply of nurses:

- The demand for nurses decreases.
- There are more nurses looking for jobs than there are jobs to fill.
- Nurses have a more difficult time finding a job and there is more competition for job openings.
- Salaries and benefits remain steady.
- Hire-on bonuses for nurse recruitment temporarily disappear.

Nursing shortages are predicted to increase as experienced nurses retire and leave the workforce. Yet not too long ago, nursing students just graduating from school had difficulty finding jobs in many parts of the country. The situation is similar in other professions such as physical therapy, radiography, and respiratory therapy where supply-and-demand cycles have shifted over recent years.

Locate websites and other resources to help you monitor the labor trends for your profession. By tracking the supply and demand for people in your field, you'll know the best time to apply for a job, and how difficult or easy it might be to find the kind of job for which you are looking.

Another important step in finding helpful employment information is identifying the **employers of choice** (companies where people like to work) in the area where you want to work. Employers of choice:

- Actively support the growth, development, and job advancement of employees.
- Provide scholarships, tuition assistance, on-site continuing education, and advanced training for employees.
- Offer flexible work schedules for employees enrolled in school.
- Host an Employee Assistance Program (EAP) to help workers resolve personal issues and overcome barriers to job retention.
- Support a work environment that fosters continual improvement and lifelong learning.

When considering where to work, keep this in mind. If an employer gave you a scholarship, a part-time job, or some other means of support while you were in school, you should show your loyalty. If the employer "took a chance" on you and invested in your education, then as a professional you have an obligation to repay that investment by working there for a reasonable period of time.

This is no time to take shortcuts on your homework. Landing your first professional job will launch your career and point it in the right direction. Making good decisions early in your career will increase your potential for a lifetime filled with satisfying and rewarding work.

Even if you're young, don't ignore the importance of retirement benefits. You probably won't think about retiring for many years, but your first job lays the foundation for your career and your life. If an employer is willing to invest in your retirement plan and perhaps even match the funds that you save yourself, you might be surprised how quickly those investments will grow over the years and provide a nice nest egg when you're ready to retire.

The Internet is the best place to find employment information and job openings. In today's world, most jobs are filled through online job postings, so you must have ready access to the Internet to find and apply for health care jobs.

- The Internet offers hundreds of websites called **job boards** where employers throughout the country post their job openings. Websites also provide information about career fairs, workshops for job-seekers, and tips on applying for jobs, writing résumés, and interviewing skills. With some websites, you can also post your résumé online for potential employers to view. Here are some examples:

  www.careerbuilder.com/Jobs
  www.monster.com
  www.healthcarejobsite.com
  www.indeed.com

- Some job boards specialize in recruiting people for specific occupations such as nursing. Here are some examples:

  www.nurse.com/jobs
  medical-assistant.jobs.net

- Many health care employers have websites that include job postings for their facilities. Here are some examples:

  Indiana University Health, www.iuhealth.org/careers/

  Mayo Clinic, www.mayoclinic.org/jobs

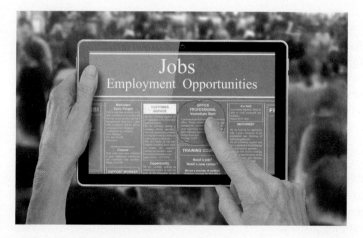

Figure 8-1 Searching for jobs online (*Pixsooz/Shutterstock*)

- Professional associations have websites to publicize job openings for people who work in those occupations. Here are some examples:

  American Association for Respiratory Care, www.aarc.org/careers
  American Society of Radiologic Technologists, www.healthecareers.com/asrt

Here are some other sources of information on job openings:

- Local newspaper advertisements; look in the Classifieds sections.
- Current health care workers; ask for opinions on the best places to work.
- **Networking** (interacting with a variety of people in different settings to exchange information and develop contacts, especially to further one's career); speak with people in your community who might know of job vacancies.
- Professional colleagues; use your contacts to learn about employment opportunities.
- Friends and relatives; you may know someone who can suggest a place to apply or introduce you to a potential employer.
- School counselors and placement coordinators; take advantage of resource people who can help you track down job openings.
- School bulletin boards; if your school has a career center or a bulletin board where job openings are listed, be sure to check it daily.

Depending on your occupation, you may want to consider using an **employment agency** (a company that connects employers and job seekers), some of whom specialize in health care. Employers list their job openings with the agency and then job-seekers review the postings to see which might be a good fit. *Public* employment agencies are funded by tax dollars and don't charge a fee for their service. *Private* employment agencies charge a fee for their services; fees are paid either by the employer or the job-seeker depending on the situation. When the supply of certain types of professionals is very limited and the demand is very high, people who meet those qualifications might be contacted directly by a **head hunter** (a recruiter hired to help an employer with its "difficult to fill" job openings) even though the professionals aren't actively involved in changing jobs.

Applying for Jobs

Once you've located websites to help you find the job for which you are searching, you can review job openings and begin applying for jobs. You can create alerts to email or text you when new jobs have been posted. You can submit a **job application** (a form used to apply for a job), post your résumé, and keep track of the places where you've applied. Sites such as these can be especially helpful when looking for job opportunities beyond your region of the country. Let's take a look at what it takes to apply for jobs.

Résumés

Potential employers need details about you and your qualifications and this is accomplished by preparing a résumé. Even if an employer doesn't require a résumé, it's still a good idea to have one. If your education and work experience are limited, you still have important information to share with potential employers. Résumés provide:

- A snapshot of your background, education, and work experience
- Experience that relates to the job for which you are applying, including your practicum experience

- The qualifications you're presenting for consideration
- Visible evidence of your written communication skills

If you've never developed a résumé, you can find examples and templates online and in reference books. (Refer to Appendix C for a Sample Résumé.) You could also ask someone who writes or reviews résumés to assist you.

Your résumé should be:

- Typed, professional in appearance, and concise (one page is best)
- Available in multiple formats (print and electronic, such as a Word document)
- Easily faxed, scanned, attached to an email, pasted in an online application, or photocopied with good quality
- Printed on plain white paper with no borders or graphics
- Well organized and formatted, using bullets and underlining

Organize the information and make sure your grammar and spelling are correct. The most current information should appear at the beginning of each section. Emphasize your educational background, skills, and abilities that match the qualifications for the job. If your education and work experience are limited:

- List some of your school accomplishments and extracurricular activities such as academic awards, sports, orchestra or choir, science fair entries, perfect attendance awards, and participation in school organizations.
- Mention leadership roles, computer skills, seminars or training sessions you've attended, certificates you've earned, and distinctions you've received.
- Include volunteer work and involvement in school and community events.

Since most jobs are filled via online postings, the format of your résumé should be very basic—no tabs, special fonts, or text boxes so the document can be easily uploaded to a job application. You may need to copy and paste portions of your résumé into sections of your job application, so formatting your résumé with this in mind will save you time later when you begin submitting job applications.

Submitting supportive documents (copies of certificates, grade transcripts, or recommendation letters from an instructor or previous employer) is usually permissible, but don't get carried away. Select one or two of the best items to submit with your application and save the others for your interview in case you get a chance to present them in person.

Cover Letters

Online job applications limit the amount of information, and the kinds of information, that you can submit. So a **cover letter** (a letter introducing a job applicant to a potential employer) can serve as your "sales letter"—a way to sell yourself to the employer in order to get an interview. (Refer to Appendix D for a Sample Cover Letter.)

Your cover letter should:

- Be neat, easy to read, and reflect appropriate grammar and spelling.
- State the job for which you are applying and how you heard about the opening.
- Give a brief overview of your education, experience, and qualifications.
- Note that your résumé is attached to your application.
- State how your employment would benefit the company.
- Request a personal interview.
- Provide your contact information and the best way and times to reach you.

References

Most employers require **references** (a list of people who can provide information about a job applicant), so before you start applying for jobs you need to line up some references. Choose your references carefully:

- One reference should be qualified to attest to your knowledge, competence, and potential for learning, such as a teacher, program director, or practicum supervisor.
- A second reference should be qualified to comment on your character, work ethic, and reliability, such as a supervisor or manager.

Consider the following when lining up references:

- Select people who are familiar with your skills, the quality of your work, and your ability to learn quickly.
- Ensure the credibility of your references; never use a spouse or a relative as a reference.
- Contact the people you've chosen ahead of time and ask for permission to list them as references.
- When asked, provide your written permission for references to disclose information about you and your performance.
- Tell people what job you're applying for and when they might be contacted by the employer.
- Make sure you have accurate contact information for each reference, including their email address.
- Choose people who have positive, insightful, and complimentary things to say about you.

If you know someone who already works for the company where you are applying, and if that person is familiar with you and the quality of your work, ask if you may list him or her as a reference. But avoid "name-dropping, pulling strings, or using connections" to try to enhance

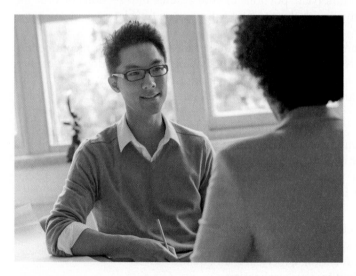

Figure 8-2 Asking a colleague to serve as a reference (*Sergey Nivens/Shutterstock*)

your chances of getting an interview and job offer. Such attempts could have a negative effect and backfire on you. Take the professional approach—stand on your own merits and get hired for the right reasons.

A frequent reason for terminating employees is poor attendance, so employers are especially interested in the attendance record of job applicants. Employers are typically impressed by job applicants who can demonstrate effective time management skills and the ability to balance school, work, and a personal life with good results. When an employer contacts your references for feedback about your performance and reliability, expect your attendance to be one of the topics brought up.

If you've already had one or more jobs, employers will probably want to contact your previous employers for recommendations. When you leave one place of employment to work for another, don't "burn your bridges." This means you should always leave your job on good terms so your employer will give you a positive recommendation when you apply for another job.

Another topic that you can expect to be raised during reference checks is your people skills. Employers need to know if you can form effective relationships, function as a team player, treat people with respect, and support patient satisfaction.

Choose the best references and make sure they're well prepared to respond when contacted. Employers may wait to check references until they're close to making a job offer. If there's more than one finalist for a job opening, the applicant with the most positive references will probably get the offer.

Job Applications

Since employers use computerized systems to manage job applications and the employment process, you will likely be required to submit your application online. Job applications convey a lot of information about you and they're an extremely important part of the employment process. (Refer to Appendix E for a Sample Job Application.)

When employers receive a surplus of applications for a particular job opening, the application is typically the first item they use to narrow down the applicant pool and screen applicants. Employers will screen your applications to:

- Determine if your qualifications match those of the job.
- Evaluate how well you read and follow instructions.
- Assess your written communication skills, spelling, and grammar.
- Decide whether or not to proceed with an interview.

If you must submit your application online, make sure you have the computer skills required to navigate the website and enter your information electronically. If necessary, ask someone who is familiar with the process to help you.

You must have an email account and it's best to set up a new, professional account with a professional name and keep it separate from your personal account. Log in to the job application website and set up your profile, username, and password. Employers can view this information, so make sure that your username and password are appropriate. Allow time to become familiar with how the computerized system works. Keep your electronic résumé handy and expect to cut and paste sections into your application. With many online systems, you can save a draft of your application and go back later to revise and complete it. Pay attention to the knowledge, skills, abilities, and qualifications that are listed in the job posting and identify some of the key words. Use these key words in your application because computerized systems search for key words to find applicants who might be a good match. If you have the opportunity, fill out a sample job application to make sure you have all of the information required.

If you aren't familiar with completing online job applications, expect to encounter some challenges until you've learned how to navigate the process. This is especially true for people with limited computer skills. If you fall into this category, take some computer classes as soon as possible. If the company where you want to work uses computers to manage job applications and the employment process, then they probably rely on computerized systems for many other aspects of their business.

If the company where you're applying still uses a paper application form, fill it out yourself and don't ask someone to do it for you. Make sure your writing is legible and neat.

Regardless of whether you complete your job application online or on paper, you should:

- Read job titles and job summaries carefully to make sure your qualifications match the jobs for which you are applying. (For example, medical assistants should not apply for physician assistant jobs; practical nurses should not apply for nurse practitioner jobs, etc.)
- Read the instructions and follow them.
- Use your best written communication skills and make sure all words are spelled correctly.
- List accurate dates for your education and work experience.
- List the job number if the employer uses a numbering system for job postings.
- Review the form to make sure you haven't left anything out before you finalize and submit it.

If the application calls for a brief statement about why you're applying for the job, take some time to think about your answer before writing it. You might be surprised how much weight your answer carries in the selection process. Convince the employer that you're familiar with the job and their company. Let them know why you believe you're a good match for the

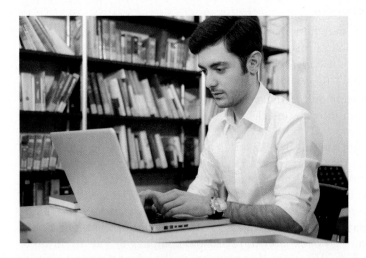

Figure 8-3 Applying for jobs online (*Minerva Studio/Shutterstock*)

qualifications they seek. If space permits, describe briefly how hiring you would benefit the company.

Your job application, résumé, and cover letter make that all-important first impression. Spend a sufficient amount of time making sure it's the impression you want to convey. These three documents plus your references will likely determine whether you get invited in for an interview or not. Present your best attributes and don't undersell yourself. Stand on your own merits and avoid exaggerating your qualifications.

Be truthful—*never* falsify your information. Lying about your qualifications is dishonest, unethical, and unprofessional. If you misrepresent your qualifications and your lies are discovered, you will be disqualified as an applicant. If your dishonesty is discovered after you've started the job, you may be dismissed from the job.

If you've had a **misdemeanor** (a minor offense with a fine and/or short jail sentence as a penalty) or a felony conviction, you must disclose it on your job application. Most employers conduct criminal history background checks to search for any misdemeanors and/or felonies as part of the employment process. A prior conviction may or may not eliminate you from consideration depending on the job you're applying for, the type of offense, how long ago it occurred, and so forth. But if you fail to disclose the conviction and your employer discovers it later on, you could lose your job and do irreparable harm to your reputation.

Employers are increasingly searching the Internet to gather additional information on job applicants. They may run a **credit report** (a review of records to assess a person's financial status), visit social media sites, and review blogs. Be very careful. Don't publish or share any personal information that you wouldn't want prospective employers to view or hear about.

Your job application and résumé provide contact information that employers will use to set up an interview. Make sure that the recorded message on your telephone reflects the image you want to convey to potential employers. Think twice about religious, political, or musical overtones in your recorded message. Refrain from having children record the message or answer your phone when you're expecting a call from a potential employer. An inappropriate, unprofessional, or confusing message may be all it takes to screen out your application.

THE MORE YOU KNOW

ORGANIZING YOUR JOB HUNT

Job hunting can lead to concerns about where you will live, how much money you will earn, and what direction your career will take. If these concerns cause you too much stress, they can affect your ability to present yourself well to prospective employers. Here are some tips to help organize your job hunt and manage your stress:

- *Stay organized.* Keep your résumé and cover letter up-to-date. Make a list of the dates and places where you have submitted job applications.
- *Plan ahead.* Get directions to the location of an interview prior to your scheduled date and visit there in advance to identify the travel time and transportation and parking options.
- *Use a schedule.* Keep an up-to-date schedule of all appointments to avoid overbooking yourself. Have your schedule in front of you when making appointments for new and follow-up meetings and interviews.

(continued)

- *Track the details*. Keep track of the details about who you speak with and who you meet during interviews and follow-up meetings. Include their names (check for correct spelling), job titles, and contact information. Keep track of follow-up phone calls, emails, and other communication.
- *Follow up*. If you've agreed to submit additional documentation regarding your skills and work experience, make sure to send the information. If an employer suggests that you contact him or her again within a certain period of time to ask about upcoming job openings, be sure to follow up.

Job hunting should be an exciting time, so use your organizational skills to manage the process and minimize your stress.

Preemployment Assessments

Expect to take some written or online **preemployment assessments** (tests and other instruments used to measure knowledge, skills, and personality traits) as part of the application and employment process. Employers need to know if your competencies and personal traits match the characteristics they're seeking. Some companies include an online assessment with their job applications. Other companies schedule half-day or full-day assessments to evaluate factors such as:

- Basic skills (reading, writing, English, and math)
- Work ethic, character, and personal values
- Personality traits and customer service skills
- Job-specific skills (computer skills, applied math, etc.)

Preemployment assessments are difficult to prepare for because they measure the accumulation of the knowledge, skills, and personal characteristics that you've developed over time. Some assessments are psychological in nature and may contain questions that seem strange and redundant. Don't try to figure out why these kinds of questions are being asked. Just try to answer all of these questions in an honest and consistent manner.

When taking preemployment assessments:

- Be well rested and ready to concentrate.
- Make sure you understand the instructions before taking the assessment.
- Try to relax and just do your best.

Some employers will share assessment results with applicants while other employers won't. When an employer is willing to share the results, ask for feedback on how well you performed to gain some insight as to your strengths and weaknesses. If your scores indicate some opportunities for improvement, work on those skills while you apply for other jobs. If you don't get an interview the first time you apply, enhance your qualifications and reapply later. Some employers require a wait period of a few months before accepting another job application from the same person.

Verifying Qualifications

Most health care jobs today require at least a high school diploma or a general equivalency diploma (GED). There are a still few jobs for people without a high school diploma or a GED, but opportunities for advancement will be very limited. Most health care jobs require successful completion of a **postsecondary** (after high school) training program or a college degree. Many jobs also require a professional license, certification, or registration.

Depending on the type of job you're seeking, you may have to submit supporting documentation such as an **official transcript** (a grade report that should be printed, sealed, and mailed directly to the recipient to prevent tampering by the applicant) from the schools you've attended; copies of diplomas, certificates of completion, or college degrees; and verification of active status of professional licenses, certifications, registrations, or other credentials required for the job.

Interviews and Job Offers

Once you've submitted your job application and survived the screening process, it's time to think about interviews and job offers.

Preparing for an Interview

Making a good impression during an interview pulls together just about everything discussed in this book. The objective is to present yourself as a competent, motivated, caring professional who is well qualified and prepared for the job. Interviewers will be looking for information about your academic achievements, occupational experience, interpersonal skills, and personal qualities to help decide if you are a good fit for the company and the position. Don't just show up for an interview. Do your homework first.

Researching the Company

Learn as much as you can about the job and the company ahead of time so you can talk intelligently about the opportunity for which you are applying. If you're applying for a job in an outpatient clinic, find out what kinds of patients are seen there, what services are provided on site, what kinds of workers are employed there, what hours the clinic is open, and so forth. If it's obvious during the interview that you aren't familiar with the company, the interviewers will wonder if you're really serious about wanting the job. If you take time to research the company first, interviewers will be impressed with your interest and may give you some extra consideration in the selection process. To research the company you should:

- Review the company's website and printed material.
- Read articles about the company online and in local newspapers and magazines.
- Find out if the company has won any recent awards or been featured in special reports.
- Speak with people who are familiar with the company such as employees, patients, and vendors.
- Spend some time on-site before your interview to observe the environment.

Even if you've already answered a question on the application form about why you're applying for the job, expect to be asked this question again during the interview. Familiarity with the company and the job will help convince interviewers that you're a good match for the opening. Someone may ask, "What did you do to investigate this job and our company to make sure this is a good match for you?" If you've done your homework, you'll have several examples to share with interviewers.

Preparing Your Portfolio

Although a **portfolio** (a collection of materials that demonstrates a person's knowledge, skills, and abilities) is not required as part of the interviewing process, it's a good idea to have one.

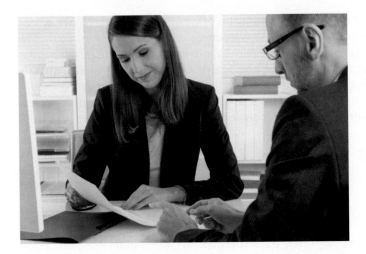

Figure 8-4 Discussing portfolio materials (*Jeanette Dietl/Shutterstock*)

Employers are typically impressed with job applicants who have taken the time to prepare samples of their school or work awards and recognitions, practicum assessments, performance evaluations, special projects, papers they've written, critical thinking exercises, etc. Gather and organize your portfolio materials and line up a professional-looking folder or briefcase in which to carry them.

Anticipating Interview Questions

To prepare for an interview, you need to anticipate the types of questions that might be asked. Interviewers use traditional and behavioral questioning techniques:

Traditional questions ask how a person would behave in a future situation (What *would* you do?)
Behavioral questions ask how a person has behaved in the past (What *did* you do?)

Many interviewers believe that past performance is the best predictor of future performance and that's why they use behavioral questions. Behavioral questions are more probing and call for more thought and specific answers. Here are some examples to illustrate the difference:

- Traditional: "What weakness would prevent you from being successful in this job?"
  Behavioral: "Describe a weakness you had in the past and explain what you did to overcome it."
- Traditional: "How would you handle stress in this job?"
  Behavioral: "Describe a previous stressful situation and how you handled it."
- Traditional: "What are your goals for the next five years?"
  Behavioral: "What were your goals when you started school and how successful have you been in accomplishing them?"

Once you've answered a behavioral question, expect more detailed follow-up questions:

- Why did you try that approach?
- What did you do or say that led to that outcome?

- How would you do things differently the next time?
- What did you learn from the experience?

Prepare for both traditional and behavioral questions since you won't know until you get there which approach the interviewers will use. It could be a combination of both types of questions.

Refresh your memory about the challenges you've faced, projects you've worked on, and goals you've achieved. Have some personal stories in mind in case you're asked for examples. Jot down this information on a notepad and take it with you to the interview. Knowing as much as you can about the job description and the skills that your interviewer seeks will help you anticipate, and prepare for, the types of questions that might be asked.

Practice at home or at school with someone firing questions at you in a mock interview setting. Be prepared to answer questions such as these:

- Why are you interested in this job?
- Have you had a job that didn't turn out as expected? What did you do about it?
- What specifically have you done to investigate this job?
- How can you be sure this is the right job for you?
- Have you ever been fired from a job? If so, why were you fired and how did you react?
- Have you experienced conflict with a former supervisor? If so, how did you resolve it?
- What do you think it would take to be successful in this job?
- What have you done to prepare for this job?
- Did you need to learn something new in your previous job? If so, how did you do that?
- What strengths would you bring to this job and this company?
- How did you support the reputation of the company you used to work for?
- What appeals to you about working for this company?
- Why should we select you over other applicants?
- Have you ever applied for a job and didn't get it? If so, what did you do?

The more questions you can anticipate in advance, the better prepared you will be. Expect some "what if?" questions such as:

- What would you do if you had to be late for work one morning?
- What would you do if you observed a coworker stealing from the company?
- What will you do if you're not selected for this job?

If you dropped out of school or have gaps in your employment history, be prepared to explain why.

Interviewing is a two-way process. At some point during the session, the interviewer will probably ask, "What questions do you have for me?" You'll need to be well prepared for this because your response will carry some weight in the selection process. Jot down some questions that you would like to ask on the notepad that you will take with you to the interview.

Here are some examples:

- Is this job full-time, part-time, or supplemental?
- What would my work schedule be?
- Would I be working as part of a team?
- Once I'm on the job, what additional training or duties should I expect?

When it comes to asking questions about how much the job pays, keep reading.

Participating in an Interview

Some employers conduct their first round of interviews by telephone. If you are scheduled for a phone interview, make sure that when you take the call, you're in a quiet place and free from interruptions. Have your résumé handy in case you need to pull information from it.

If your interview is in person:

- Get plenty of sleep and eat a good breakfast or lunch before your appointment.
- Make sure you know exactly where to go, how to get there, and where to park.
- Plan to arrive at least 15 minutes early.
- If you get delayed, call the contact person to let them know why you can't be there on time, apologize for any inconvenience, and ask if you need to reschedule.

Allow plenty of time for the interview itself. Other applicants may be scheduled for interviews during the same time period as you, so interviewers could be running late and you might be kept waiting.

It should go without saying but must be mentioned: Don't bring children with you to your interview. Having children present is disruptive and an indication that you lack reliable childcare. If your childcare plans fall through, it's better to reschedule your interview than to arrive with your children.

Once you've arrived at the right time and place, it's important to make a positive and professional first impression. Your appearance "will speak louder than words." Interviewers could be your age or younger, but it's more likely they'll be older than you and perhaps about the same age as your parents. What type of clothing and personal image will they consider professional and appropriate for an interview? This is no time to think about styles and fashion trends or to wear something outrageous in order to be remembered or "stand out in the crowd." You definitely want to make a lasting impression, but it should be based on your qualifications and friendly personality, not an unconventional appearance.

Interviewers are going to "size you up" by assessing how well their patients, employees, leaders, and business associates might react to you and your appearance if you were to get the job. So it's important to look your very best. The importance of wearing appropriate clothing cannot be stressed too much. Men should wear a suit or a jacket and tie. Women should wear a business suit

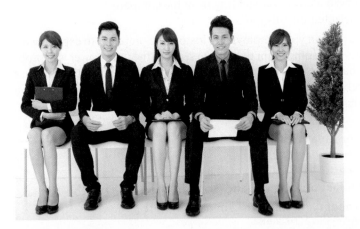

Figure 8-5 Dressed for success for their interviews (*Tom Wang/Shutterstock*)

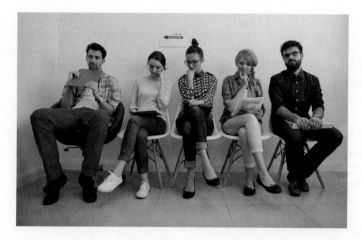

Figure 8-6 Dressed inappropriately for their interviews (*Gpointstudio/Shutterstock*)

or a professional-looking skirt, blouse, and jacket. Appropriate shoes and accessories are important. Avoid tight clothing, low necklines, sagging pants, and evening wear. "Dress for success," even if you have to borrow clothes.

Here are some things to remember:

- Be on your best behavior from the moment you arrive on the property until you leave the property; treat everyone you encounter at the site with respect and use good manners.
- Don't talk on your phone while waiting to be interviewed.
- Before your interview, silence your phone (or turn it off) and put it away to avoid any distraction or interruption.
- Have your notepad handy, with the information you've jotted down in advance, and bring a pen to take notes during the interview.

Here are some documents to have ready:

- Copies of your résumé.
- Your list of references with their contact information.
- Your portfolio, if you prepared one.
- Thank-you notes from coworkers, patients, or doctors.
- Awards or honors that you've received.
- Transcripts from courses, classes, and continuing education.
- Copies of professional certificates and other evidence of your performance and professional growth.

Bring copies of the most relevant items to your interview but don't overwhelm the interviewer with papers. Select just a few items that relate most closely to the job for which you are applying and have them ready in case you need them.

Smile! Smiling is one of the easiest ways to make a good first impression. As soon as you are called into the room, thank the person for the interview. Don't sit down until shown a seat and until the person conducting the interview has been seated. Offer a firm handshake. Never hug the interviewer! Try to remember the names of the people to whom you are introduced. Apply your best interpersonal communication skills and personality traits. Remember the importance of customer service in health care. All health care employers seek job applicants with pleasant personalities who can relate well to other people. Practice your best people skills during the interview. It's okay to be nervous. In fact, interviewers might wonder what's wrong with you if you aren't nervous. But try to maintain your composure and self-confidence.

During your interview:

- Describe the skills and abilities you would bring to the job.
- Convince interviewers that you would make a positive contribution to their organization and serve as an effective member of their team.
- Remember why you chose a career in health care; let your enthusiasm and commitment to helping people show.
- Be sincere; don't just make up answers that you think interviewers want to hear.
- Share some brief personal stories as examples of how you've overcome challenges and achieved your goals in the past.
- Be yourself; don't pretend to be someone you *think* would be more appealing to the interviewers.
- Trust the interviewers to recognize a good match when they see one; you want to be a good match for the job, and you want the job to be a good match for you.
- Be honest; if you're asked why you left school or terminated employment, tell the truth.
- Be prepared to answer questions about your attendance, transportation, and back-up plans if things don't go as expected.

Here are some more things to think about:

- Sit up straight, don't chew gum or bite your fingernails, and try to relax.
- Pay attention to your body language and the nonverbal messages you are sending.
- Convey a positive attitude; don't express anger about a former teacher, job, or supervisor.
- Don't "carry baggage" from your past into what could become a new situation and fresh start.
- Display self-confidence and a genuine interest in what's being discussed.
- Don't ramble; stay on track and focus on the message you want to convey.
- Don't let your guard down; everything you say and do will be taken into account.

Even if you decide early in the interview that you aren't interested in the job, continue to "put your best foot forward." A few years from now you may want to apply there again. The person who interviews you at one company may know the people who do the hiring at other companies. Never pass up an opportunity to make a good impression.

Some interview sessions are quite formal whereas others are more conversational and informal. If you're invited to lunch or dinner and it feels like a social setting, you are still being sized up as a potential employee. Don't be surprised if you're interviewed by more than one person, perhaps at the same time. Having one person fire questions at you can be intimidating enough without having two or three people doing the same thing during the same session. Sometimes employers have no choice but to have multiple people interview an applicant at the same time. Occasionally, it's done intentionally to see how well an applicant performs under pressure.

Answer questions thoughtfully. Concentrate on each question and think before you answer. Don't just blurt out the first thought that pops into your head, but don't ponder too long either. Employers need to know if you can think and respond quickly. Let your interviewer know that

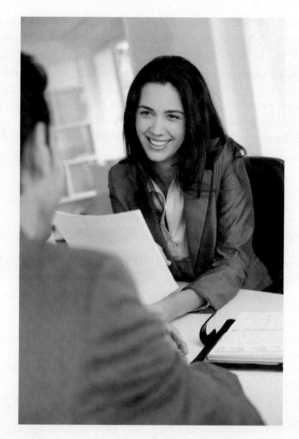

Figure 8-7 Making a positive impression (*Goodluz/Shutterstock*)

you're always eager to learn new things. If you present yourself as someone who resists change, you'll likely lose points in the selection process.

Some interviewers ask intimidating, strange, or confusing questions just to see how applicants perform under stress. Don't let these kinds of questions shake your confidence. Some questions are inappropriate and illegal to ask during an interview, such as, "Do you have any disabilities?" or "Have you ever been arrested?" These types of questions probe for personal information such as:

- Age, race, ethnicity, and religious or political beliefs
- Marital status, number and age of children, and pregnancies
- Sexual preference and gender identity

Unfortunately, some interviewers will ask inappropriate and/or illegal questions and use the information to discriminate against job applicants during the selection process. So it's important to be prepared for these kinds of questions and have some responses in mind. For example, an interviewer might ask a young female applicant questions such as: When do you plan to start a family? How many children do you plan to have? How old are your children? Who takes care of your children while you're at work? With questions such as these, interviewers are concerned about the applicant's ability to manage parenthood and a job at the same time. Which of the following responses do you think would be most appropriate?

- "You aren't supposed to ask questions like that so I'm not going to answer."
- "I think that most people find balancing their personal and professional lives a challenge. But I've been working part time and taking care of my grandmother and my younger brother and sister for the past two years while enrolled in school full time. So I'm sure I have the skills and the support it takes to manage my family and my job successfully."

It should be obvious which of these two responses would be best received by the person asking the questions.

PROFESSIONALISM ONLINE

ESTABLISHING A PROFESSIONAL ONLINE PRESENCE

Potential employers may conduct online searches to find information about you. If you don't have a presence on social media, employers may think you aren't up to date with digital communication. So it's important to have a presence online; just make sure it reflects your image and reputation as a health care professional.

Using a site such as LinkedIn is a good way to establish your professional identity online. You can search for jobs, learn about employers, and gain helpful information and advice to further your career. You can meet and keep in touch with colleagues and connect with people who already work for the companies where you plan to apply.

Keep your profiles on professional sites up-to-date. Avoid posting personal information or other content that could distract from your professional efforts.

As part of the interviewing process, some health care employers ask applicants to log in to their social media sites and allow interviewers to see what is posted there. If the applicant refuses, the interview may be cut short with no job offer extended. This may seem extreme, but it's occurring more frequently. Interviewers want insight as to how your personal life might impact your employment with their company. If you've posted photos, videos, or other content that could be considered inappropriate, or if you've made negative comments about health care companies, coworkers, doctors, or patients, your application for employment could be quickly screened out.

Make sure *everything* that's posted about you online supports your professional identity, and don't be surprised if a potential employer finds your content or asks you to share it with them.

Remember that interviewing is a two-way process. When the interviewer says, "What questions do you have for me?" you should already have some jotted down on your notepad. Here are two more questions to consider:

- "What characteristics are you looking for in an ideal applicant?" (Gather some important information and create an opportunity to describe how your qualifications match what the interviewer is seeking.)
- "What is the potential for growth and advancement within your company?" (This conveys that you are ambitious and seeking a company with which you can grow.)

Jot down the responses to your questions along with any other information that you don't want to forget. Interviewers will notice that you're organized, pay attention to details, and record important information. Avoid asking for information that's already available in printed materials or on the company's website. Interviewers will wonder why you didn't do your homework.

Not everyone agrees on whether or not to ask questions about pay and benefits during the first interview. Although pay and benefits are important, it's best to focus on the primary responsibilities of the job and the qualifications being sought by the employer first. If you know there's going to be a second follow-up interview, wait for that appointment to ask about pay and benefits. Or, let the interviewer take the lead in bringing up the discussion during your first interview. Here are some sample questions:

- Does this job include employment benefits and, if so, where could I get information about the benefits? How soon would I become eligible for the retirement plan?
- Do you offer tuition assistance or other types of support for employees who want to get more training or work on a college degree?

Give some thought ahead of time to what your pay and benefit requirements would be in case you're asked those questions during your first interview. Saying, "I don't know" or "I haven't really thought about it" indicates you haven't done your homework. Before your interview, investigate average pay ranges for the job you are seeking by tapping into online resources or speaking with a placement adviser at school or a personnel department representative where you would be working. Keep in mind that pay ranges are based on the geographical location of the health care facility and many other factors.

How much pay do you need? It is okay to say "The salary is negotiable," but have an acceptable range in mind in case you get pinned down or a job offer is extended. If you've done your homework, you've already identified what is most important in selecting the best offer. Instead of focusing on starting pay and benefits, new graduates should be more concerned about the job itself, support for continuing education, and opportunities to gain new skills and valuable work experience.

TRENDS AND ISSUES

HOW MUCH DOES THE JOB PAY?

Compensation for jobs varies according to the region of the country where you work. Investigate the *average pay range* ($37,000 to $62,000 per year, for example) for the occupations of interest to you, based on where you plan to live and work.

Positions are labeled as exempt or nonexempt:

- **Exempt positions** are jobs that involve management or other advanced functions or skills and that provide a guaranteed salary but are exempt from (do not offer) additional pay for overtime hours.
- **Nonexempt positions** are jobs that do not involve management or other advanced functions or skills and that pay a salary or wage plus an additional hourly rate for overtime hours.

Compensation is either an hourly rate (such as $18.00/hour) or an annual rate (such as $37,440/year.) A full-time employee with a 40-hour/week schedule will work about 2,080 hours per year. In addition to

(continued)

base pay, nonexempt employees are paid for *overtime* and receive a higher rate of pay for those hours. Nonexempt employees who work holidays or the evening, night, or weekend shifts may also be paid at a higher rate for those hours.

As a new employee with little or no work experience, you will likely start in a nonexempt position at or near the bottom of the pay range. As time passes and you gain more experience, you will earn pay raises and move toward the midpoint of your pay range. If you remain employed with the company for a significant period of time and earn high performance evaluations, your rate of pay will move toward the top end of your pay range. If you secure a job promotion, your responsibilities will increase along with your pay.

Investigate the *average cost-of-living* for the area of the country where you plan to live and work. If the cost of living is especially high, you'll need a higher rate of pay than if you live in a region where the cost of living is low. For this reason, pay rates are often higher in large cities than in small towns or rural areas. Employers base their compensation rates on *market factors*, which often take the average cost of living for their area into consideration.

After the Interview

Regardless of whether you want the job or not, you should follow up the interview with a letter thanking the employer for the opportunity to interview. This demonstrates courtesy and good manners and it also puts your name and communication skills in front of the decision-makers one more time. Delivering a handwritten thank-you letter or sending a thank-you email message within 24 hours after your interview will make a good impression since the majority of job applicants fail to follow up. Your thank-you correspondence also provides an opportunity to restate how excited you are about joining the company and to follow up on something discussed or forgotten during the interview. (Refer to Appendix F for a Sample Interview Follow-Up Letter.)

If you want the job:

- Contact the interviewer and ask if there is anything else you can do to verify your qualifications or answer any remaining questions.
- Try to wait patiently. It can take several weeks before employment decisions are finalized and offers are made.
- Avoid calling the interviewer to ask if a decision has been made yet. You don't want to become an annoyance or appear desperate. Most companies will notify all applicants when a position has been filled.

Expect some competition with other job applicants. When employers face shortages of qualified workers, it's easier to get a job and you may have several from which to choose. But when there's a surplus of qualified job applicants for the number of positions available, competition can be fierce. If you've mastered everything so far in this book, you should be in good shape to land the job you desire.

Considering Job Offers

Once you receive a job offer, it is decision-making time. You may even have the luxury of considering more than one job offer at the same time. To help ensure that this is the right job for you at this stage of your career, compare the offer with your list of occupational preferences. How well does the job match what you're looking for? Is the pay that you've been offered sufficient considering the cost of living in the area where you plan to live and work? If the pay is too low, or if you believe

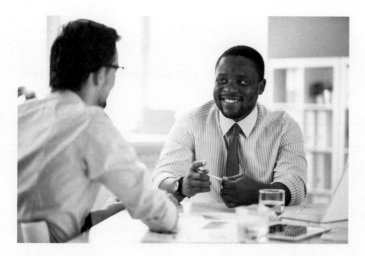

Figure 8-8 Discussing a job offer (*Pressmaster/Shutterstock*)

you deserve a higher rate of pay, you will need to negotiate with the company to see if they would increase their offer. Confer with your parents, instructors, advisers, or role models to help you analyze the situation and make the right decision. If this is your first health care job, you might not get everything you want. Identify your top priorities and consider making some compromises if the job might move you closer to what you're looking for in the future.

Once you've accepted a job offer, the offer will probably be conditional based on completing a preemployment physical exam and passing a drug screen and a criminal history background check. Employers can ill afford to hire people with substance abuse issues or problems related to a criminal history.

If you don't get selected, you'll know you did your best and will have learned something of value in the process. If you believe you are well qualified, don't give up; employers value perseverance. Ask for feedback on how to enhance your qualifications, follow the advice, and reapply. It's not unusual for applicants to be turned down the first time and then hired later on. If you reapply and are turned down a second time, work with an adviser or mentor to revisit your goals and identify ways to increase your qualifications.

If you're seeking employment in a large or specialized facility or in a city or town where the competition for jobs is formidable, consider applying for a job in a smaller facility or in another city or town first and then making a move later on. Gaining work experience with a good reference someplace else may be the key to securing the job you really want. Graduating from school and landing your first job isn't the end of your journey, it's really just the beginning.

Professional Development

Once you've secured a good job and started working, it's time to point your career in the right direction. It's never too early to plan ahead. Regardless of what profession you're in or where you work, you need to start thinking about:

- Engaging in **professional development** (education for people who have begun their careers and wish or need to continue growing in that profession).

- Building leadership skills.
- Participating in professional associations.
- Developing a plan for career advancement.

All of these activities are critical for health care professionals who want a **dynamic** (in motion, energetic, and vigorous) career.

CASE STUDY

Carla couldn't believe what she had just witnessed. Using his cell phone, a male student on practicum at her site had just taken an embarrassing photo of an elderly female wearing only a patient gown with the back side flapping open. She immediately called the student into her office, took his cell phone from him, and left him there while she tried to calm herself down in the room next door. She called the student's program director and told her they had a serious problem that required immediate attention. The program director arrived in a matter of minutes and met briefly with Carla, who was still in shock. The program director took possession of the student's phone and quietly escorted him from the building.

Carla barely had time to report the incident to her manager before she got a call from the dean of the School of Health Sciences where the student was enrolled. The dean was calling to apologize on behalf of the school for the student's behavior. He assured Carla and her manager that the embarrassing photo had not been shared with anyone and had been deleted from the student's phone. He further stated that the student had violated the school's policy and would therefore be expelled from the program. Carla never saw or heard from the student again. She chalked it up to just one more example of how doing something stupid can ruin your career.

Speaking of one's career, Carla was starting to think more about hers. She had always viewed her work as a career, not just a series of jobs. She wanted each step in her career to be well thought-out and planned in advance. Her commitment and hard work had paid off so far, but where was she headed next? Ever since Carla had earned her bachelor's degree she had thought about continuing her education but hadn't made any decisions yet. Her passion had always been in patient care. The opportunity to serve patients and help people live happy, healthy lives

meant a great deal to Carla, and it defined who she was as a person. But she also loved being a supervisor, helping her staff members grow personally and professionally as they developed their skills.

The more she thought about her future, the more she realized she was increasingly intrigued by the business side of health care. So much was changing as a result of health care reform, technological advancements, and the evolving medical needs of the American population. Over the past couple of years, she'd spent a significant amount of time working alongside her practice manager, learning about finance and budgeting, strategic planning, insurance contracts, and the legal aspects of running a medical practice. Perhaps becoming a practice manager herself would be a good next step.

Given what was going on in her personal life, she thought it might be time to relocate to another part of the country and take on some new challenges and adventures. After all, she was still young and had her whole life and career ahead of her. But lots of questions popped up. What qualifications would she need to become a practice manager and what would the duties involve? What would it take to gain more leadership skills and learn more about the business side of health care? What would she need to know about the job market and cost of living if she moved someplace else? How much income would she need and where could she start in finding employment opportunities in other states? So many questions!

Is it time for Carla to take some well thought-out risks and resume climbing the career ladder again? She isn't sure yet where she might be headed, but she's excited about the prospects of making a change in her health career.

What should Carla do? What would you do if you were in Carla's place? Stay tuned . . .

The Need for Professional Development

Lifelong learning is a vital part of working in health care. You must expand your knowledge and skills at every stage of your career and focus on professional development.

Here are several reasons why health care professionals must engage in professional development:

- *Ethical behavior demands it.* To provide the best, most up-to-date care for your patients, you need to be aware of the latest developments in your field. Providing outdated, sub-standard care would be unethical and dangerous. This is why many licensed and certified professionals such as doctors, nurses, and EMTs must complete a specific number of continuing education hours over a period of time to maintain the active status of their credentials.
- *Technology and medical procedures advance rapidly.* Equipment that was unavailable just a few years ago is part of routine medical care today. New procedures can result in better outcomes for patients but only when professionals know how to use the technology and perform the procedures safely and effectively.
- *The needs of patients change.* The needs of the population that you serve are constantly changing. As more patients become elderly, you'll need to learn more about geriatrics and the health care needs of seniors. If you work in direct patient care and a new micro-organism or virus emerges, you'll need to learn how to treat your patients and protect yourself.
- *Your job description will change.* Nothing stays the same when it comes to job duties in health care. Employers constantly reorganize departments, redesign work, and reassign staff members. As the organization changes, so do job titles and duties. When jobs become obsolete, they're replaced by new jobs. Two jobs might be merged into one, with employees cross-trained to work in both areas.
- *Your responsibilities will increase.* As you advance in your career, you'll need to gain additional knowledge and skills to handle new responsibilities. For example, you might have to prepare budget reports, interview job applicants, develop a strategic plan, or measure productivity and patient satisfaction.

Here are some resources for professional development:

- *Professional associations.* Professional associations provide conferences, courses, workshops, online modules, and other opportunities for professional development.
- *Employer training.* Employers offer training to help employees develop and enhance their skills. This may include classes on customer service, communication skills, computer skills, and how to use new equipment and software programs.
- *College courses and degree programs.* Colleges and universities offer courses and degree programs to support the professional development of health care workers. Each year, more courses are offered online to provide convenience for working professionals. Employers may offer tuition assistance and flexible work schedules for employees who wish to return to school and work on advanced degrees and professional certifications.
- *Professional journals.* Online and printed professional journals help alert people to the latest developments in their fields. Journals also provide opportunities for health care professionals to write articles and become published authors.

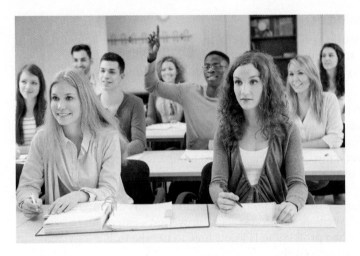

Figure 8-9 Taking a class for professional development (*Robert Kneschke/Shutterstock*)

Developing Leadership Skills

Like most other kinds of businesses, health care companies need people with effective leadership skills. Working in a leadership role as a supervisor, coordinator, manager, or director can be stressful but the rewards often outweigh the negatives. Successful leaders have the ability to articulate a **vision** (a mental image; to imagine what the future could be), outline a plan of action, and direct individuals and groups toward common goals. Effective leadership is crucial in health care where the pace of change is rapid, the challenges are difficult, and the stakes are high. Health care is a complex life-and-death business. Its leaders must be capable, strong, dedicated, compassionate, empathetic, and sensitive to the needs of others. Leadership means providing the guidance, encouragement, and support that people need to achieve success.

CONSIDER THIS

LEADERSHIP STYLES AND TEAMWORK

In today's world, highly effective health care leaders are in great demand to help navigate the rapid change within the health care industry. Improving productivity, quality of care, and cost effectiveness while enhancing patient and employee satisfaction are the primary challenges for people moving into leadership positions. Having a cadre of competent leaders is extremely important in strengthening the financial status of companies and in recruiting and retaining highly skilled professionals.

People display different leadership styles and each style has a unique impact on teamwork. Here are three examples:

- A *democratic* leader makes the final decisions but invites other team members to contribute to the decision-making process. This usually supports job satisfaction because team members feel appreciated and respected. This style can also help develop the leadership skills of team members. A democratic leader may result in better outcomes because everyone's suggestions have been taken into account.

- An *autocratic* leader exercises authority over the team. Members have little opportunity to offer suggestions and may resent being treated in this manner. This style may be acceptable when supervising routine work performed by lower-skilled employees. But autocratic leadership often results in low morale and high turnover.
- A *laissez-faire* (French for "let it be") leader leaves team members alone to do their work. This loose style of leadership works best with an experienced staff that routinely gets good results. Workers who need direct supervision and more support may feel abandoned by a *laissez-faire* leader. This style can lead to a lack of respect for the leader and less than desirable outcomes.

The **perks** (benefits that come with status) associated with leadership jobs might look attractive, but there are good reasons why leaders often report stress and burnout. Effective leadership requires:

- Working long hours (without overtime pay) to complete your own work while facilitating the work of other people.
- Maintaining your technical and patient care skills while strengthening your leadership skills.
- Communicating effectively to resolve disagreements and conflicts among adults who really ought to behave better.
- Managing stress while meeting tight deadlines and attempting to do more, with less, and get better outcomes.
- Exercising care and caution in everything you say and do.
- Mastering new software, tracking emerging trends, and keeping up with industry developments.

Unless you've been in a leadership position yourself, it's hard to imagine the stress involved in keeping so many different things in balance. It's easy to be critical of leaders who do things that you don't agree with or who don't respond as quickly as you would like. The next time you encounter leaders in your school or company, think about what it must be like to walk in their shoes and consider giving them a break. Leaders are just like the rest of us, human beings trying to do their very best each and every day. No one is perfect and sometimes our leaders fall short.

Aside from the drawbacks of leadership roles, there are lots of benefits to being a leader. Leaders typically:

- Function in exempt positions without having to **clock in and out** (use a time clock or electronic system to record hours worked).
- Receive higher pay than nonexempt employees working at lower levels of the organization.
- Have more flexibility in their work schedules.
- Receive more paid time off and work fewer (or no) weekends and holidays.
- Have offices or cubicles, helpful assistants, and clerical support.
- Get to attend workshops, conferences, and company-paid business trips.

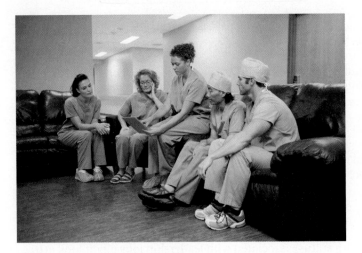

Figure 8-10 Leading a surgical team meeting (*Tyler Olson/Shutterstock*)

People who experience high levels of job satisfaction working in leadership roles often say it's not the pay or benefits that make them look forward to coming to work each day. They appreciate having the opportunity to:

- Articulate a vision, lay out a plan, and stimulate a collaborative effort.
- Help the organization fulfill its mission and reach new heights.
- Encourage people to learn, grow, and achieve their goals.
- Make improvements to benefit the company, the employees, and the patients.

Creating and maintaining an environment that fosters excellence is an important aspect of leadership, especially in health care where quality outcomes are so important. Employees who work in an environment geared for excellence are more likely to take pride in their work, perform at high levels, and continually seek ways to improve patient care and customer service. Leaders:

- Facilitate excellence among individuals and the group as a whole.
- Provide the resources and tools employees need to do their work.
- Act as advocates for individuals and the group within the organization.
- Monitor the performance and outcomes of individuals and the group.
- Adapt their leadership style to meet the needs of the group at any given time.

In addition, effective leaders:

- Respect the rights, dignity, opinions, and abilities of others.
- Display self-confidence and a willingness to take a stand.
- Practice good listening skills and respect the opinions of those who disagree with them.
- Display competence in cultural diversity and embrace the benefits of individual differences.
- Communicate effectively and state instructions and ideas clearly.
- Devote as much effort to their work (or more) as the people who report to them.

- Complete assignments on time and according to expectations.
- Display optimism and a can-do attitude.
- Remain open-minded and willing to change and compromise.
- Praise others and give credit where credit is due.

Effective leaders don't expect subordinates to do something they aren't willing to do themselves. They openly support the company's mission, vision, and values and encourage others to do the same. When they disagree with a company policy or action, they discuss the matter privately with the appropriate people.

Ways to Develop Leadership Skills

Health care employees who earn high performance evaluations and who demonstrate potential leadership skills may be offered leadership roles even before acquiring a full set of leadership skills. If this happens to you, you'll need to ramp up quickly. But if you have time to prepare before moving into a leadership position, there are lots of ways to gain leadership skills. Consider the following:

- Enroll in leadership classes and programs at school and at work.
- Read books and articles; review online resources.
- Work alongside an experienced, skilled leader and observe his or her behavior.
- Function as part of a team and observe other people's leadership skills as you develop your own.
- Volunteer to serve on committees at school, at work, and in your community.
- Participate in clubs and athletics at school.
- Help organize special events, fundraisers, health fairs, and other projects.

All of these activities provide valuable experience in working with other people and collaborating to achieve desired results. Don't overlook the importance of being an effective follower. When you collaborate with other people, you'll switch between leading and following based on the needs of the group at any particular time.

If you set your sights on gaining a leadership position, make sure you tell people so they can support your efforts. Learn as much as you can about the business side of health care as well as the technical aspects of your profession. Take some assessments to identify your strengths and areas for improvement. Become aware of how your image and behavior are perceived by the people whom you may someday lead.

Becoming an effective leader will take some time and patience. Here are a few places to start:

- Become well skilled and experienced in your health care discipline.
- Develop your critical thinking skills and learn to make thoughtful decisions.
- Strengthen your verbal and written communication skills and focus on conflict resolution and negotiating skills.
- Learn about other cultures and develop respect and appreciation for people who are different from you.
- Become active in your professional associations.

Participating in Professional Associations

Becoming an active member in one or more professional associations is one of the best ways to develop and practice your leadership skills and engage in professional development.

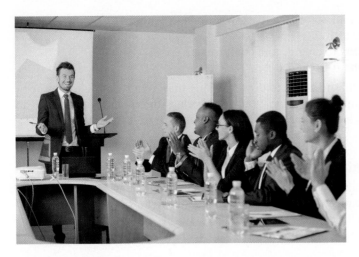

Figure 8-11 Participating in a professional association committee meeting
(*Vgstockstudio/Shutterstock*)

Membership in a student organization or in a health care professional association provides the opportunity to gain knowledge and practical experience in working with a wide variety of other people.

Health care has numerous professional associations to help workers remain current with emerging trends. Most of these organizations are discipline-specific (nursing, radiography, physical therapy, medical assisting, etc.) and have local, state, and national chapters working together on common goals.

Participating in a health care professional association provides:

- Opportunities to develop leadership skills through elected offices and committee work
- Updates on technological advances and new medical procedures
- Current information on salary ranges, labor trends and projections, and job postings
- Reports on **legislative issues** (topics involving local, state, and national law-making)
- Interaction with other health care professionals
- Pooled funding to support improvements in the profession
- Influence as a united group to encourage positive change

You can find information about professional associations by checking websites, reading professional journals, attending continuing education sessions, and speaking with colleagues about the profession. Consider participating in professional social media sites such as LinkedIn to connect with other people who share common interests and goals.

Planning for Career Advancement

Planning for career advancement requires thinking ahead about where you want to be in a few years and what it's going to take to get there. Developing a **career plan** (a step-by-step strategy for a person's professional growth and development) is important for health care workers who want to advance in their professions.

Some health care employers encourage, or even require, their employees to have a career plan. The plan is developed by the employee in conjunction with his or her manager to make sure that the individual's goals align with the company's goals. The plan outlines the knowledge and skills the employee should acquire, and identifies a timeline and a set of measurable goals. When it's time for the employee's annual performance evaluation, his or her performance will be rated in part by how well he or she achieved the goals that were set.

RECENT DEVELOPMENTS

TAKING ADVANTAGE OF RETIREMENTS

An increasing number of health care employers are actively engaged in **succession planning** (a proactive approach to identifying and preparing employees to fill positions as other workers retire). As the health care workforce ages and more employees retire, employers will need a steady supply of well-qualified people to step in and take their place. Retirements create opportunities for advancement. So it's important to plan ahead and be ready when these opportunities arise. Including your manager in career planning can help pave the way for your next career move.

Even if your employer doesn't require a career plan, you should still have one. Many health occupations have career ladders for workers to climb. You can move from an entry-level job up to a higher-skilled job or a specialist role by completing more education and earning additional credentials. In some occupations you can move laterally (sideways, as opposed to "up") by broadening your knowledge and skills in the same discipline. Identify the career ladders for your occupation and think about what direction you might like to head in the future. Whether you develop your own career plan or work in conjunction with your manager, it's important to monitor your progress and make adjustments as needed.

As time passes, you might find that your interests are moving in a different direction than you had expected. You might discover that you really enjoy training people and decide to pursue teaching as the next step in your career. Or perhaps you enjoy research projects and decide to pursue research as a career track. People change careers for different reasons. Working in patient care for a prolonged period of time can be emotionally and physically exhausting for some people, so switching careers might provide some relief. Sometimes people just get restless and need a change, or they discover an interesting occupation that they didn't know existed. If you decide to make a change, you'll need to do some occupational research and revise your career plan.

HOT TOPICS

OCCUPATIONAL RESEARCH AND CAREER PLANNING RESOURCES

A variety of online resources are available providing up-to-date information to assist with occupational research and career planning. Here are some examples:

- *O*NET Online* (www.onetonline.org). A major source of occupational information on hundreds of different jobs. It will take some work on your part to explore the entire website and learn how to find the detailed information you need, but your time and effort will be worth the investment.

(continued)

- *Dictionary of Occupational Titles* (www.occupationalinfo.org). Lists job titles, tasks, and duties for thousands of occupations.
- *Occupational Outlook Handbook* (www.bls.gov/oco/). Discusses the nature of the work, employment outlook, training and qualification requirements, earnings, and working conditions for a variety of occupations.
- *Career One Stop* (www.careeronestop.org). Provides tools for career exploration including assessments and helpful information to create career goals, explore career options, gain skills, and find a job. You can also access assessments and view videos that describe different occupational clusters.

As you proceed with career planning, keep your priorities in mind and strike a healthy balance between your personal and professional lives. Take things one step at a time and avoid overloading yourself. It's not unusual for people to wonder if the time they spend at work and school might have a negative impact on their families. They may be setting a good example for their children through hard work, self-discipline, and perseverance, but balancing career goals with the demands of a busy personal life can be very challenging. Make sure to set aside time to enjoy your life and spend quality time with family and friends.

Fulfilling your career plan may require some adjustments along the way. Don't be surprised if your goals change or if you become discouraged when things take longer than you had anticipated. Adjustments and delays are part of the process as you learn more about yourself, what you want from your career, and what works best for you and your family. The important thing is to have a career plan and be somewhere on the road to where you eventually want to be.

THINK ABOUT IT

SUPPORTERS AND NONSUPPORTERS

Everyone needs some help at some point in their life and this is especially true for young people who are planning and preparing for their future. Who can *you* turn to for help when you need it?

Identifying a *network of supporters* is a good strategy to make sure you'll have the help you need, when and where you need it. Parents, family members, and friends are a good place to start. Also consider your program director, instructors, and people you've met through your practicum experience. Mentors and role models are part of your network of supporters, so put them on your list. If you've had a job, you might want to include your supervisor or a coworker who was especially helpful.

Choose people who know you well and who take an interest in your growth and development. Include people whom you admire and respect, and whose opinions and advice you value. Share your goals and career plan with each person and ask if he or she would be willing to provide some encouragement and advice along the way. If you've chosen wisely, most of them will be happy to help.

The topic of nonsupporters must also be addressed. There may be people in your life who are not supportive of your efforts. They may be envious, overly competitive, or threatened by the thought of your success. Some people may question your goals or your abilities and claim you're *reaching too high*. Others may try to hold you back or even sabotage your efforts. Watch out for these negative forces and don't let them derail your plans.

Keep your eyes open for new opportunities when you least expect them. If options arise to train in a different discipline, move from an inpatient to an outpatient setting, transfer to a new clinic or hospital, or advance into a leadership role, seize the opportunity and let it work to your advantage. You never know what might be out there, just waiting for you around the next corner. It's all a part of lifelong learning and your journey in health care.

Expect to take some risks along the way. Risk-taking *does not* mean being foolish or haphazard in decision making, but it *does* mean taking some well thought-out steps that force you to stretch a little bit. If you don't try, you'll never know what you could have accomplished.

If the going gets tough, don't give up. Talk with your network of supporters for encouragement. You'll probably hear that just about everyone has gone through what you are going through. Most people think about giving up at one point or another in their careers. If your goals are worth achieving, they're worth fighting for. So hang in there.

REALITY CHECK

When filling out job applications, developing a résumé, and participating in interviews, it's absolutely essential to be honest with everything you say and do. There are plenty of examples of people who lied about their identity, education, work experience, credentials, or criminal history and got caught. Some of these people got caught prior to receiving a job offer. Others were already on the job before their dishonesty was discovered. In some cases, it might take an employer several months to realize that an employee had falsified information on his or her job application. If you lie about your identity or qualifications or fail to disclose personal information that might have disqualified you from employment, it really doesn't matter how long you're on the job before someone finds out. You can be fired at any time for fraud and dishonesty. In most health care companies, once you've been fired under conditions such as these, you won't get a second chance and you'll never be eligible for rehire by the same company.

It's a small world. More than likely, your manager networks with leaders from other companies in your area. Once you've developed a reputation for dishonesty and fraud, word spreads quickly. This is especially true in small towns or in geographical areas with a limited number of health care employers. All it takes is one dishonest act to make a negative, and sometimes permanent, impact on a person's future employment opportunities. Don't let this happen to you.

For More Information

Job Boards
>www.careerbuilder.com/Jobs
>www.monster.com
>www.healthcarejobsite.com
>www.employmentguide.com

Occupational Information
>O*NET Online
>www.onetonline.org
>*Dictionary of Occupational Titles*
>www.occupationalinfo.org

Career One Stop
>www.careeronestop.org
>*Occupational Outlook Handbook*
>www.bls.gov/oco/

Labor Trends and Employment Projections
>Bureau of Labor Statistics, U.S. Department of Labor
>www.bls.gov

Resources and Tips for Job Applications, Cover Letters, Résumés, etc.
>www.jobsearch.about.com

KEY POINTS

- Identify your occupational preferences and the labor trends for where you want to work.
- Look for the best job opportunities that match your qualifications and interests.
- Make sure your résumé and cover letter convey a professional image.
- Identify appropriate references and ask if they would be willing to serve.
- Be honest and accurate when describing your qualifications.
- Disclose any misdemeanors or felonies on job applications.
- When applying online, allow time to learn how to navigate the computerized system.
- Expect to take some preemployment assessments as part of the job application process.
- Prepare for a job interview by having answers ready for the questions you expect to be asked.
- Present a professional image during your interview, including your appearance and behavior.
- Establish a professional presence online; make sure that everything that is posted about you on social media sites supports your professional image and reputation.
- Expect a criminal history background check and drug screen as part of the employment process.
- Adopt the philosophy of lifelong learning and engage in professional development activities.
- Build your leadership skills and become active in a professional association.
- Develop a career advancement plan and expect it to change over time.

LEARNING ACTIVITIES

Using information from Chapter Eight:
- Answer the Chapter Review Questions
- Respond to the What If? Scenarios

Chapter Review Questions

Using information presented in Chapter Eight, answer each of the following questions.

1. List four questions to answer when identifying your occupational preferences.

2. Explain the value of researching labor trends and projections.

3. Identify three places on the Internet to find job openings.

4. Describe four characteristics of a professional résumé.

5. Name five things you should do when filling out a job application form.

6. Explain why employers use preemployment assessments.

7. Describe five ways to present a professional image during a job interview.

8. Explain the importance of having a professional presence online.

9. List two reasons why health care workers must engage in professional development.

10. Describe four characteristics of effective leaders.

11. Identify two ways to develop leadership skills.

12. Describe the benefits of participating in a health care professional association.

13. Explain the importance of having a career advancement plan.

What If? Scenarios

Think about what you would do in the following situations and record your answers.

1. You're graduating from school in a few months and plan to move out of state. You need to find a good job but aren't familiar with health care employers in the city where you expect to live.

2. Your manager says she thinks you have leadership potential but you have no idea how to gain leadership skills.

3. You have a job interview at 8:00 A.M. on Saturday morning. Your friends are having a party Friday night that starts at 9:00 P.M. and they want you to join them.

4. The job you want requires five years of previous work experience. You have three years of work experience in a large hospital that, to you, seems comparable to five years in a smaller hospital. A small change on your résumé would make you appear eligible even though it wouldn't be totally accurate.

5. After deciding to apply for a job in an outpatient clinic, you find out your mother knows the clinic's personnel manager. Just a few months ago, your mother helped him refinance his home mortgage and your mother has offered to make a phone call to the manager on your behalf.

6. You've applied for the same job twice and have yet to be selected.

7. A few years ago you were charged with disorderly conduct resulting from a situation that occurred in a local bar. After an investigation, the charges were dropped. But you're afraid that if you mention the situation on your job application you won't be considered for the opening.

8. A close friend of yours is applying for health care jobs via online websites and she has asked for your assistance. Her personal email address and username reflect her interest in exotic dancing, her résumé is printed on pink paper with fancy borders, and the message on her phone was recorded by her 5-year-old daughter.

9. One hour prior to leaving for your interview appointment your mother calls to say she is sick and can't watch your two children while you're gone. You have no back-up plan and consider taking your children with you to the interview along with an iPad to keep them occupied.

10. You're a manager preparing to interview a job applicant. You notice a man outside your office window cleaning out his car. He dumps his ashtray, plastic bottles, and other trash on the ground and then walks away and enters your building. Within a few minutes the same man knocks on your door and announces that he's here for his interview.

Closing Thoughts

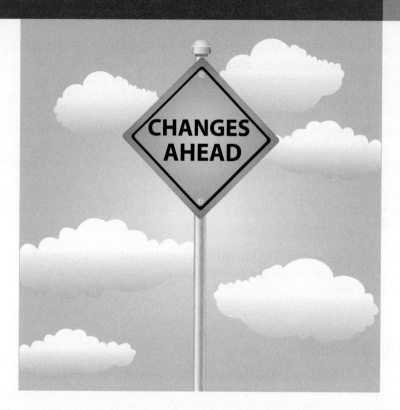

There's time left for one last Reality Check and some closing thoughts.

You'll soon be joining an industry that's undergoing rapid change. As the demand for health care grows, you and your colleagues will be challenged to *do more, with less, and get better outcomes*. Obesity is reaching a crisis level, caring for aging baby boomers is consuming more resources, and emerging medical technology is raising new moral, ethical, and legal dilemmas. With so many demands on the U.S. health care system, the only thing you can know for certain is that even more change is on the horizon.

Your life is about to change as well. You'll soon be entering the job market as a health care worker, focused on earning the reputation of a health care professional. Change can be a good thing in life if you can anticipate what's coming your way and prepare for it. The future can be exciting and unsettling at the same time. Just think about this quote:

Life is unsafe at any speed, and therein lies much of its fascination.

(Journalist Edgar Ansel Mowrer, 1892–1977)

Let's take one last look at things to do, thoughts to remember, and next steps to take.

Things to Do

1. *Have a career plan and expect it to change.* Know where you're headed and how you're going to get there. Expect things to change, but stay on the right track and take advantage of unexpected opportunities when they arise. Keep your goals up-to-date and share them with people who can help you succeed.

2. *Set yourself up for success.* Use good judgment and make thoughtful decisions. When you need some help, don't hesitate to ask for it. Don't let other people discourage you or prevent you from reaching your goals. If your goals are worth achieving, they're worth fighting for, so hang in there. Keep an optimistic attitude and surround yourself with people who have a positive influence on your life.

3. *Keep your priorities straight.* Your job and career should be high on your list, along with your personal health and wellness and your commitment to spending quality time with your family and friends. Reliability, dependability, accountability, and trustworthiness are the keys to earning self-respect and the respect of other people.

4. *Never stop learning.* If you expect to excel in health care, you must always be a student. Continually sharpen your skills, maintain your competence, and participate in professional development activities every chance you get. Remember that knowledge is the key to just about everything.

5. *Develop your leadership skills.* No matter where life takes you, your ability to articulate a vision and make it a reality through collaboration with other people will serve you well.

Thoughts to Remember

1. *Who you are as a person makes a difference.* If you want to be seen by others as a professional, you must earn that honor every day you come to work. Demonstrating a strong work ethic, meeting legal and ethical responsibilities, and displaying good character traits are the keys to a professional reputation. Treat people with compassion and respect, and represent your profession and your employer with dignity and pride. Always *do the right thing* because *it's the right thing to do.*

2. *Your patients come first.* When you work in health care, it's not about you or your job title or your schedule for the day. It's always about the patient. How your patients feel about their health care experience can have a significant impact on your company's success. *High tech* drives advancement in health care and medicine, but it can never replace the importance of *high touch.*

3. *Care about quality and safety.* Health care is an extremely complex industry with life and death hanging in the balance. It's easy for things to *fall through the cracks* and cause problems. Pay attention to the details, and watch for ways to improve quality and safety. Help create and maintain an environment where patients, coworkers, and others feel safe and in good hands.

4. *Keep up with current events.* This is *your* career, so be aware of what's going on in health care, in your profession, and in your place of employment. Get involved in your professional associations and help shape the future.

5. *Make positive ripples with everything you say and do.* Stop and think before you act. Be present in the moment, and act with intention and self-awareness. Consider the impact that your attitude, behavior, and appearance have on other people. Respect other people's opinions and values, and do your best to improve the lives of those around you.

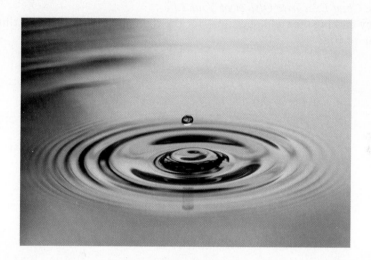

Next Steps to Take

1. *Graduate from school and secure your professional credentials.* These are the first two steps in laying the foundation for your career and your future. Earn high grades, complete graduation requirements, and pass your certification, licensure, or registration exams.

2. *Strengthen your skills.* Focus on soft skills as well as your hard skills. Improve your ability to communicate, resolve conflict, and solve problems through critical thinking. Learn new computer skills and enhance your ability to manage your time, personal finances, and stress. Embrace diversity and learn to appreciate and value people who are different from you.

3. *Accept responsibility.* Adopt the attitude, "The buck stops here." Make your own decisions with the support of your family and friends, and then accept the consequences. Admit when you've made a mistake and learn from it. This is your life, so seize control of it. Take some calculated risks to stretch a bit and develop your full potential. When the going gets rough, hang in there.

Becoming the CEO of Your Life

Whether you provide direct patient care or serve in a support role behind-the-scenes, you'll be part of a nationwide workforce that strives to improve the lives of others. Today's amazing health care system was built by those who came before you—the scientists, inventors, doctors, nurses, and others who devoted their work and their lives to improving medical science and the health and wellness of those they served. Perhaps one day *you* will be among those who will change the course of medicine and health care for the better.

Become the *Chief Executive Officer of Your Life.*
Start now by making the right decisions, for the right reasons, at the right times.
It's really up to you.

Spruce Family Medicine Clinic
567 Spruce Street
Greentree, IN 47202

Job Title: Certified Medical Assistant
Job Code: B254
Job Family: Clinical
Job Status: Nonexempt
Supervisory Responsibility: No
Reports to: Office Manager
Pay Range: MB7
Effective Date: January 1, 2015

Summary

In addition to demonstrating core behaviors and standards of service expected of all employees, incumbent performs routine patient care and administrative procedures to assist physicians and nurses in examining and treating patients in a medical office setting.

Essential Duties

Essential duties include but are not limited to:

1. Greets patients, answers telephones, schedules appointments
2. Provides care to patients, prepares patients for examinations
3. Assists the physician during the examination
4. Explains treatment procedures to patients
5. Takes medical histories, records vital signs
6. Performs ECGs, removes sutures, changes dressings
7. Instructs patients about medications and special diets
8. Collects laboratory specimens, performs basic laboratory tests
9. Forwards prescriptions to a pharmacy
10. Updates and files patient medical records
11. Complies with HIPAA and confidentiality requirements
12. Performs clerical functions and insurance billing
13. Maintains medical equipment and inventory of supplies
14. Maintains a clean, safe, orderly environment

Qualifications

Education: Graduation from an accredited Medical Assistant program. Proof of high school diploma or GED. Associate of Science Degree in Medical Assisting.

Experience: No experience required. One year relevant work experience preferred.

Certification: Certification by the American Association of Medical Assistants or the American Registry of Medical Assistants required.

Knowledge/Skills/Abilities

Incumbent will demonstrate the ability to:

- Perform and assist with diagnostic and therapeutic procedures
- Conduct medical office procedures and operate medical office equipment
- Communicate and document clinical and administrative information
- Apply knowledge of sterile technique, infection control, and safety precautions
- Apply age-specific competencies
- Establish and maintain effective working relationships with patients and staff
- Demonstrate good customer service and conflict resolution skills
- Establish priorities, organize tasks, and manage time efficiently
- Allocate and utilize resources cost-effectively
- Remain calm in stressful situations
- Display effective interpersonal and team skills
- Ensure patient privacy and the confidentiality of patient information
- Present a professional image as a representative of the practice

Computer skills:

- Demonstrate proficiency in Microsoft Word, Excel, Access, and Outlook
- Ability to perform clinic-specific computer applications and learn new applications and procedures

Additional qualifications may be required for any particular position. Employees may be expected to perform duties in addition to those presented in this description.

Sample Performance Evaluation

Performance Evaluation
Certified Medical Assistant

Employee Name _____   Employee Number _____

Job Title/Job Code _____   Department/Unit _____

Supervisor Name _____   Supervisor Title _____

Time period covered by evaluation: From _____ To _____

Date of supervisor meeting with employee (evaluation date) _____

This Performance Evaluation form may be completed by the:

- Employee, for his or her self-evaluation as part of his/her performance review
- Employee's supervisor, as part of the employee's performance review
- Employee's coworkers, as part of the employee's 360-degree feedback review

Rating Scale

Evaluate each performance factor using the following 1 to 5 scale:

5 Consistently exceeds expectations
4 Frequently exceeds expectations
3 Consistently meets expectations
2 Inconsistently meets expectations
1 Consistently fails to meet expectations

Part 1: Core Behaviors   Rating

1. Communication Skills   _____
2. Teamwork/Interpersonal Skills   _____
3. Problem-Solving Skills   _____
4. Organizational/Time Management Skills   _____
5. Respect for Diversity   _____
6. Service Excellence/Customer Service   _____
7. Support for Quality Improvement   _____
8. Support for Cost-Effective Operations   _____
9. Support for Corporate Mission and Values   _____

Comments:

Part 2: Personal Characteristics   **Rating**

1. Appearance ———————
2. Attitude ———————
3. Initiative ———————
4. Adaptability, flexibility ———————
5. Reliability, trustworthiness ———————
6. Judgment ———————
7. Ethics, integrity ———————
8. Stress management ———————
9. Accountability ———————

Comments:

Part 3: Job-Specific Competencies   **Rating**

1. Greets patients, answers telephones, schedules appointments ———————
2. Provides care to patients, prepares patients for examinations ———————
3. Assists the physician during the examination ———————
4. Explains treatment procedures to patients ———————
5. Takes medical histories, records vital signs ———————
6. Performs ECGs, removes sutures, changes dressings ———————
7. Instructs patients about medications and special diets ———————
8. Collects laboratory specimens, performs basic laboratory tests ———————
9. Forwards prescriptions to a pharmacy ———————
10. Updates and files patient medical records ———————
11. Performs clerical functions and insurance billing ———————
12. Maintains medical equipment and inventory of supplies ———————
13. Maintains a clean, safe, orderly environment ———————

Comments:

Part 4: Overall Performance   **Rating**

    Attendance/punctuality   _____
    Technical knowledge   _____
    Quality of work   _____
    Quantity of work, productivity   _____

Comments:

Part 5: Improvement Plans (if applicable)
Identify improvement plans for each performance factor rated 2 or below:

Part 6: Achievements and Recognition
List special achievements, awards, designations, or other types of recognition during this evaluation period:

Part 7: Goals and Professional Development Activities
List at least one measurable goal and a self-development activity for the upcoming evaluation period:

OVERALL COMMENTS:

_____

SIGNATURES

The person who completed the form:

Name _____   Job Title _____

Relationship to the employee undergoing review   _____

Signature _____   Date Completed _____

The employee undergoing review:

Name _____   Job Title _____

Signature _____   Date Signed _____

(Signature does not necessarily indicate agreement with evaluation ratings.)

EMPLOYEE COMMENTS:

Performance Evaluation Approval:

Name _____   Job Title _____

Signature _____   Date Approved _____

Sample Résumé

Jane Jones, A.S., CMA (AAMA)

---

123 Maple Street • Greentree, IN 47202
812/333-4444 • jjones@mail.net

Professional Experience

January 15 to March 25, 2016 • Poplar Grove Family Practice Center, Poplar Grove, IN

Student Extern—160 hours

- Scheduled and managed appointments
- Performed accounts receivable and billing and collections procedures
- Performed procedural and diagnostic coding
- Performed venipuncture, electrocardiography, urinalysis, and respiratory testing
- Obtained vital signs, recorded patient history
- Prepared patients for and assisted with procedures, treatments, and minor office surgeries

June 1 to August 31, 2014 • Greentree Baptist Hospital, Greentree, IN

Hospice Unit Volunteer—30 hours/week

- Answered telephones
- Delivered flowers
- Staffed the information desk
- Filed paperwork

January 3 to May 15, 2014 • Shady Dell Rehab Center, Elm City, IN

Nursing Assistant—20 hours/week

- Served meals and fed patients
- Bathed and showered patients
- Lifted, repositioned, moved, and transported patients
- Created and led recreation activities

Education And Certification

A.S. degree in Medical Assisting • Greentree Community College, Greentree, IN
April 3, 2016

Certified Medical Assistant • American Association of Medical Assistants
April 20, 2016

References available upon request.

123 Maple Street
Greentree, IN 47202
812/333-4444
jjones@mail.net

May 1, 2016

Mr. John Johnson
Office Manager
Spruce Family Medicine Clinic
567 Spruce Street
Greentree, IN 47202

Dear Mr. Johnson:

In response to your posting for a Certified Medical Assistant on careerbuilder.com, I am pleased to submit my application for the CMA position at the Spruce Family Medicine Clinic. My skills and medical experience closely match your qualifications. After serving as a nursing assistant in the Shady Dell Rehab Center and doing volunteer work in Greentree Hospital's hospice unit, I decided to pursue a career in medical assisting and enrolled in Greentree Community College's program.

While working as a Student Extern at the Poplar Grove Family Practice Center, I performed and assisted with a variety of clinical and administrative procedures. My college grades and extern evaluations placed me at the top in my class of 25 students. My program director, Vanessa Smith, and Poplar Grove's Medical Director, Dr. James Sullivan, volunteered to serve as professional references.

If you are looking for an enthusiastic medical assistant who learns quickly and displays exceptional communication, interpersonal, and customer service skills, I would be proud to join your team at the Spruce Family Medicine Clinic.

My résumé is attached and I am available for a personal interview at your convenience. Please contact me at 812/333-4444 or jjones@mail.net.

I'm looking forward to meeting you and learning more about employment opportunities with the Spruce Family Medicine Clinic. Thank you for considering my application.

Sincerely,

Jane Jones, A.S., CMA (AAMA)

Sample Job Application Form

Spruce Family Medicine Clinic
Greentree, Indiana

It is our policy to comply with all applicable state and federal laws prohibiting discrimination in employment on race, age, color, sex, religion, national origin or other protected classification.

Instructions: Print clearly in black or blue ink. Answer all questions. Sign and date the form.

Personal Information

First Name _____

Middle Name _____

Last Name _____

Street Address _____

_____

City, State, Zip Code _____

Telephone Number (_____) _____

Email Address _____

Are you over 18 years old?   Yes _____ No _____
Are you a U.S. citizen or otherwise authorized to work in the U.S. on an unrestricted basis?

Yes _____ No _____

Have you ever been convicted of, or pleaded no contest to, a felony?
(Conviction will not necessarily disqualify an applicant for employment.)

Yes _____ No _____

If yes, describe conditions: _____

Position and Availability

Position Applied For _____

Job Number _____

Are there any hours, shifts or days you cannot or will not work?

No _____ Yes _____

Preferences:

Status   Part time _____ Full time _____ Supplemental _____

Shift   Day _____ Evening _____ Night _____ Weekends _____

Are you available to work overtime as required? Yes _____ No _____

What date are you available to start work? _____

Education

High School/GED Education:

Have you earned a high school diploma or GED? Yes _____ No _____

Awarded by _____

Date awarded _____

Postsecondary Education (List all schools attended; use a separate sheet of paper if necessary)

School Name   _____

School Address   _____

                  _____

Field of Study   _____

Degree/Diploma   _____

Graduation Date   _____

Other Postsecondary Education:

School Name   _____

School Address   _____

                  _____

Field of Study   _____

Degree/Diploma   _____

Graduation Date   _____

Professional License/Certification/Registration:

Title/Date _____

Awarded by _____

Expiration date _____

Other Training and Skills: _____

_____

_____

_____

Awards/Recognition: _____

_____

Employment History

(List all employment during the past five years; use a separate sheet of paper if necessary)
Present or Last Position:

Employer: _____

Address: _____

_____

Supervisor:

Name _____

Title _____

Phone _____

Email _____

Your Position:

Job Title _____

Employment dates From:_____ To: _____

Responsibilities _____

Reason for leaving _____

Previous Position:

Employer: _____

Address: _____

_____

Supervisor:

Name _____

Title _____

Phone _____

Email _____

Your Position:

Job Title _____

Employment dates   From:_____ To: _____

Responsibilities _____

Reason for leaving _____

May We Contact Your Present Employer?

Yes _____ No _____

How did you learn of this opening? _____

Have you ever worked here before? No _____ Yes _____

If yes, dates of employment: From _____ To _____

Job title _____

References:

1. Name _____ Title _____

   Address _____ Phone _____

   Email _____

   Relationship to you _____

2. Name _____ Title _____

   Address _____ Phone _____

   Email _____

   Relationship to you _____

3. Name _____ Title _____

   Address _____ Phone _____

   Email _____

   Relationship to you _____

I certify that information contained in this application is accurate and complete.
I understand that false information may be grounds for not hiring me or for immediate
termination of employment at any point in the future if I am hired.
I authorize the verification of any or all information listed above.

Printed Name _____

Signature _____

Date Signed _____

Ms. Jane Jones, A.S., CMA (AAMA)
123 Maple Street
Greentree, IN 47202

June 10, 2016

Mr. John Johnson, Office Manager
Spruce Family Medicine Clinic
567 Spruce Street
Greentree, IN 47202

Dear Mr. Johnson:

Thank you for the opportunity to interview with you and Dr. Seymour yesterday for a CMA position. Having met you and your colleagues and toured the facility, I am very excited about the prospect of joining the Spruce Family Medicine team.

I believe that my education, experience, and commitment to quality care and service excellence make me well qualified for the CMA position.

Thank you again for the interview and I look forward to hearing from you soon.

Sincerely,

Jane Jones

Jane Jones, A.S., CMA (AAMA)
812/333-4444
jjones@mail.net

Externship Journal

Student's Name: Jane Jones

Student's School: Greentree Community College

Externship Dates: January 15 to March 25, 2016

Externship Site: Poplar Grove Family Practice Center

456 Walnut Lane

Greentree, IN

Week One/January 15–19

Day One

- I arrived at my extern site for my first day at 7:45 AM
- Got a tour of the facility and met the doctors and staff
- Met with the practice manager and learned about protocol for student externs
- Spent the rest of the day shadowing Dawn, the medical assistant to Dr. Sullivan
- Dawn showed me where everything is kept
- I observed how Dawn prepares the rooms for the doctor
- This is a very busy office. I observed many different procedures and so far I am really impressed with how the back office and front office work together as a team.
- I observed Dawn's technique at drawing blood. Her technique is a little different than our instructor showed us, but she still used all the same equipment.
- Left the office at 5:00 PM

Day Two

- I arrived at 7:45 AM
- Escorted all of Dr. Sullivan's patients to their rooms
- Observed how Dawn assists the doctor with different procedures such as pap smears and skin tag removals
- I did my first blood draw on a patient and was successful on my first attempt!
- Left the office at 5:00 PM

Day Three

- I arrived at 7:45 AM
- Jumped right in and starting escorting patients to their rooms and preparing the rooms
- Performed 2 EKGs in the morning

- Ate lunch with two of the medical assistants in the break room. One said she was unhappy about having to change her hours and work a Saturday morning each month. She tried to get the other MA to join her in complaining to management. I just listened and stayed out of the conversation.
- Gave 3 injections and drew blood on several patients in the afternoon
- Left the office at 5:00 PM

Day Four

- I arrived at 7:45 AM
- Helped out in the medical records department since one of the women there called in sick
- Prepared and filed charts
- Left the office at 5:00 PM

Day Five

- Arrived at the office at 7:45 AM
- Today we didn't have any morning appointments until 10:00 AM
- I was invited to their staff meeting. The practice manager said she's developing a new policy about social media because one of the employees had posted comments about the practice on his Facebook page. She said she wouldn't hesitate to fire someone if they committed a HIPAA violation or damaged the practice's reputation.
- For the rest of the morning, I escorted patients to their rooms and assisted Dr. Sullivan
- Worked in the lab in the afternoon
- Performed blood draws and UAs
- Left the office at 5:00 PM
- Wow, I can't believe a whole week has gone by already!

H Sample Practicum Thank-You Letter

123 Maple Street
Greentree, IN 47202

March 27, 2016

Dr. James Sullivan, Medical Director
Poplar Grove Family Practice Center
118 N. Maple Street
Poplar Grove, IN 47201

Dear Dr. Sullivan and Staff:

I am writing to thank all of you for taking time out of your busy work schedules to allow me to complete the extern portion of my education in your office. I have learned so much by working with you. Having a student extern in the medical office can be a strain on everyone, but I know the experience I have received will make me a much better medical assistant.

In just a few days I will graduate from school with an associate's degree. The knowledge and skills I gained while working with you will really help when I sit for the MA certification exam next month.

I really appreciate all of the encouragement and support you have given me.

Thank you again for your time and patience during my externship.

Sincerely,

Jane Jones

Jane Jones, Student Extern
jjones@mail.net

Glossary of Terms

360-degree feedback a performance evaluation procedure in which people who have worked with the employee during the past year are asked to provide input for the evaluation. (2)

abuse improper, cruel, or violent treatment. (3)

accountability accepting responsibility and consequences of one's actions. (1)

accountable care organizations networks of health care providers that work together and share responsibility and accountability for a large group of patients. (1)

accreditation certified as having met standards. (Intro)

acute severe but of short or limited duration. (1)

adaptive skills ability to adjust to change. (6)

advance directive a written instruction such as a living will recognized under state law relating to the provision of health care when the individual is permanently or temporarily impaired by a mental and/or physical condition. (5)

advanced practice providers (APPs) advanced health care providers such as physician assistants, certified nurse practitioners, certified nurse midwives, clinical nurse specialists, and certified registered nurse anesthetists. (1)

adverse effects unfavorable or harmful outcomes. (1)

adversity hardships; misfortune. (6)

advocates people who speak or write in support of something or someone. (5)

aggressive likely to confront or attack. (4)

alternative medicine healing arts that are not part of traditional medical practice in the United States. (1)

apps applications; software programs that perform specific functions on smartphones and hand-held computer devices. (1)

assault a threat or an attempt to injure another person. (3)

assertive confident and self-assured. (4)

attachment a file linked to an email message. (4)

attitude manner of acting, feeling, or thinking that shows one's disposition or opinion. (Intro)

Baby Boomers people born in the United States between 1946 and 1964. (1)

baseline data information gathered before a change begins to form a basis for analyzing subsequent changes. (1)

battery the unlawful touching of another person without his or her consent, with or without an injury. (3)

behavorial questions questions that ask how a person has behaved in the past. (8)

biased favoring one thing, person, or way over another based on some prior experience. (4)

blog an online personal journal available to the public. (1)

body language nonverbal messages communicated by posture, hand gestures, facial expressions, and so forth. (4)

body mass index (BMI) measure of body fat based on height and weight for adult men and women. (6)

body mechanics proper body movements such as safe lifting techniques to prevent or reduce injuries. (6)

breach a break, failure, or interruption. (1)

callous insensitive and emotionally hardened. (3)

career plan a step-by-step strategy for a person's professional growth and development. (8)

caregivers health care workers who provide direct, hands-on patient care. (Intro)

certification a credential from a state agency or a professional association awarding permission to use a special professional title to a person who meets pre-established competency standards. (Intro)

character a person's moral behavior and qualities. (3)

cheating deceiving by trickery. (3)

chronic occurring frequently over a long period of time. (1)

civility politeness and consideration. (4)

cliques small, exclusive circles of people. (4)

clock in and out use a time clock or electronic system to record hours worked. (8)

clone a group of cells that is genetically identical to the unit from which it was derived. (3)

cloud a network of remote servers on the Internet used to store, manage, and process data. (2)

code of ethics standards by which a group decides the difference between right and wrong; behavioral expectations for people who practice in a given profession. (3)

cognition knowing, understanding. (1)

colleagues fellow workers in the same profession. (4)

common sense using good judgment and thinking and behaving in a reasonable way. (2)

competence possessing necessary knowledge and skills for a given occupation or task. (Intro)

complementary medicine combining alternative medical approaches with traditional medical practices. (1)

compliance acting in accordance with laws and with a company's rules, policies, and procedures. (2)

conduct behavior or standard of behavior. (3)

confidentiality maintaining the privacy of certain matters. (1)

conflict of interest an inappropriate relationship between personal interests and official responsibilities. (2)

conflict resolution overcoming disagreements among two or more people. (4)

confrontation facing boldly and defiantly. (4)

conscience moral judgment that prohibits or opposes the violation of a previously recognized ethical principle. (3)

consensus a decision accepted by all participants in a group. (4)

consent permission given for something to happen. (2)

constructive criticism positive and negative comments and opinions offered to help another person improve. (2)

consumers purchasers or users of a product or service. (1)

contingency plans back-up plans prepared in case original plans don't work. (2)

continuity the quality of being continuous, uninterrupted, and connected. (1)

continuous quality improvement (CQI) using methods and tools to identify, prevent, and reduce the impact of process failures. (1)

cooperation acting or working together for a common purpose. (4)

corporate mission the special duties, functions, or purposes of a company. (2)

corporate values beliefs held in high esteem by a company. (2)

corrective action steps taken to overcome a problem. (2)

courtesy polite behavior, gestures, and remarks. (4)

cover letter a letter introducing a job applicant to a potential employer. (8)

credentials a letter or certificate given to a person to show that he or she has the right to exercise a certain authority. (Intro)

credit report   a review of records to assess a person's financial status. (8)

critical thinking   using reasoning and evidence to make an analysis or reach a decision. (2)

cultural competence   the ability to interact effectively with people from various cultures. (5)

cultures   groups of people who share the same values and norms. (5)

de-escalate   to reduce intensity or difficulty. (4)

diagnostic   deciding the nature of a disease or condition. (Intro)

dialect   language that is distinct to a culture. (4)

dictate   to read aloud and record patient information for medical records. (5)

digital communication   the use of computers, software, and networks to store and share information including data, video, and voice. (1)

dignity   worth, merit, honor. (Intro)

diligent   careful and conscientious in one's work. (2)

disabled   having a condition that damages or limits a person's physical or mental abilities. (1)

discipline   a branch of knowledge or learning such as nursing, medical assisting, surgical technology, and so forth. (1)

discretion   taking care and using good judgment about what one says or does. (2)

discrimination   unfair treatment of a person or group on the basis of prejudice. (5)

dismissal   involuntary termination from a job. (2)

diverse   differing; varied. (1)

diversity   differences, dissimilarities, variations. (4)

dress code   standards for attire and appearance. (6)

drug screen   lab test to detect illegal substances. (7)

duty to act   the obligation to care for a patient who requires it. (3)

dynamic   in motion, energetic, and vigorous (as characterizing a career, for example). (8)

electronic health record (EHR)   computerized health record. (1)

emancipated   legally considered an adult; a status granted to some minors under the age of 18 who, for example, are married, serving in the military, living independently, or undergoing treatment for certain conditions for which the law permits minors to consent to their own care. (5)

emoji   pictures or characters representing facial expressions, objects, places, or other concepts. (1)

emoticons   combinations of keyboard characters used to convey the sender's emotions, such as :-) to represent a smile. (4)

emotional intelligence quotient (EQ)   the ability to perceive, assess, and manage your own emotions and other people's emotions. (1)

empathetic   able to relate to another person's emotions and situation. (5)

employers of choice   companies where people like to work. (8)

employment agency   a company that connects employers and job-seekers. (8)

employment benefits   employer-paid insurance and retirement savings. (8)

employment status   full-time, part-time, or supplemental employment. (8)

empowered   given authority, enabled, or permitted. (1)

error   something done incorrectly through ignorance or carelessness. (1)

ethics   standards of conduct and moral judgment. (3)

etiquette   acceptable standards of behavior in polite society. (4)

exempt positions   jobs that involve management or other advanced functions or skills and that provide a guaranteed salary but are exempt from (do not offer) additional pay for overtime hours. *See also* nonexempt positions. (8)

expressed consent   consent for care that is given in writing or verbally. (5)

extenders people whose job is to assist other workers who have more education or higher credentials. (5)

extroverts people who predominantly focus outwardly. (5)

false imprisonment the holding or retaining of a person against his or her will. (3)

felony a serious criminal offense that carries a penalty of imprisonment for more than one year and possibly the death penalty. (3)

fraud intentional deceit through false information or misrepresentation. (2)

front-line workers employees who have the most frequent or direct contact with a company's customers. (2)

gatekeepers people who monitor the actions of other people and/or control access to something. (1)

generalizations facts, patterns, and trends about groups of people that are backed up by statistics and research findings. (5)

geriatric elderly; a medical specialty or service for older adults. (1)

goals aims, objectives, or ends that one strives to attain. (2)

Golden Rule a rule, held in most religions, that you should treat other people the way you would like to be treated. One familiar form of the Golden Rule is "Do unto others as you would have them do unto you." *See also* Platinum Rule. (4)

grammar the system or structure of a language; the generally accepted rules of speech and writing. (6)

gross domestic product (GDP) the total market value of all goods and services produced in one year in a nation. (1)

gross misconduct unacceptable behavior of a serious nature often leading to dismissal from a job. (3)

group norms expectations or guidelines for group behavior. (4)

hacked being the victim of unauthorized access gained by a computer. (2)

harassment any verbal or physical abuse of a person because of race, religion, age, gender, or disability. (3)

hard skills hands-on technical skills and duties. (1)

HCAHPS (pronounced H-caps) Hospital Consumer Assessment of Healthcare Providers and Systems; a standardized survey for hospitals to use in collecting and publishing patient-satisfaction data in which patients recently released from the hospital are asked to comment on their experience and satisfaction with their hospital stay. (5)

head hunter a recruiter hired to help an employer with its "difficult to fill" job openings. (8)

healing environments physical spaces designed to reduce stress, ensure safety, and uplift the spirits of patients, visitors, and staff. (5)

health care exchanges open marketplaces through which buyers and sellers of health insurance can come together to help consumers compare and shop for health insurance coverage. (1)

health disparities unfair misdiagnosis and treatment of some groups, generally minority groups. (5)

health risk assessments questionnaires that identify which health issues a person needs to focus on based on medical history and lifestyle. (6)

health screenings tests or examinations to find a disease or condition before symptoms may have appeared. (6)

hierarchy a group of people or units arranged by rank. (Intro)

HIPAA Health Insurance Portability and Accountability Act of 1996. The law's goals are to make it easier for people to keep health insurance, protect the confidentiality and security of their health care information, and help to control health care administrative costs. (2)

hire-on bonus extra compensation for accepting a job offer. (8)

HITECH Health Information Technology for Economic and Clinical Health signed into law in 2009 as part of the American Recovery and Reinvestment Act (ARRA). The law addressed the confidentiality of health information transmitted electronically. (2)

hoard to resist giving something up. (4)

hospice services care provided for the terminally ill that focuses on comfort and quality of life instead of a cure. (1)

hostile workplace an uncomfortable or unsafe workplace. (2)

immunizations vaccinations to protect against getting a disease. (6)

impaired having a reduced ability to function properly. (2)

implied consent consent for care that is expressed by a patient's actions, such as removing clothing and putting on a patient gown. (5)

incapacitated permanently or temporarily impaired by a mental and/or physical condition. (5)

inclusive a tendency to include everyone. (4)

inconsistent at variance with one's principles; not staying the same throughout. (3)

individual mandate the requirement that everyone must have health insurance or be subject to a penalty tax. (1)

infant mortality rate the number of infants that die during the first year of life. (1)

infectious diseases conditions caused by viruses, bacteria, fungi, or parasites that can be passed from person to person. (6)

inferior lower or less worthy. (4)

insubordination refusal to do an assigned task or to follow established rules. (2)

integrity the quality of being honest and of sound moral principle. (3)

intelligence quotient (IQ) the mental ability to learn and understand. (1)

intentional done on purpose. (2)

interdependence mutual dependence between things, people, or parts of an organization. (2)

interpersonal relationships connections between or among people. (4)

interpersonal skills the ability to interact with other people. (1)

introverts people who predominantly focus inwardly. (5)

invasion of privacy unlawfully making public knowledge of any private or personal information without the consent of the wronged person. (3)

invincible incapable of being overcome. (6)

job application a form used to apply for a job. (8)

job boards websites where employers post job openings. (8)

job description a list of the essential duties of and qualifications for a job. (2)

journal a written record of personal thoughts and experiences. (7)

judgment ability to make considered decisions and choices and reach reasonable conclusions. (3)

labeling describing a person with a word that limits him or her, such as "lazy" or "mean." (4)

labor projections estimates of the number of positions that will need to be filled in the future. (8)

labor trends the general direction or development over time of workforce supply and demand. (8)

Lean Sigma the combination of two quality improvement approaches known as Lean and Six Sigma. Lean initiatives aim to streamline processes, reduce or eliminate waste, and increase speed and efficiency. Six Sigma initiatives, used successfully for many years in the manufacturing industry, aim to reduce variations and defects as a means of improving quality and reducing costs. (1)

legibility the ability of handwriting to be read and interpreted accurately by others. (1)

legislative issues topics involving local, state, and national law-making. (8)

liable legally responsible. (3)

libel a written false statement that damages a person's good reputation. (3)

license a credential from a state agency awarding legal permission to practice to a person who meets pre-established qualifications. (Intro)

life expectancy the statistical number of years of life remaining at any given age. (1)

literacy the ability to read and write. (4)

loyalty demonstrating allegiance to people that one is under obligation to defend or support. (3)

malnutrition poor nutrition caused by an insufficient or poorly balanced diet or by a medical condition. (6)

malpractice failure to meet the standard of care or conduct prescribed by a profession. (3)

manners standards of behavior based on thoughtfulness and consideration of other people. (4)

Medicaid a government program that provides health care for low-income people and families and those with certain disabilities. (1)

medical homes organizations that provide comprehensive, coordinated health care to patients who are members. (1)

Medicare a government program that provides health care primarily for people age 65 and older. (1)

mentors wise, loyal advisors. (7)

metrics a set of measurements that quantify results. (1)

mindfulness awareness of what is happening or of one's surroundings. (2)

misdemeanor a minor offense with a fine and/or short jail sentence as a penalty. (8)

mistake to understand, interpret, or estimate incorrectly. (1)

moral convictions strong or absolute beliefs about what is right or wrong. (3)

morale the general mood or spirit of a person or group. (3)

morals standards of behavior or belief based on differentiating between right and wrong. (3)

multiskilled cross-trained to perform more than one function, possibly in more than one discipline. (1)

negligence failure to perform or give care in a reasonably careful and cautious manner. (3)

netiquette standards for appropriate conduct on the Internet. (4)

networking interacting with a variety of people in different settings to exchange information and develop contacts, especially to further one's career. (8)

noncompliant refusing or failing to follow instructions. (5)

nonexempt positions jobs that do not involve management or other advanced functions or skills and that pay a salary or wage plus an additional hourly rate for overtime hours. *See also* exempt positions. (8)

norms expectations or guidelines for behavior. (5)

obese weighing more than 20% above a person's ideal weight. (1)

objective real or actual; not affected by feelings. (2)

observations opportunities to view a "real-life" setting to take note of what happens there. (7)

occupational preferences the types of work and work settings that an individual prefers. (8)

office politics clique-like relationships among groups of coworkers that involve scheming and plotting. (7)

official transcript a grade report that should be printed, sealed, and mailed directly to the recipient to prevent tampering by the applicant. (8)

opioid a narcotic with opium-like effect but not derived from opium. (3)

optimist one who looks on the bright side of things. (2)

organizational chart an illustration of the components of a company and how they relate to each other. (2)

out-of-pocket expense costs not covered by insurance that patients have to pay themselves. (1)

outcome data information gathered after a change has taken place to examine the impact or results of the change. (1)

outpatient describes care or a facility outside of a hospital. (Intro)

palliative care care designed to reduce pain and suffering and to improve the quality of life. (1)

passive accepting without resistance. (4)

passive-aggressive acting in an aggressive manner while appearing to be passive. (4)

patient portals secure online websites that give patients access to personal health information. (5)

payer a person or group that covers the expense of received goods or services. (Intro)

peers people at the same rank within a company or society. (2)

people skills personality characteristics that enhance one's ability to interact effectively with other people; also called *soft skills*. (1)

performance-based pay a system in which pay levels and pay increases are tied to a performance evaluation. (2)

performance evaluation a measurement of success in executing job duties. (2)

perks benefits that come with status. (8)

personal financial management the ability to make sound decisions about personal finances. (6)

personal image the total impression created by a person. (6)

personal management skills the ability to manage one's time, personal finances, stress, and change. (6)

personal skills the ability to manage aspects of one's life outside of work. (6)

personal space the amount of space a person requires between him- or herself and another person in order to feel comfortable. (4)

personal values things of great worth and importance to a person. (3)

personality distinctive qualities of a person; patterns of behavior and attitudes. (1)

perspective the manner in which a person views something. (1)

pessimist one who looks on the dark side of things. (2)

plagiarize to use another person's work and claim credit for it. (4)

Platinum Rule a rule that you should treat other people the way *they* want to be treated, in contrast to the Golden Rule that you should treat other people the way *you* would like to be treated. *See also* Golden Rule. (4)

polite having good manners. (4)

political correctness eliminating language or practices that could offend social sensibilities about cultural groups such as race and gender. (5)

portfolio a collection of materials that demonstrates a person's knowledge, skills, and abilities. (8)

postsecondary after high school. (8)

posture the position of the body or parts of the body. (6)

practicum a "real-life" learning experience obtained through working on-site in a health care facility while enrolled as a student; also known as a clinical, an externship, an internship, a hands-on experience, or the like. (Intro)

preemployment assessments tests and other instruments used to measure knowledge, skills, and personality traits. (8)

preexisting condition a medical condition a patient has prior to applying for health insurance. (1)

prejudiced having judged or formed an opinion before the facts are known. (4)

prenatal before birth. (1)

preventive actions taken to avoid contracting a medical condition. (1)

primary care the initial or basic medical care provided to a person within the health care system. (1)

priorities things having precedence in time, order, or importance. (3)

probationary period a period of time during which an organization closely monitors an employee's attendance and performance. (2)

problem solving a systematic process to find solutions to difficult issues and situations. (2)

process a set of actions or steps that must be accomplished correctly and in the proper order. (1)

procrastinate to postpone or delay taking action. (6)

profane improper and contemptible, usually with regard to language. (7)

professional associations organizations composed of people from the same occupation. (Intro)

professional development education for people who have begun their careers and wish or need to continue growing in that profession. (8)

professionals people with experience and skills who are engaged in a specific occupation for pay or as a means of livelihood. (Intro)

protocol a prescribed policy or procedure. (3)

provider one who performs or enables a service such as a doctor, health care worker, or health care organization. (Intro)

prudent careful and cautious. (3)

punctual arriving on time. (2)

rational based on reason; logical. (2)

readmission quick return to a hospital after discharge. (1)

reasonable care use of the degree of caution and concern while providing care that a prudent and rational person would use in similar circumstances. (3)

reasoning forming conclusions based on logical thinking. (2)

references a list of people who can provide information about a job applicant. (8)

reimbursement paying back or compensation for money spent. (2)

reliable can be counted upon; trustworthy. (2)

reportable conditions situations wherein health care workers are required to file a confidential report to the county health department, such as suspected child or adult abuse or the diagnosis of certain diseases. (3)

reportable incident any event that can have an adverse effect on the health, safety, or welfare of people in the facility or organization. (3)

reputation a person's character, values, and behavior as viewed by others. (Intro)

resilience the ability to adapt and recover from stress and difficulty. (6)

respect a feeling or showing of honor or esteem toward another. (Intro)

responsibility an obligation or a sense of duty binding someone to a course of action. (2)

résumé document summarizing one's qualifications for a job. (3)

retirement benefits employer-funded pension contributions. (8)

role models people that others aspire to be like. (5)

root cause the factor that led to a problem and that, when fixed, will solve the problem and prevent it from happening again. (1)

samples room a place where health care facilities keep samples of drugs and medical supplies. (7)

scope of practice boundaries that determine what a worker may and may not do as part of his or her job. (Intro)

self-care the actions people take to establish and maintain their own physical, mental, and emotional health. (6)

self-esteem belief in oneself; self-respect. (Intro)

self-worth   a sense of one's own importance and value. (Intro)

selfie   a photograph of a person taken by him- or herself using a smartphone. (4)

sentinel event   an unexpected occurrence involving death or serious physical or psychological injury, or the risk thereof, with serious injuries including the loss of a limb or function. (1)

sexual harassment   unwelcome sexual advances, requests for sexual favors, and other verbal and physical contact of a sexual nature. (2)

single-payer system   a universal health care system where a single-payer fund, rather than private insurers, pays for health care costs. (1)

slander   a spoken false statement that damages a person's good reputation. (3)

slang   the informal language of a particular group. (4)

smartphones   cell phones that also function as hand-held computers. (1)

social media   electronic communication that enables users to establish online communities for the purpose of sharing content, ideas, personal messages, and other information such as videos and photographs. (1)

soft skills   *see* people skills. (1)

specialists   people who are devoted to a particular occupation or branch of study. (1)

staffing level   the number of people with certain qualifications who are assigned to work at a given time. (1)

stagnant   without motion; dull, sluggish. (2)

stakeholders   people with a keen interest in a project or organization; may be end-users of a product or service. (1)

standards of care   care that would be expected to be given to a patient by a similarly trained person under similar circumstances. (3)

stereotypes   beliefs that are mainly false about a group of people. (5)

stress management   means of dealing with stress and stressful situations. (6)

subjective   affected by one's state of mind or feelings. (2)

subordinates   people at a lower rank or under someone's supervision. (2)

succession planning   a proactive approach to identifying and preparing employees to fill positions as other workers retire. (8)

surrogate   a person designated to exercise the patient's rights when the patient is unable to act on his or her own behalf. (5)

synergy   people working together in a cooperative action to produce an effect greater than their separate efforts. (4)

systematic   methodical. (2)

systems perspective   standing back, viewing an entire process, and understanding how one's role fits into that process. (2)

taboo   banned from social custom. (6)

therapeutic   an activity or method of treating or curing a disease or condition. (Intro)

time management   the ability to organize and allocate one's time. (6)

torts   wrongful acts that result in physical injury, property damages, or damages to a person's reputation for which the injured person is entitled to compensation. (3)

traditional questions   questions that ask how a person would behave in a future situation. (8)

traits   characteristics or qualities related to one's personality. (1)

transferable skills   skills acquired in one job that are applicable in another job. (1)

transparency   in online postings, revealing clearly who is making the statements in the post. (5)

trust   confidence in the honesty, integrity, and reliability of another person. (Intro)

trustworthiness   the quality of deserving others' confidence in one's honesty, integrity, and reliability. (3)

unethical   violating standards of conduct and moral judgment. (2)

up-code modify the classification of a procedure to increase financial reimbursement. (2)

vendor a person or company with whom your company does business. (Intro)

vision a mental image; to imagine what the future could be. (8)

well groomed personally clean and neat. (6)

whistleblower a person who exposes the illegal or unethical practices of another person or of an organization or company. (2)

work ethic attitudes and behaviors that support good work performance. (1)

workplace bullies employees who intimidate and belittle coworkers. (4)

Index

Note: Page numbers with f indicate figures.